Diagnostic Advances in Precision Medicine and Drug Development

AF858423

Edited by
Emmanuel Kwaku Ofori, Seth Kwabena Amponsah,
and Yashwant V. Pathak

CRC Press
Taylor & Francis Group
Boca Raton London New York

CRC Press is an imprint of the
Taylor & Francis Group, an **informa** business

First edition published 2025
by CRC Press
2385 NW Executive Center Drive, Suite 320, Boca Raton FL 33431

and by CRC Press
4 Park Square, Milton Park, Abingdon, Oxon, OX14 4RN

CRC Press is an imprint of Taylor & Francis Group, LLC

ISBN: 9781032781716 (hbk)
ISBN: 9781032782324 (pbk)
ISBN: 9781003486909 (ebk)

DOI: 10.1201/9781003486909

Typeset in Times
by Deanta Global Publishing Services, Chennai, India

I dedicate this book to my two biological sisters, Eunice and Portia, who I believe would take pleasure in my achievements, and to my mother, Mabel Ofori, who imparted the principles of resilience and tenacity to me from the outset.

To my wife Irene and my three exceptional children, Michelle, Janelle, and Adom: you are my wellspring of strength and inspiration.

Emmanuel K. Ofori

I dedicate this book to my close friends who continuously encourage me: Christian, Nana Dwumfour, Daniel, Kojo, Gideon, Joseph, Emmanuel, and Michael.

Seth K. Amponsah

To the loving memories of my parents and Dr. Keshav Baliram Hedgewar, founder of Rashtriya Swayamsevak Sangh (RSS) in Bharat, who gave proper direction to my life. To my beloved wife Seema, who gave positive meaning, and my son Sarvadaman, who gave a golden lining to my life.

I want to dedicate this book to Prof. Ved Nanda, Prof. Radheshyam Dwivedi, Prof. Manohar Shinde, and Shri Baburam Guptajee, my mentors and role models; I learned a lot from them.

Yashwant V. Pathak

Contents

About the Editors

Emmanuel Kwaku Ofori is currently an Associate Professor and Head of the Department of Chemical Pathology at the University of Ghana Medical School. He obtained his PhD in July 2018 from the University of Lausanne in Switzerland. He teaches several disciplines in the health sciences (medical, nursing, veterinary, and laboratory sciences, among others). He has supervised and mentored many undergraduate and postgraduate students. His research focuses on lipidomics, metabolic medicine, and steroidal adaptations to diet and exercise. He aims to become an international expert on translational research into metabolic diseases. He has about 38 publications to his credit. He has also presented several abstracts at global conferences. He is the Academic Editor for *PLOS One* and the *Journal of Diabetes Research.*

Seth Kwabena Amponsah is Associate Professor of Medical Pharmacology at the University of Ghana Medical School. He has had post-doctoral fellowships under the BANGA-Africa Project and BSU III (DANIDA – Denmark). He has over 13 years experience in teaching and research. His research focus includes Clinical Pharmacology (infectious disease and antimicrobial stewardship): prudent use of antimicrobials, antimicrobial level monitoring, and efficacy of antimicrobials in patients. He has experience in population pharmacokinetic modeling, non-compartment pharmacokinetic estimation, and pharmacokinetic evaluation of new drug formulations. He has published over 60 research articles, four books, 20 book chapters, and several conference abstracts. He is Academic Editor for *PLOS One* and Associate Editor for *Pan African Medical Journal.*

Yashwant V. Pathak has over 15 years of versatile administrative experience in an institution of higher education as a dean (and over 30 years as a faculty member and researcher in higher education after his PhD). Presently holds the position of Associate Dean for Faculty Affairs and Tenured Professor of Pharmaceutical Sciences. Prof. Yashwant Pathak is an internationally recognized scholar, researcher, and educator in health care education, nanotechnology, drug delivery systems, and nutraceuticals. He has received many international and national awards, including four Fulbright Fellowships, Endeavour Executive Fellowship by Australian Government, four outstanding faculty awards, and he was selected as a Fellow of the American Association for Advancement of Science (AAAS) in 2021 for his contribution toward the advancement of science. He has published over 350 research publications, reviews, and chapters in various books. He has edited over 60 books in various fields, including nanotechnology, nutraceuticals, conflict management, and cultural studies. He is also actively involved in many non-profit organizations, to mention a few: Hindu Swayamsevak Sangh, USA, Sewa International USA, International Accreditation Council for Dharma Schools and Colleges, International Commission for Human Rights and Religious Freedom, and Uberoi Foundation for Religious Studies, among others.

Contributors

Godwill Acquah
Department of Radiography
School of Biomedical and Allied Health Sciences
University of Ghana
Accra, Ghana

Nathaniel Ebo Aidoo
Department of Chemical Pathology
University of Ghana Medical School
Accra, Ghana

Rosemary Ampofo
Department of Radiography
School of Biomedical and Allied Health Sciences
University of Ghana
Accra, Ghana

Richmond Owusu Ateko
Department of Chemical Pathology
University of Ghana Medical School
Accra, Ghana

Seth Kwabena Amponsah
Department of Medical Pharmacology
University of Ghana Medical School
Accra, Ghana

Avni Bhambure
MIT School of Bioengineering Sciences and Research
MIT Art, Design and Technology University
Pune, India

Chandni Chandarana
Department of Pharmaceutical Quality Assurance
SSR College of Pharmacy
Silvassa, India

Megha Chavda
Department of Pharmacognosy
SSR College of Pharmacy
Silvassa, India

Deborah Clotworthy
Department of Medical Pharmacology
University of Ghana Medical School
Accra, Ghana

Benedicta Obenewaa Dankyi
Department of Medical Pharmacology
University of Ghana Medical School
Accra, Ghana

Aarohi Deshpande
MIT School of Bioengineering Sciences and Research
MIT Art, Design and Technology University
Pune, India

Funmilola Adesodun Fisusi
School of Applied Sciences
University of Brighton
Brighton, United Kingdom

Mansa Fredua-Agyeman
Department of Pharmaceutics and Microbiology
School of Pharmacy
College of Health Sciences
University of Ghana
Accra, Ghana

Blay Kwofie
Department of Medical Pharmacology
University of Ghana Medical School
Accra, Ghana

Elikem Kumahor
Laboratory Sub-BMC
Korle-Bu Teaching Hospital
Accra, Ghana

Lalit Kumar
Department of Pharmaceutics
National Institute of Pharmaceutical Education and Research
Hajipur, India

Mawusi Adepa Mawuli
Department of Chemical Pathology
University of Ghana Medical School
Accra, Ghana

Shama Mujawar
MIT School of Bioengineering Sciences and Research
MIT Art, Design and Technology University
Pune, India

Refat M. Nimer
Department of Medical Laboratory Sciences
Jordan University of Science and Technology
Irbid, Jordan

Christian Obirikorang
Department of Molecular Medicine
Kwame Nkrumah University of Science and Technology
Kumasi, Ghana

Emmanuel Kwaku Ofori
Department of Chemical Pathology
University of Ghana Medical School
Accra, Ghana

Hubert Owusu
Department of Molecular Medicine
Kwame Nkrumah University of Science and Technology
Kumasi, Ghana

Hiba Parveen
Gyani Inder Singh Institute of Professional Studies
Dehradun, India

Akhilesh Patel
NIMS Institute of Pharmacy
NIMS University
Jaipur, India

Yashwant V. Pathak
USF Health Taneja College of Pharmacy
University of South Florida
Tampa, USA
and
Faculty of Pharmacy
Airlangga University
Surabaya, Indonesia

Bhupendra G. Prajapati
Department of Pharmaceutics and Pharmaceutical Technology
Shree S. K. Patel College of Pharmaceutical Education & Research
Faculty of Pharmacy
Ganpat University
India

Parixit Prajapati
Department of Pharmaceutical Chemistry
SSR College of Pharmacy
Silvassa, India

Nii Boi-Doku Prepra-Ameyaw
Laboratory Sub-BMC
Korle-Bu Teaching Hospital
Accra, Ghana

Louisa Quainoo
School of Medicine and Dentistry
Kwame Nkrumah University of Science and Technology
Kumasi, Ghana

Benedicta Quaye
Department of Clinical Anatomy
Faculty of Health and Medicine
Lancaster University
UK

Anas M. Abdel Rahman
Department of Biochemistry and Molecular Medicine
College of Medicine
Alfaisal University
Riyadh, Saudi Arabia

Sheila A. Santa
Department of Medical Laboratory Sciences
School of Biomedical and Allied Health Sciences
University of Ghana
Accra, Ghana

Sajeeda Shaik
Department of Pharmaceutical Chemistry
Manipal College of Pharmaceutical Sciences
Manipal Academy of Higher Education
Manipal, India

Rupesh K. Shirodkar
Department of Pharmaceutics
Goa College of Pharmacy
Panaji, India

Derick Seyram Sule
Department of Radiography
School of Biomedical and Allied Health Sciences

University of Ghana
Accra, Ghana

Benjamin Tagoe
Department of Pharmaceutical Sciences
North Dakota State University
Fargo, USA

Emmanuel A. Tagoe
Department of Medical Laboratory Sciences
School of Biomedical and Allied Health
University of Ghana
Accra, Ghana

Junaid Tantray
NIMS Institute of Pharmacy
NIMS University
Jaipur, India

Ruchi Verma
Department of Pharmaceutical Chemistry
Manipal College of Pharmaceutical Sciences
Manipal Academy of Higher Education
Manipal, India

Foreword

The field of diagnostic medicine has gained prominence over the years; nonetheless, there seem to be limited publications that explore the methodologies and tools employed in this discipline. Technology integration into diagnostic care is revolutionizing the healthcare industry by enhancing the precision, efficiency, and accessibility of diagnostic processes. The new book presents content on modern advancements in diagnostic medicine utilizing technologies such as artificial intelligence (AI) and telemedicine.

Because the field of medicine is constantly changing, information concerning new developments must be thoroughly preserved. This book includes comprehensive yet concise information on various diagnostic devices and methods utilized in medical practice. This book will be highly popular among both primary and secondary audiences. The book comprises 20 chapters. These chapters provide essential data along with practical and clinically pertinent information. The book examines contemporary trends, prospective benefits, and the capacity of these technologies to revolutionize diagnostics.

The book ends with ethical enquiries regarding AI, challenges, and potential future directions in diagnostic medicine, along with prospective strategies and recommendations for optimizing the capabilities of emerging technology in health diagnostics. I can attest that the chapters in this book are well-crafted, and the text integration is exemplary. The themes in the chapters are straightforward, uncomplicated, and understandable. This book will benefit students, researchers, and professionals in pharmaceutical industries, laboratory medicine, clinical sciences, and allied health disciplines. As a doctor and consultant, I strongly recommend this book to healthcare professionals who want to stay current on the latest advances in diagnostic medicine.

I would like to congratulate the editors, Emmanuel K. Ofori, Seth K. Amponsah, and Yashwant V. Pathak, as well as the chapter contributors, on this outstanding resource.

Prof. Timothy D. Osafo
Consultant in Laboratory Medicine
MBChB, DCP, DPath, MRCPath, FGCP, FRCPath

Preface

Over the years, scientists have made significant technological efforts in chemistry, biochemistry, laboratory science, and biotechnology to improve disease diagnosis and patient management. Further, drug developers have utilized novel diagnostic methods during preclinical and clinical trials, improving their development processes.

Before the 18th century, medicine was based on the narrative of a patient's symptoms. In addition to this subjective portrait of the illness, the physician observed the patient's appearance (behavior) and any signs of disease. During the 18th and 19th centuries, medical instrumentation was an essential arm of medicine. This aided the physical examination of patients and made the physician less dependent on subjective narration.

The introduction of machines such as the X-ray, electrocardiogram (ECG), and chemical laboratory analyzers during the 19th and 20th centuries further enhanced the objectivity of medicine. Biological matrices such as blood, sweat, saliva, urine, and stool, all of which are naturally discharged, can today, thanks to technology, provide information that can indicate one's health and/or sickness. Indeed, health diagnostics is substantially transforming due to technological advancements and evolving medical paradigms. These technologies are anticipated to improve diagnostic accuracy, customize patient treatment, and elevate healthcare outcomes.

This book will provide an overview of diagnostic procedures, their underlying principles, and the tools utilized to perform them. In this book, we will emphasize recent developments in automated techniques such as mass spectrometry, high-performance liquid chromatography (HPLC), polymerase chain reaction (PCR), and immunohistochemistry, as well as several imaging techniques that include magnetic resonance imaging (MRI), bone density scan (DEXA), and ultrasound scan that aid in precision medicine and the drug development process. Recent advancements in digital health (using artificial intelligence) will also be highlighted.

The book has the following key features:

- Describes recent developments in molecular diagnostics, imaging techniques, spectroscopic and chromatographic methods
- Discusses innovative methodologies for diagnostic testing
- Gives a comprehensive overview of the integration of artificial intelligence in digital health

The editors are grateful to all contributing authors who continue to have a positive influence in their roles as researchers and academicians. The editors also thank CRC Press (Taylor and Francis) for facilitating all processes involved in producing and publishing this book.

1

Improving Diagnostic Care through Technology

Emmanuel Kwaku Ofori, Seth Kwabena Amponsah, and Yashwant V. Pathak

1.1 Introduction

Technology has been intricately tied to the evolution of healthcare since the beginning of time. Numerous innovations, ranging from the stethoscope to imaging machines, have significantly contributed to the development of diagnostic treatment and the enhancement of diagnostic accuracy and outcomes. Artificial intelligence (AI), machine learning (ML), and telemedicine are examples of cutting-edge technologies being incorporated into modern medicine, causing a revolution in diagnostic treatment, increasing precision, and making healthcare more accessible [1, 2]. Personalized medicine can improve the quality of medical decision-making by providing information that informs patient-specific treatment decisions, which benefit patients and national healthcare systems.

This chapter will investigate how these technologies are comprehensively revolutionizing diagnostic care. We will explore the applications of AI and ML, as well as telemedicine, wearable technology, genomics, and big data analytics, and we will analyze their current applications, potential benefits, and associated challenges. We intend to highlight these technologies' considerable influence on diagnostic therapy and the future of healthcare by analyzing several case studies and practical examples.

1.1.1 Advances in Point-of-Care Diagnostics

Advancements in soft materials, lab-on-a-chip technologies, nanotechnology, and biotechnology, along with the emergence of drone-mounted diagnostic devices, have created novel and efficient point-of-care (POC) molecular diagnostic platforms suitable for resource-limited environments. Point-of-care diagnostics provides the opportunity to provide rapid, sensitive, and user-friendly analysis in settings that are not laboratories and have limited resources. POC is beneficial when real-time on-site diagnosis is limited, allowing diagnostic support [3].

Recent developments in nanotechnology, polymers, and smartphones have produced diagnostics devices that are practical POC approaches. These devices have found widespread application in the medical profession. Applications of POC diagnostic techniques for identifying infectious diseases in resource-limited settings and settings in the developing world have gained much attention in global health monitoring and management. POC tools based on smartphones can monitor a wide range of physical and molecular processes. It can now carry out complex biomedical examinations thanks to incorporating two high-resolution cameras, computational capacity, and a wireless internet network connection [3, 4].

Further, the implementation of smartphones in settings with low resources, where there is still a demand for biomedical technologies that are portable, rapid, and precise, has the potential to revolutionize the public healthcare system. Some smartphone communication capabilities include near-field communication (NFC), infrared, Bluetooth, Wi-Fi, and global positioning systems (GPS). These capabilities contribute to an improvement in the performance of smartphone-based testing. The NFC technology

DOI: 10.1201/9781003486909-1

enables radio tags to name items and can be employed for close-range monitoring and control. If a digital versatile disc (DVD) and spectroscopy attachments are utilized with a smartphone, achieving a wavelength resolution of less than one nanometer is feasible [5, 6]. Using a wide range of computer platforms based on smartphones makes it possible to detect biological targets such as proteins, DNA, and cells. The use of a quantitative phase microscope that is based on a smartphone and is handheld allows for the observation of blood cells as well as squamous cells that are found in Pap smears [7].

It is common knowledge that glucose tests are reliable POC self-test assessment methods. Continuous glucose monitoring (CGM) platforms that are non-invasive are becoming increasingly popular in the field of glucose self-monitoring. Enzyme-free patch biosensors are also utilized to monitor glucose levels without causing discomfort [8, 9]. Dipstick biosensors are a straightforward diagnostic tool that offers qualitative detection and contain chemicals that have been pre-deposited. These examples include pH, uric acid, pathogen detection, and antioxidant strips. It is simple to manufacture them, and they are simple to include in commercial productions.

1.1.2 Telemedicine and Remote Diagnostics

Telemedicine involves transmitting clinical information remotely through technological communications. Some technologies used in telemedicine include the internet, videoconferencing, store-and-forward imaging, streaming media, and wireless communications [10]. Several subspecialties within telemedicine include telepathology, teleradiology, teledermatology, telesurgery, and telepsychiatry [11]. The application of AI will be a significant component of many of the diagnostic improvements applied to the medical field over the next few years. Telemedicine can significantly improve diagnostic procedures and treatment methods on a global scale. There will also be an impact on neurological evaluations and examinations brought about by AI. Patients can receive real-time diagnostic information regarding a range of illnesses, including sepsis, mental disorders, stroke, and immunological dysfunction, through the use of smart monitoring devices that they wear [12].

The divide that had previously existed between patients and healthcare practitioners has been bridged through the utilization of telemedicine, particularly in areas that were either underserved or rural. Through the utilization of technology created explicitly for communication, patients can receive consultations, diagnoses, and treatment plans without the necessity of their physical presence. Telemedicine has evolved beyond consultations to encompass diagnostic tools like digital stethoscopes and portable ultrasound machines, making it possible for medical practitioners to undertake physical examinations remotely. This method has proven particularly useful during the COVID-19 pandemic, as it was vital to reduce participants' interaction with the virus. It is now possible for people to obtain medical attention without leaving the convenience of their homes, thanks to the availability of virtual consultation platforms. These systems combine video conferencing, digital diagnostic tools, and electronic health records (EHRs), which enable medical personnel to make decisions based on correct patient information using the information available [13].

1.1.3 The Role of AI and ML in Diagnostics

AI refers to computer-coded programs or algorithms that can make judgments and predictions by analyzing the data, rules, and instructions programmed into them [14]. One further approach to AI is ML. This computer program can train us to analyze and comprehend data and recognize patterns even our brains cannot identify [15]. ML can generally be classified into two categories: supervised learning, in which the computer can view the end data, and unsupervised learning, in which the computer is not given any outcome data [16]. AI and ML have exhibited a tremendous amount of potential in terms of further improving diagnostic precision. Algorithms can evaluate large datasets much faster than humans, leading to discovering patterns and links that may not be immediately apparent to medical professionals. Indeed, knowing about individuals who are more likely to develop a condition or disease in the future is vital for early detection.

When imaging data, genetic information, and clinical history are all combined, for example, it is possible to arrive at diagnoses that are more accurate and specific to the individual. Big data platforms capable of processing data in real time can also significantly improve diagnostic procedures' accuracy and speed. For instance, real-time analysis of patient data can facilitate the delivery of choices and diagnoses more expediently, ultimately resulting in improved outcomes for patients in emergency care settings. Hospitals' use of big data platforms is becoming increasingly popular. These platforms allow hospitals to better integrate and analyze patient information from various sources, eventually leading to more comprehensive and timely diagnoses [17]. Implementing AI in medical operations has been hampered by delays and impediments in low and middle-income countries (LMICs), particularly in sub-Saharan Africa (SSA), making it more difficult for these countries to embrace and implement AI in medical procedures [18].

1.1.4 AI in Diagnostic Imaging

Diagnostic imaging has dramatically advanced with digital modalities led by computed tomography (CT), computed radiography (CR), and ultrasound (US) [18, 19]. Image quality has constantly seen improvements. Advancements in magnetic resonance imaging (MRI) have made excellent resolution of soft tissues possible, particularly in the brain, joints, and spine [20]. AI in radiology represents a significant advancement in the profession. Evaluation of X-rays, CT scans, and MRIs has been accomplished by developing deep learning algorithms [15]. AI algorithms can diagnose illnesses like lung, breast, and brain tumors more accurately, significantly reducing errors during the diagnostic process [21].

Compared to a CT scan, an MRI can provide a more precise resolution of neuronal structures of the brain. There are no radiation side effects associated with MRI modalities. Portable MRI scanners are now available for use in operating rooms and ambulance services. Positron emission tomography (PET) employs radioactive substances to investigate the metabolic activities of various body tissues. Gamma rays are produced when positrons mix with electrons in the body's cells. Gamma cameras can detect these gamma rays, resulting in three-dimensional image formation. The discovery of such molecular tracers that target-specific cancer cells is the focus of the future of PET. AI also plays a significant part in managing chronic diseases. It is possible for individuals who suffer from illnesses such as diabetes, hypertension, and heart disease to reap the benefits of having their vital signs and other health indicators monitored through the utilization of remote monitoring. Glucose monitors, blood pressure cuffs, and intelligent scales are examples of gadgets that make it feasible for healthcare professionals to receive real-time data [22].

1.1.5 AI in Pathology

The field of pathology is also making advances with AI. Telepathology refers to the practice of pathology that is carried out remotely through the use of macroscopic and microscopic pictures and the utilization of telecommunication links for remote interpretations, second opinions, consultations, and educational reasons [23, 24]. Pathologists can reap the benefits of these systems since they can identify malignant cells and other abnormalities with a high degree of precision. This gives pathologists a second opinion and reduces the number of diagnostic errors that occur. Pathologists could devote more time to more complex activities, such as evaluating predictive or prognostic biomarkers in the context of particular clinical findings, if they delegated time-consuming and repetitive screening chores to AI algorithms.

Histopathological analysis based on AI has shown tremendous potential in detecting breast cancer. Using AI, it is possible to identify between breast cancer and healthy breast parenchyma with 98.8% accuracy in numerous benchmark datasets [25]. In addition to the capability of predicting molecular or clinical factors based on histomorphological data, AI applications will play an increasingly essential role in interpreting molecular pathological data within the coming years. One example is the classification of deoxyribonucleic acid (DNA) methylation profiles of squamous cell carcinomas of the lung using deep learning (DL). This classification is done to differentiate between a metastasis of a head and neck carcinoma and primary lung cancer [26].

Similarly, AI techniques are becoming increasingly significant in multiomics-based genetic tumor classifications. This has the potential to improve both the accuracy and the speed of the diagnosis. However, even though AI and ML can completely transform the pathology field, a significant obstacle in deploying such models in routine clinical diagnosis is that, up until this point, only a relatively small number of pathology laboratories have built an entirely digital workflow. Cost, technological limitations (such as limited resolution), opposition from pathologists (such as reluctance and skepticism), a lack of standards, and the possible danger of competition for pathology services are some drawbacks associated with the widespread use of telepathology [27]. In addition, electricity availability, dependable telecommunications bandwidth in remote or underdeveloped regions, and cultural considerations may also hinder international telepathology [28].

1.1.6 Predictive Analytics in Disease Management

Identifying the likelihood of future events based on patterns that have occurred in the past is the goal of predictive analytics (PA), which involves the utilization of historical data, statistical algorithms, and ML approaches [29]. The use of PA in managing chronic diseases allows for the analysis of massive amounts of patient data, which may be used to forecast the evolution of the condition, anticipate future problems, and tailor individualized treatment strategies. These algorithms can process vast volumes of patient data, including electronic health records, test findings, and data from wearable devices, to forecast the disease's evolution, identify high-risk patients, and suggest individualized interventions. In managing diabetes mellitus, PA allows for the prediction of blood glucose levels, the recommendation of insulin dosages, and the suggestion of dietary alterations to enhance glucose control [30]. By analyzing patient data, such as lifestyle habits and medical history, predictive models can foresee an illness's severity and recommend preventative measures. The structure of the human brain inspired these models, which are particularly effective at recognizing intricate patterns within data. Detecting early indicators of diabetic retinopathy, for instance, is accomplished through utilizing convolutional neural networks (CNNs) in medical imaging [31]. In contrast, recurrent neural networks (RNNs) can analyze time series data to track the evolution of chronic diseases [32]. Incorporating AI into managing chronic diseases involves substantial regulatory and ethical challenges, even though it offers promising benefits. The landscape of legislation governing AI in healthcare is still developing, and various issues are associated with data privacy and security and compliance with existing healthcare laws and regulations.

Continuous monitoring and upgrading of AI models are done to ensure compliance with regulatory standards [33]. However, this requires significant resources and a comprehensive understanding of regulatory standards and artificial intelligence technology. In addition, compliance problems include concerns over data privacy and security. Ethical questions also remain paramount when incorporating AI-powered predictive analytics into managing chronic diseases.

1.1.7 AI in Genomics

Genetic information about an individual in treatment for diagnostic or therapeutic purposes, as well as the associated health outcomes and policy consequences, is the primary focus of genomic medicine, a relatively emerging medical speciality. Genetic medicine is an interdisciplinary medical speciality that incorporates genomic information, and it has experienced rapid expansion in recent years. Genomics can advance oncology, pharmacology, infectious disease, and unusual and previously unknown ailments [34, 35]. The term "Whole-Genome Sequencing" (WGS) has emerged as a prominent topic in medical diagnosis. The classic Sanger sequencing approach required more than ten years to complete human genome sequencing [36].

On the other hand, next-generation sequencing (NGS) has become a topic of discussion that encompasses the contemporary DNA sequencing technique and high-throughput sequencing that enables scientists to sequence the entire genome quickly. These technologies simultaneously allow for the sequencing of hundreds of millions of DNA molecules, making them handy tools for genomic research. The application of NGS to large-scale genomics has caused an increasing level of precision and success in medical practice, which has been observed over the past years [37]. The genome-wide association study, also known as GWAS, is a method that has gained popularity for its application to genomic data. It aims to research the relationship between genetic variants, such as single-nucleotide polymorphisms (SNPs), and phenotypes, defined as a particular characteristic or disease [38].

Genomics relies heavily on AI since it assists in comprehending otherwise complex genetic data. By analyzing vast amounts of gene data, algorithms powered by AI can identify patterns that point to genetic predispositions to particular diseases. This ability is crucial in cancer genomics, where AI plays a role in identifying mutations that certain drugs can target, enabling the customization of treatment plans. ML techniques, integral to AI technology, employ computers to learn from genetic data to make predictions or choices autonomously. It is becoming increasingly possible to cure a genetic disease before it spreads to other patients if one can analyze a database with information on genetic diseases and then cross-reference that information with patient records. The sequencing of the genome has revolutionized oncology. Oncologists can deliver targeted therapies that are more effective and less harmful than traditional chemotherapy approaches. This is because targeted therapies can identify specific genetic abnormalities present in tumors. Drugs like imatinib's success in successfully treating chronic myeloid leukemia (CML) is a tribute to the promise of genetics in diagnosing and treating the disease [39].

1.1.8 AI and Electronic Health Records

Increasing data repositories throughout the healthcare sector has led to a significant increase in the digitization of health data. Due to the advantages of secondary data reuse over original data collection, the clinical research community has shown an increasing interest in developing efficient methods to reuse clinical data from EHRs [40]. Compared to traditional clinical research, researchers who reuse EHR data may not be required to recruit patients or collect fresh data, which could reduce costs. On top of that, electronic health record data frequently include essential longitudinal information about a patient's condition, medical care, and disease progression. The reuse of EHR data, on the other hand, has its challenges, notably due to the complexity and heterogeneity of the data [41]. Each EHR system record corresponds to a specific healthcare incident a patient has experienced. The data is maintained in a collection of tables. Including demographic data (age, gender, address, etc.) and a wide range of clinical information, EHR offers a rich information source.

The use of AI in conjunction with electronic health records has the potential to revolutionize the diagnostic care process completely. Algorithms powered by AI can examine patient information to identify patterns and trends that may indicate the beginning of diseases. Health professionals can utilize the knowledge retrieved from EHR in various contexts, including clinical decision support, epidemiological, improvement of population care, and pattern identification. However, phenotyping based on EHR is challenging because of the heterogeneity and incompleteness of EHR data.

1.1.9 Wearable Technology and Personal Health Monitoring

It is becoming increasingly common for the healthcare industry to recognize the value of wearables as valuable instruments for monitoring and controlling patients' health. Introducing wearable technology into the medical field has ushered in a new era of profound changes. These changes have made it possible to improve patient outcomes and make treatments more individualized. There are implications for preventative care, the treatment of chronic diseases, and the overall delivery of healthcare that are associated with the incorporation of wearables into healthcare ecosystems [42]. Smartwatches' original purpose was to keep track of the time, but they have since developed into sophisticated health monitoring gadgets. As a result of its incorporation of sensors, accelerometers, and heart rate monitors, smartwatches can deliver real-time information regarding vital signs. Many users can effortlessly monitor their heart rate, identify any anomalies that may occur, and enhance their understanding of their cardiovascular health. Smartwatches also contribute to medication adherence and general health management, in addition to their monitoring capabilities. Individuals can receive timely messages on medication schedules and other health-related events. The constant flow of real-time data makes identifying irregularities easier and promotes the timely implementation of medical interventions [43].

Medical wearables are an essential component in improving the level of connectedness between patients and healthcare professionals. These wearables ensure that real-time patient data is accessible to medical professionals by linking with medical databases, making it possible for medical professionals to make educated decisions and provide personalized healthcare to these individuals. Because of the constant nature of wearable monitoring, there is the possibility of detecting health issues at an earlier stage. The analysis of patterns and trends in vital sign data over time enables the identification of minor changes that may precede the start of a medical problem. Wearable devices make a significant contribution to the reduction of hospital readmissions [44]. These devices offer a seamless method of continuous monitoring after release from the hospital. It is possible to remotely monitor patients fitted with wearables for any indicators of deterioration or difficulties, allowing for timely interventions and the prevention of unnecessary visits to the hospital. Patients conveniently check their vital signs, track their progress, and receive insights into their health using mobile applications and user-friendly interfaces. Wearables give consumers a thorough understanding of their daily routines by monitoring their nutrition, sleep patterns, and physical activity [45]. Because of this awareness, positive behavioral adjustments are encouraged, which result in better lives and the prevention or progression of chronic diseases.

Although wearable technology has great potential to revolutionize healthcare, several concerns have been raised regarding the privacy and security of sensitive information due to wearables' ongoing data collection. Because wearables can transmit and store data, stringent security measures to prevent unauthorized access must be implemented. Data encryption and secure transmission methods are necessary to guarantee patient information security. The ethical considerations surrounding wearables include ensuring that individuals consent to data acquisition and addressing questions around data ownership. It is critical to ensure that sensitive data is not abused or misused, and realistic processes must be followed to prevent unauthorized access to specific health information.

1.1.10 Pharmacogenomics

Pharmacogenomics explores how an individual's genetic makeup can affect their reaction to prescribed medications [46]. Genetic testing is now possible to determine whether or not a patient is likely to respond to various antidepressants or whether or not they are at risk of experiencing severe adverse effects from specific medicines. When medical specialists comprehensively understand these hereditary traits, they can better modify prescription regimens to enhance effectiveness while limiting undesired consequences. Our understanding of the genetic basis of individual drug responses has advanced as a result of research that has been conducted on diseases and treatments. Single-nucleotide polymorphisms (SNPs), genomic insertions and deletions, and genetic copy number variations (CNVs) are some of the prevalent genetic variants found in research [47]. SNPs are the most common among the inherited sequence differences. Even if there is not a significant amount of variation in the concentration of the drug at the target location, drugs can nonetheless generate highly variable effects. Pharmacological activities can vary depending on the variations that occur in several genes. These variants typically influence the drug's pharmacokinetics or pharmacodynamics.

Although a pharmacogenomic link has been identified and verified, other challenges must be overcome before implementation in clinical settings. A translation of this kind necessitates the availability of beneficial alternative therapies for individuals with high-risk genotypes and changes to healthcare infrastructure. Currently, the most well-known examples of genetic polymorphisms that influence medication response in humans are monogenic (single gene) characteristics that affect drug metabolism [48]. As an illustration, consider the case of thiopurine S-methyltransferase (TPMT) and the impact it has on the thiopurine medications mercaptopurine and azathiopurine in patients who inherit TPMT alleles that are not functioning [49]. In clinical settings, these medications are employed as immunosuppressants for neoplasias. Patients who inherit a TPMT deficiency amass high amounts of the active thioguanine nucleotides in their blood cells when treated with mercaptopurine or azathiopurine. This is because TPMT is the major inactivation pathway for these medicines in hematopoietic tissues. This can result in severe hematopoietic toxicity, which has the potential to be fatal with severe consequences. Although clinical diagnostic assays are now available for detecting inactivating SNPs in the human TPMT gene, the utilization of TPMT genotyping for making treatment decisions is still restricted. The hepatic cytochrome P450 gene CYP2D6 is a candidate gene. This gene is responsible for catalyzing the metabolism of various medicines [50]. Based on the fact that genetic variants are inherited as haplotypes, the design of GWAS allows for the evaluation of SNPs that tag a haplotype, which eliminates the requirement to genotype all variants that are present in the haplotype. However, GWAS should only be regarded as the first stage because the SNPs revealed to be related to particular traits by GWAS are not necessarily causal variations; the latter must be discovered through complete resequencing. Although there are several obstacles that clinicians must overcome to integrate pharmacogenomics in clinical practice successfully, the ultimate consequence is that patients are prescribed medications for which the relevant genotype is unknown. There is also the limited availability of pharmacogenomics education for health practitioners. A further obstacle is the expense involved. Assessing drug response phenotypes (such as drug toxicity and drug response) in pharmacogenomics is frequently more challenging than measuring genetic variability. This is because drug response phenotypes are complicated to detect. Consequently, clinical studies must incorporate the practice of obtaining informed consent from patients to acquire genomic DNA samples.

1.1.11 Technological Challenges to Diagnostic Care

Even though technology possesses enormous potential, it also poses obstacles regarding ethics and practicality. Algorithmic bias and data privacy are issues that need to be addressed to guarantee that everyone has equal and fair access to advanced diagnostic tools. Data privacy and security protection have become paramount due to digitizing diagnostic data and digital medical records [51]. Installing robust cybersecurity measures and complying with legislation requirements is essential. Encryption, secure access controls, and continuous monitoring of data systems are all vital components in protecting sensitive health information and staying one step ahead of cyber threats. It is possible for algorithms that use AI to inherit biases from the training data, which can lead to disparities in diagnostic accuracy between different populations. Ensure that training datasets are varied and that AI systems are regularly monitored. This will mitigate the effects of bias and render diagnostics more equitable.

A significant barrier still stands in the way of the equal distribution of diagnostic technologies. People who live in rural locations and areas with low socioeconomic status may have restricted access to new diagnostic technology, which can make the health disparities that already exist much worse. Efforts are being made to bridge this gap by investing in telemedicine infrastructure, supplying diagnostic gadgets at inexpensive prices, and training healthcare providers in these places.

1.2 Future Directions

The path that will lead diagnostic care providers into the future is the seamless integration of various technological innovations. The combination of genetics, telemedicine, wearable technologies, and artificial intelligence is projected to develop a patient-centered and holistic approach to healthcare [52]. Developing more robust and reliable systems that can scale well, are energy efficient, and can be easily incorporated into healthcare systems should be the focus of study in the future. They should address privacy, security, scalability, seamless connectivity, interoperability, accuracy, and precision that can be attained in anticipating and treating disease attacks. Emerging mechanisms and novel medicines for therapy will simultaneously demand cutting-edge molecular diagnostics as the landscape of illness diagnosis continues to advance. However, this will be the case simultaneously. By utilizing molecular and artificial intelligence technologies, we can better understand how these factors influence human health and how they may be manipulated for treatment.

The potential to continuously monitor a greater variety of health markers is one of the characteristics projected to be included in the next generation of wearable technology, which is expected to become even more complex. Future wearables are anticipated to integrate sensors that can identify biomarkers for various diseases. This would make it possible to diagnose health problems at an earlier stage and address them personally. Among the potential applications of wearable biosensors are monitoring inflammation markers, predicting flare-ups in autoimmune diseases, and facilitating preventative medication. Telemedicine is growing due to several factors, including improvements in internet connectivity and the development of increasingly sophisticated remote diagnostic tools. In the future, telemedicine systems may mix virtual reality (VR) and augmented reality (AR) to provide immersive and interactive consultations [53]. This will further bridge the gap between in-person and remote therapy. The subject of genomics is making tremendous advancements, with an increased emphasis on epigenetics, which is the study of how human behavior and environmental variables can impact the expression of genetic material. We can improve our understanding of disease mechanisms by integrating epigenetic data with genetic information, ultimately leading to more accurate diagnosis and treatment approaches.

1.3 Conclusion

The healthcare landscape is transforming because of the increased use of technology in diagnostic therapy. Big data analytics is helping to improve the management of illnesses, AI and ML are helping to improve diagnostic accuracy, telemedicine is helping to make healthcare more accessible, wearable technology is providing continuous health monitoring, genomics is helping to pave the way for personalized medicine, and telemedicine is helping to make healthcare more accessible. On the other hand, these accomplishments are followed by several challenges, such as discrimination based on algorithmic bias, data privacy protection, and equal access to technology. To effectively solve these challenges, it will be necessary for stakeholders including healthcare providers and technologists to work together on their respective endeavors. Through the promotion of a mindset that is both collaborative and ethical, we will be able to fully harness the potential of technology to develop a healthcare system that is more efficient and centered on the patient. Diagnostic care has a bright future ahead of it as a result of the fact that technology is prepared to play a significant role in improving the results for patients and bringing about changes in the delivery of healthcare.

REFERENCES

1. Qayyum MU, et al. Revolutionizing healthcare: the transformative impact of artificial intelligence in medicine. *Bull Informatics*. 2023;1(2):71–83.
2. Thacharodi A, et al. Revolutionizing healthcare and medicine: the impact of modern technologies for a healthier future—a comprehensive review. *Health Care Sci*. 2024;3(5):329–349.
3. Heidt B, et al. Point of care diagnostics in resource-limited settings: a review of the present and future of PoC in its most needed environment. *Biosensors*. 2020;10(10):133.
4. Zarei M. Portable biosensing devices for point-of-care diagnostics: recent developments and applications. *TrAC Trends Anal Chem*. 2017;91:26–41.
5. Scheeline A. Smartphone technology–instrumentation and applications. In: Crocombe, R., Leary, P. and Kammrath, B. (eds.). *Portable spectroscopy and spectrometry*; 2021; volume 2; John Wiley and Sons: Hoboken, New Jersey, USA: . p. 209–35.
6. Peveler WJ, Algar WR. Toward clinical applications of smartphone spectroscopy and imaging. In: Crocombe, R., Leary, P. and Kammrath, B. (eds.) *Portable spectroscopy and spectrometry*; 2021; volume 2; John Wiley and Sons: Hoboken, New Jersey, USA. p. 199–226.
7. Ayardulabi R, et al. Point-of-care applications of smartphone-based microscopy. *Sens Actuators A Phys*. 2021;331:113048.
8. Pullano SA, et al. Glucose biosensors in clinical practice: principles, limits and perspectives of currently used devices. *Theranostics*. 2022;12(2):493.
9. Zafar H, et al. Comprehensive review on wearable sweat-glucose sensors for continuous glucose monitoring. *Sensors*. 2022;22(2):638.
10. Alenoghena CO, et al. Telemedicine: a survey of telecommunication technologies, developments, and challenges. *J Sensor Actuat Netw*. 2023;12(2):20.

11. de Araújo Novaes M. Telecare within different specialties. In: Shashi Gogia; *Fundamentals of telemedicine and telehealth*. Elsevier publishers, NewYork, USA; 2020. p. 185–254.
12. Mukherjee S, et al. State of the art in smart portable, wearable, ingestible and implantable devices for health status monitoring and disease management. *Sensors*. 2022;22(11):4228.
13. Zhang X, Saltman R. Impact of electronic health record interoperability on telehealth service outcomes. *JMIR Med Inform*. 2022;10(1):e31837.
14. Gaur K, Jagtap MM. Role of artificial intelligence and machine learning in prediction, diagnosis, and prognosis of cancer. *Cureus*. 2022;14(11):e31008.
15. Janiesch C, Zschech P, Heinrich K. Machine learning and deep learning. *Electron Markets*. 2021;31(3):685–95.
16. Sarker IH. Machine learning: algorithms, real-world applications and research directions. *SN Comput Sci*. 2021;2(3):160.
17. Habeeb RAA, et al. Real-time big data processing for anomaly detection: a survey. *Int J Inf Manage*. 2019;45:289–307.
18. Ephraim RKD, et al. Application of medical artificial intelligence technology in sub-Saharan Africa: prospects for medical laboratories. *Smart Health*. 2024;33:100505.
19. Abhisheka B, et al. Recent trend in medical imaging modalities and their applications in disease diagnosis: a review. *Multimed Tools Appl*. 2024;83(14):43035–70.
20. Sneag DB, et al. MRI advancements in musculoskeletal clinical and research practice. *Radiology*. 2023;308(2):e230531.
21. Khalifa M, Albadawy M. AI in diagnostic imaging: revolutionizing accuracy and efficiency. *Comput Methods Programs Biomed*. 2024;5:100146.
22. Alfian G, et al. A personalized healthcare monitoring system for diabetic patients by utilizing BLE-based sensors and real-time data processing. *Sensors*. 2018;18(7):2183.
23. Bashshur RL, et al. The empirical foundations of telepathology: evidence of feasibility and intermediate effects. *Telemed e-Health*. 2017;23(3):155–91.
24. Farahani N, Pantanowitz L. Overview of telepathology. *Surg Pathol Clin*. 2015;8(2):223–31.
25. Försch S, et al. Artificial intelligence in pathology. *Dtsch Arztebl Int*. 2021;118(12):199.
26. Weusthof C, et al. Establishment of a machine learning model for the risk assessment of perineural invasion in head and neck squamous cell carcinoma. *Int J Mol Sci*. 2023;24(10):8938.
27. Jahn SW, Plass M, Moinfar F. Digital pathology: advantages, limitations and emerging perspectives. *J Clin Med*. 2020;9(11):3697.
28. Adelakun O, Garcia R. Technical factors in telemedicine adoption in extreme resource-poor countries. In: Mildred M.G. Olivier, Clarisse C. Croteau-Chonka; *Global health and volunteering beyond borders: a guide for healthcare professionals*. Springer; New York, USA; 2019. p. 83–101.
29. Razzak MI, Imran M, Xu G. Big data analytics for preventive medicine. *Neural Comput Appl*. 2020;32(9):4417–451.
30. Vettoretti M, et al. Advanced diabetes management using artificial intelligence and continuous glucose monitoring sensors. *Sensors*. 2020;20(14):3870.
31. Tsiknakis N, et al. Deep learning for diabetic retinopathy detection and classification based on fundus images: a review. *Comput Biol Med*. 2021;135:104599.
32. Zhu Y, et al. Prediction of chronic kidney disease progression using recurrent neural network and electronic health records. *Sci Rep*. 2023;13(1):22091.
33. de Almeida PGR, dos Santos CD, Farias JS. Artificial intelligence regulation: a framework for governance. *Ethics Inf Technol*. 2021;23(3):505–25.
34. Shendure J, Findlay GM, Snyder MW. Genomic medicine–progress, pitfalls, and promise. *Cell*. 2019;177(1):45–57.
35. Roth SC. What is genomic medicine? *J Med Libr Assoc*. 2019;107(3):442.
36. Shendure J, et al. DNA sequencing at 40: past, present and future. *Nature*. 2017;550(7676):345–53.
37. Berger MF, Mardis ER. The emerging clinical relevance of genomics in cancer medicine. *Nat Rev Clin Oncol*. 2018;15(6):353–65.
38. Uffelmann E, et al. Genome-wide association studies. *Nat Rev Methods Primers*. 2021;1(1):59.
39. Banerjee S, Amin SA, Jha T. Therapies of hematological malignancies: an overview of the potential targets and their inhibitors. *Curr Chem Biol*. 2021;15(1):19–49.

40. Meystre SM, et al. Clinical data reuse or secondary use: current status and potential future progress. *Yearb Med Inform.* 2017;26(01):38–52.
41. Tayefi M, et al. Challenges and opportunities beyond structured data in analysis of electronic health records. *Wiley Interdiscip Rev Comput Stat.* 2021;13(6):e1549.
42. Smuck M, et al. The emerging clinical role of wearables: factors for successful implementation in healthcare. *NPJ Digit Med.* 2021;4(1):1–8.
43. Izu L, Scholtz B, Fashoro I. Wearables and their potential to transform health management: a step towards sustainable development goal 3. *Sustainability.* 2024;16(5):1850.
44. Bonacaro A, Rubbi I, Sookhoo D. The use of wearable devices in preventing hospital readmission and in improving the quality of life of chronic patients in the homecare setting: a narrative literature review. *Professioni Infermieristiche.* 2019;72(2):143–51.
45. Del-Valle-Soto C, et al. A comprehensive review of behavior change techniques in wearables and IoT: implications for health and well-being. *Sensors.* 2024;24(8):2429.
46. Cacabelos R, Cacabelos N, Carril JC. The role of pharmacogenomics in adverse drug reactions. *Expert Rev Clin Pharmacol.* 2019;12(5):407–42.
47. Almal SH, Padh H. Implications of gene copy-number variation in health and diseases. *J Hum Genet.* 2012;57(1):6–13.
48. Zhang G, Nebert DW. Personalized medicine: genetic risk prediction of drug response. *Pharmacol Ther.* 2017;175:75–90.
49. Evans WE. Pharmacogenetics of thiopurine S-methyltransferase and thiopurine therapy. *Ther Drug Monit.* 2004;26(2):186–91.
50. He ZX, et al. Impact of physiological, pathological and environmental factors on the expression and activity of human cytochrome P450 2D6 and implications in precision medicine. *Drug Metab Rev.* 2015;47(4):470–519.
51. Kiran N, et al. Digital pathology: transforming diagnosis in the digital age. *Cureus.* 2023;15(9):e44620.
52. Ognjanović I, Zoulias E, Mantas J. Progress achieved, landmarks, and future concerns in biomedical and health informatics. MDPI *Healthcare.*; 2024;12(20):2041.
53. Worlikar H, et al. Mixed reality platforms in telehealth delivery: scoping review. JMIR Biomed Eng. 2023;8:e42709.

2

Electrolyte Potentiometers in Medical Diagnosis: From Bench to Bedside

Elikem Kwami Kumahor and Nii Boi-Doku Prepra-Ameyaw

2.1 Potentiometry

Potentiometry is an application of electrochemistry and has been used clinically in the measurement of electrolytes (Na, K, Cl, Ca, Mg, and Li) as well as blood pH and pCO_2 measurements [1]. This technique measures these analytes across several sample matrices, including whole blood, plasma, serum, and urine. The technique has been developed and improved over several decades and is currently the basis for modern biosensors used in point-of-care devices [2].

2.1.1 Historical Background

Historically, electrolyte measurement was done using flame photometry (flame atomic emission spectrometry). The principle underlying this technique is the emission of radiation at a specific wavelength when atoms are excited by heat (flame) [3].

2.1.2 Flame Photometry

A serum spray is injected into a flame, where the high temperature excites some atoms generated as electrons transition into higher energy shells. As these atoms cool down, the electrons return to their ground state by emitting energy at a specific wavelength. The emitted radiation is measured spectrophotometrically [4]. In practice, this technique is technically cumbersome because it requires dilution and protein precipitation, which increases the analysis time and makes it error-prone [5]. Interference from elements emitting similar wavelengths can be a source of error. In addition, some excited atoms emitted radiations with very different wavelengths, introducing imprecision to the measurements [6].

2.1.3 Early Development of Electrochemical Techniques

In 1906, Max Cremer invented the hydrogen ion-responsive glass electrode. M. Cremer's electrode was composed of silica and an alkali metal oxide. Fritz Haber and his student Klememsiewicz further described and improved his work to develop the first glass pH electrode capable of measuring the acidity or alkalinity of chemical solutions [7]. Glass electrodes have an inherent sensitivity to alkali metal cations (Na, Mg, Ca) which manifested as an "alkaline error" at a high pH. It was discovered that electrodes with selectivity for several elements could be produced by varying the composition of silicon and metal oxides. However, only Na and H glass electrodes are used in current clinical practice.

DOI: 10.1201/9781003486909-2

2.2 The Galvanic Cell

The galvanic electrochemical cell demonstrates the basic concepts of modern potentiometric measurement techniques. It consists of two electrodes that are connected by an electrolyte solution. Each electrode is a half-cell composed of a single electrolyte solution that is in contact with a metal conductor that serves to conduct ions. The indicator electrode is one-half of the cell, which makes contact with the sample containing the measured analyte [8]. The reference electrode is the other half of the cell, which makes contact with the reference solution.

The force which drives electrons from one electrode to the other is the electromotive force [9]. It describes the maximum potential difference between the two electrodes when no current runs through the cell. To measure the ionic activity of an unknown sample, the measuring electrode is introduced to the test sample and the potential difference between the reference electrode and the measuring or indicator electrode is measured using a potentiometer. The ionic activity of an electrochemical cell can be calculated from the Nernst equation [10].

2.2.1 Nernst Equation

$$E = \frac{RT}{nF} log_e \frac{a_1}{a_s}$$

Where E is the potential difference of the cell, a_1 and a_2 are the ionic activity in the two solutions. F is the faraday's constant, R is the universal gas constant and T is the absolute temperature. According to the Nernst equation, the potential difference of an electrochemical cell (E) is directly proportional to log of the ionic activity at the measuring electrode (a_1). Since the ionic activity of the reference electrode is known, the ionic activity of the measuring electrode can be calculated. This closely approximates the concentration of ions or analytes measured.

2.3 Types of Electrodes

Several types of electrodes have been designed to be used in potentiometric measurement. The most common principles on which electrodes are based include redox, ion-selective (Figure 2.1), and carbon dioxide (CO_2) electrodes.

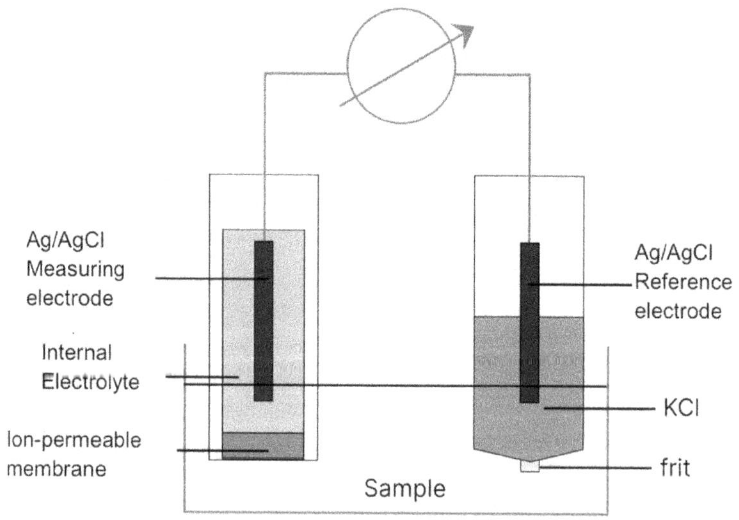

FIGURE 2.1 Diagram of an ion-selective membrane electrode.

2.3.1 Redox Electrodes

Redox electrodes operate on the principle of redox reactions. These are electrochemical reactions where electrons are transferred from one compound to another. Any substance that accepts electrons is an oxidant and any substance that donates electrons is a reductant. In a homogenous electrochemical reaction, electrons are transferred between two redox couples. Thus a reductant produces its conjugate oxidant and vice versa. The reaction can go in both directions to reach electrochemical equilibrium [11]. In an electrochemical cell, a redox electron is composed of a metal conductor dissolved in an electrolyte solution. The metal electrode may be an inert metal or maybe an ionic metal, which can participate in the redox reaction [12].

2.3.2 Inert Metal Electrodes

Gold (Au) and Platinum (Pt) are commonly used as metal electrodes because they are inert and do not participate in the overall redox reaction. They are typically used as reference electrodes and can be modified into pH meters [13].

2.3.3 Metal Electrodes Participating in Redox Reactions

The silver-silver chloride electrode (Ag/AgCl) and mercury-mercurous chloride ($Hg/HgCl_2$) are metal electrodes in the redox reaction.

$$AgCl_{(solid)} + e^- \leftrightarrow Ag^o{}_{(solid)} + Cl^-$$

$$Hg_2Cl_2 + 2e^- \leftrightarrow 2Hg^o + 2Cl^-$$

These electrodes become ionized, thus providing a sustained supply of metal ions in the solution. Ag/AgCl electrodes are often used as reference and electrode elements in ion-selective electrodes (ISE) [14]. $Hg/HgCl_2$ are also called calomel electrodes, which are frequently used as reference electrodes for pH measurement. They are however not frequently used in clinical instruments.

2.3.4 Ion- Selective Electrodes

Ion-selective electrodes are defined as electrodes that selectively interact with a single ionic species. They incorporate certain types of membranes that select specific anions or cations. The electrical potential produced at the interface between the membrane and sample solution is directly proportional to the log of ionic activity or concentration of the measured ion [15]. ISEs deliver a simple, rapid, and versatile analytical method applicable to a wide range of analytes. Examples of selective membranes include glass, crystalline, and polymeric materials. The chemical composition of these materials is designed to achieve optimal selectivity toward the ion of interest. There are three basic types of membranes: solid-state membranes, liquid ion exchange electrodes, and neutral carrier membranes.

2.4 Solid Ion Exchange Membranes

2.4.1 Glass Electrode

The glass membrane electrode was the first ion-selective electrode to be invented by Cremer in 1906. It is mainly used as a sensor to detect and measure H^+ and Na^+ concentration in serum and is an integral component of pCO_2 sensors. Glass electrode membranes are produced from melting varying percentages of silicon and aluminium oxide and oxides of elements such as sodium or calcium. Electrons with selectivity for H^+, Na^+, K^+, Li^+, Ag^+, NH_4^+ are produced by varying the composition of aluminium oxide and silicon.

2.4.2 The Glass pH Electrode (Hydrogen Electrode)

This thin glass membrane consists of three layers separating two solutions of different hydrogen ion activity. The two outer layers are hydrated, while the middle layer remains dry. Hydrogen ions from the internal and external solutions exchange with the two hydrated layers, creating a membrane potential (Figure 2.2). With the ionic activity of the internal solution remaining constant, the concentration of H^+ in the outer solution can be calculated from the Nernst equation.

2.4.3 The Sodium Glass Electrode

When a glass electrode is introduced into a solution with low H^+ concentration relative to sodium, the sodium component of the membrane potential of the glass electrode becomes significant. This effect is known as the "alkali error". This error has been taken advantage of in fabricating a glass electrode which has increased sensitivity to sodium ions. A typical clinical sensor for Na^+ has 71% Silicon, 11% Na_2O and 18% Al_2O_3.

2.5 Liquid Ion Exchange Electrodes

Liquid ion exchange electrodes consist of a hydrophobic solvent containing ionizable compounds. This lipid membrane forms the selective membrane separating the inner electrode solution from the outer sample solution. The prototype electrode using this system is the calcium electrode.

2.5.1 The Calcium Electrode

The calcium selective electrode is composed of a calcium salt of an alkyl phosphate dissolved in di-n-octyl phenyl phosphate, impregnated into an inert matrix such as PVC.

The calcium electrode is strongly selective for ionized calcium over magnesium, sodium, and potassium.

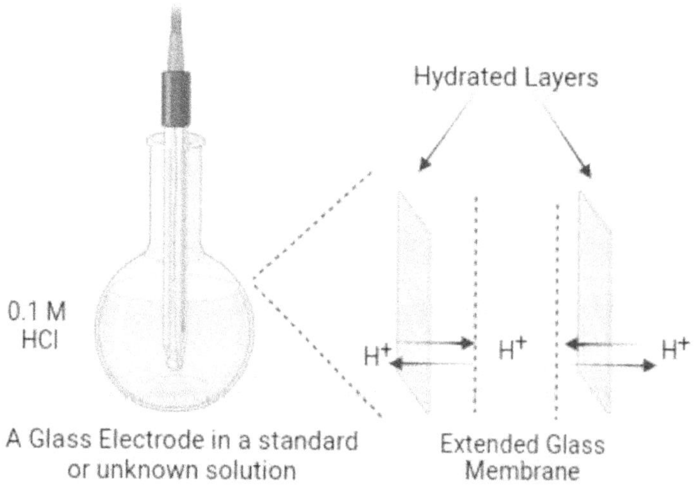

FIGURE 2.2 A glass pH electrode.

2.6 Neutral Carrier Electrodes (Ionophore)

2.6.1 Potassium Electrode

Neutral carrier electrodes mimic living cell membranes' ability to transport specific ions and molecules through dedicated channels in opposition to their concentration gradient. This system was achieved in vitro by discovering macro-cyclic antibiotics that caused increased permeability of cell membranes to specific ions. This antibiotic is valinomycin. It consists of a ring compound containing several ring oxygen atoms. Cations like potassium are selectively transported from an aqueous solution through a hydrophobic matrix by binding to this compound. The compound is electrically neutral and carries potassium (K^+) in the complex form. Valinomycin can be incorporated into an inert polymer like PVC or silicone rubber. However, the membrane has a limited lifespan because valinomycin slowly leaches out into the aqueous phase. The potassium selective electrode using neutral antibiotic valinomycin was the first polymer membrane electrode to be developed. Following this, polymer membrane electrodes are becoming increasingly popular in clinical chemistry because of their versatility as selective membranes (Table 2.1). They are used to measure electrolytes, including K, Na, Cl, Ca, Li, Mg, and carbonate.

2.7 Gas Permeable Membranes/Gas Dialysis Electrodes

2.7.1 Electrodes for the Partial Pressure of Carbon Dioxide

The development of the pCO_2 electrode by Stow and Severinghaus in 1958 marked a significant advancement in blood gas analysis. Utilizing a CO_2-permeable Teflon membrane, this sensor facilitates the diffusion of CO_2 from the sample to an aqueous bicarbonate solution on the surface of a conventional pH glass electrode. The resulting pH change is directly proportional to the log of pCO_2, enabling measurement of this critical respiratory parameter.

$$CO_2 + H_2O \rightleftarrows H_2CO_3 \leftrightarrow H^+ + HCO_3^-$$

$$\Delta \log pCO_{2(\mathrm{sample})} \approx \Delta \mathrm{pH}_{(\mathrm{internal\ layer})}$$

An ammonium (NH_4) electrode from measuring the partial pressure of ammonia dissolved in the plasma is very similar in design to the CO_2 electrode.

TABLE 2.1

Polymer membrane electrodes (ionophore)

Analyte	Ionophore
Potassium (K^+)	Valinomycin
Hydrogen (H^+)	Tridodecylamine
Ammonium (NH_4^+)	Nonactin
Sodium (Na^+)	ETH 227
Sodium (Na^+)	Methyl monensin
Magnesium (Mg^{++})	ETH 1117
Potassium (K^+)	Bis(benzyl-15-crown-5)-heptanedioate
Sodium (Na^+)	ETH 157
Calcium (Ca^{++})	ETH 1001

2.7.2 Oxygen Electrode

Compared to the potentiometric technique employed by pH meters, the Clark oxygen electrode, developed in the 1950s, utilizes an amperometric approach based on polarographic detection. This method measures the current generated by an electrochemical reaction at the electrode surface, rather than the potential difference between two half-cells. Oxygen in the sample solution disrupts the current flow, leading to a linear response. This contrasts with the Nernstian behavior observed in potentiometry.

$$O_2 + 2H_2O + 2e^- \rightarrow H_2O_2 + 2OH^-$$

The electrochemical response facilitates the quantification of dissolved oxygen within a solution by measuring the current at a constant voltage. The measured current demonstrates a linear relationship with oxygen consumption, which is directly proportional to the sample's pO_2.

2.7.3 Arterial Blood Gas Analyzer

The invention of the glass pH electrode, pCO_2 electrode, and pO_2 electrode laid the foundation for developing the three-way blood gas analyzer. These analyzers have benefited from progressive miniaturization, facilitating their implementation in point-of-care settings such as satellite laboratories, intensive care units (ICUs), and emergency departments. This widespread deployment enables rapid blood gas analysis, leveraging the established principles of these electrodes. Consequently, critical care settings can now evaluate patient samples swiftly, yielding vital information regarding acid–base balance. A typical blood gas panel includes: pH, partial pressure of carbon dioxide (pCO_2), partial pressure of oxygen (pO_2), bicarbonate (HCO_3^-).

Bicarbonate is calculated from the Henderson-Hasselbalch's equation:

$$\log c\, HCO_3^- = \text{pH-pK'} + \log [PCO_2 \times \alpha CO_2(P)]$$

Modern arterial blood gas analyzers may incorporate electrodes for measuring ionized Ca^{++} and lactate to give a complete picture of the patients' acid–base status.

2.8 Enzyme Electrodes

An enzyme electrode is similar to a gas permeable membrane electrode. However, in addition to being a selectively permeable membrane; they have enzymes impregnated into the membrane to facilitate the conversion of substances to products, which are then detected by electrochemical means [16]. A classical example of this type of electrode is the glucose electrode.

2.8.1 Glucose Electrode

The electrochemical measurement of glucose forms the basis of modern glucometers and point-of-care glucose measuring devices. The glucose oxidase enzymes catalyze the conversion of glucose to gluconic acid in water and oxygen.

$$\text{Glucose} + O_2 + H_2O \rightarrow \text{gluconic acid} + H_2O_2$$

There are two mechanisms through which the glucose electrode functions. Both are amperometric. The first records the consumption of oxygen, while the second records the generation of H_2O_2. This method is available in both wet and dry chemistry analyzer setups. This glucose measurement method is rapid but suffers from poor precision compared to spectrophotometric methods.

2.8.2 Urea Electrode

Like the glucose electrode, the urea electrode utilizes an electrode composed of ammonium with a cellophane envelope coating a thin layer of the urease enzyme behind it. It was the first of the enzyme electrodes to be manufactured; however, it never transitioned to clinical use because of the poor selectivity of ammonium electrode. In addition, the spectrophotometric measurement is more accurate and precise compared to this.

2.9 Factors Affecting Ion-Selective Electrode Measurements

Many factors influence the accuracy and precision of potentiometric measurement. These may lead to results significantly different from those obtained by other methods. Device manufacturers usually control for technical factors like junction potentials and interfering ions to minimize their impact on the analytical system.

2.9.1 Selectivity

Majority of electrodes used in clinical practice must have very high selectivity toward a target ion in biological fluids, particularly serum and whole blood. All electrodes can respond in varying degrees to more than a single ion. Various techniques have been adopted to reduce the contribution of interfering ions by modifying some of the measurement conditions or remove the interfering ions. The membrane potential of an electrode is the sum total of potentials from all the ions the electrode responds to. Each ion's potential is based on the membrane's selectivity to that ion [17]. The Nicolsky-Eisenman equation describes this relationship:

$$EMF = E_O + \frac{RT}{nF} log_e \left(Ai + Sij1 * Aj1 + Sij2 * Aj2.... \right)$$

Where Ai is the activity of the major ion being measured, Aj1, Aj2, etc. are activities of interfering ions of the same charge, Sij1, Sij2 etc. The contribution of each ion to the membrane potential is the product of the activity of the ion and the selectivity constants are relative to the major ion (Ai), the selectivity constant of the major ion being unity.

2.9.2 Junction Potentials

This is the potential that arises at the junction of two solutions of different physical or chemical properties, where the mobility of ions in the solutions differs. This results in a charge separation at the interface of the two fluids.

In clinical practice, the junction potential may arise between serum and the electrode as well as plasma and erythrocytes. The issue of junction potentials can be approached in several ways to minimize its effects on the accuracy of measurement. This can be achieved by calculations which correct for errors from junction potentials and changing the concentration of the electrolyte solution [18].

2.9.3 Temperature

The Nernst equation shows that the ionic activity measured by an electrode is temperature dependent. An increase in the temperature of the solution increases the sensitivity of the measurement and the response rate of the electrode [19].

2.9.4 Chemical Interferences

2.9.4.1 *Endogenous Chemical Interference*

Chemical compounds in plasma can bind to ions of interest and affect the accuracy of potentiometric measurements. A classic example is calcium which has a high percentage of plasma calcium bound to albumin. In such cases, spectrophotometric methods are preferred to potentiometric methods for measuring total calcium, since they can estimate both bound and unbound calcium concentrations. However, potentiometry is reserved for the measurement of ionized calcium [20]. Many other compounds in blood bound to proteins and cell membranes, examples are Cu, Zn, Pb, etc. The free ion concentration for these compounds is easily measurable, thus the ions need to be liberated before estimations are made.

2.9.4.2 *Exogenous Chemical Interference*

Anticoagulants such as EDTA, citrate, and oxalate act by removing calcium from plasma thus they may interfere with potentiometric calcium measurement. Heparin inhibits antithrombin III; however, there is some minimal calcium binding. To correct the heparin-binding error, very low volumes of heparin are used as anticoagulant, or the heparin is pre-saturated with calcium [21].

2.9.5 Protein-Lipid Dilution Effects

Electrochemical measurements are routinely performed on whole blood, plasma, or serum samples. Ideally, the presence of red blood cells, proteins, and fats (lipids) shouldn't interfere with the electrode's ability to detect the target ions. This assumption is based on the concept of the electrolyte exclusion effect (Figure 2.3) [22]. Imagine a sponge soaked with water (representing the watery part of plasma, where electrolytes reside) and tiny balls (representing proteins and lipids). Squeezing the sponge (adding more protein/lipid) reduces the available space for water. Similarly, high protein or fat content in blood can condense the water volume where electrolytes are found. There are two main methods for electrolyte analysis: direct ISE measurement and indirect ISE measurement. In healthy individuals, plasma is about 93% water and 7% protein and lipids combined. Direct ISE measures electrolytes directly in the sample without dilution, assuming this 93% water content. While this assumption leads to slightly higher readings than reality due to the exclusion effect, manufacturers have already incorporated corrections into their instruments [23].

However, things get more complex when the analysis involves diluting the sample before using the ISE (indirect ISE measurement). This might be necessary if the blood has abnormally high protein (e.g., in multiple myeloma) or fat (e.g., high cholesterol) levels. As mentioned earlier, these extra proteins or fats act like the squeezing action on the sponge, reducing the water content where electrolytes reside [23].

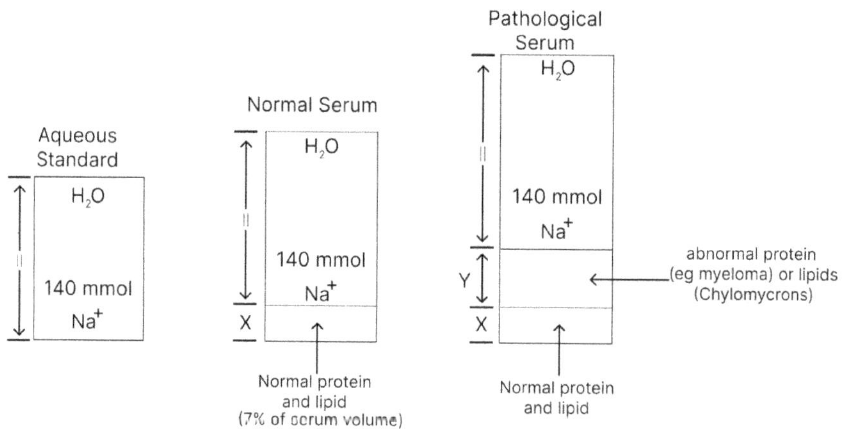

FIGURE 2.3 Electrolyte exclusion effect.

The problem with indirect ISE in such cases (hyperlipidemia or hyperproteinemia) is that the measurement still assumes the same fixed water content. Since the sample is diluted, this leads to an underestimation of the electrolyte levels, even though they might actually be high.

Healthcare providers can opt for direct ISE measurement or alternative methods like flame photometry to avoid this issue. Flame photometry directly measures the light emitted by excited elements like sodium and potassium, bypassing the need for assumptions about water content and avoiding the exclusion effect. Additionally, advanced ISE methods have been developed that can account for the exclusion effect, making them reliable even with abnormal protein or lipid levels.

2.10 Advantages and Disadvantages of Ion-Selective Electrodes

2.10.1 Advantages

1. The technique allows for very rapid analysis of samples, significantly reducing the turnaround times (TAT).
2. The instrumentation is simple and this allows portable and affordable point-of-care devices to be manufactured.
3. This technique offers sample versatility since optically clear solutions are not required. Thus, whole blood may be used in the analysis.
4. The integrity of the sample is preserved throughout the analysis, thus subsequent measurements of the same or different analytes can be made.

2.10.2 Disadvantages

1. Analysis may be influenced by ionic or chemical interferences.
2. Electrodes have a limited half-life and may be subject to contamination leading to systematic errors.
3. Electrode response becomes non-linear at very high or low concentrations.
4. Junction potentials in different sample media may vary and create imprecise measurements.
5. Primary calibration is difficult because calibrators are usually aqueous and must be corrected for biological solutions before running patient samples.

2.11 Biosensors

2.11.1 Introduction

The field of electrochemistry has given rise to a fascinating new era of miniaturized devices capable of detecting molecules within biological samples. This began with Clark's invention of the oxygen electrode [24]. He subsequently combined this innovation with the enzyme glucose oxidase within a special converter (transducer) to create the very first biosensor for detecting glucose levels [25]. Building on this initial success, researchers continued to push the boundaries. The development of fiberoptic sensors with special indicators allowed for the detection of various blood gas parameters like pH, carbon dioxide pressure (pCO_2), and oxygen pressure (pO_2) [26]. Today, we have implantable devices with needle-like electrodes placed under the skin for continuous glucose monitoring. This technology has significantly improved diabetes management for many patients [27].

These innovations continue with extensive research and development in immunosensors and nucleic acid biosensors. These advancements are revolutionizing the landscape of molecular diagnostics and medicine, promising even more exciting possibilities for the future.

TABLE 2.2

Types of transducers and their application

Type of transducer	Application
Potentiometric (ion-selective electrodes, gas sensing electrodes, field effect transistors)	pH, pCO_2, Na, K, Cl occasional enzymes, and immunological analytes
Amperometric (enzyme electrodes)	Glucose, urea, creatinine, and immunological analytes
Fiber-optic devices	pH, certain enzymes, and immunological analytes
Calorimetric (thermistors)	Subcellular organelles, enzymes, vitamins, and antibiotics
Conductance (conductimeters)	Enzyme substrates
Acoustic (piezoelectric crystals)	Volatile gases, antibodies

2.11.2 Definition

Biosensors can be described as small devices that make use of biological and biochemical reactions to detect an analyte of interest [28].

There are two essential components of a biosensor:

1. Biocatalyst: these are biological elements that interact with the target analyte being measured to generate a specific response. Examples are enzymes, cells, tissues, or nucleotides [29].
2. Transducer: these are devices that convert the biological or biochemical signal produced from the biocatalyst into a measurable signal response. Most common transducers (Table 2.2) generate light signals (optical) and/or electrochemical signals (potential difference or current) [30].

2.11.3 Classes of Biosensors

Biosensors are classified based on the principle of operation of the biocatalyst. There are two main groups:

1. Bioaffinity Biosensors

   These operate on the principle of selective binding of the analyte of interest to a specific ligand-partner. Examples of this ligand – receptor pairings are antigens, antibodies, nucleotides, DNA, and cells [31].
2. Biocatalytic Biosensors

   These devices make use of enzymes that catalyze the target substrate (analyte) into products, which can be measured. An example of this is the glucose oxidase sensor popularly used for glucose measurement and monitoring in the management of diabetes mellitus [30].

2.12 Enzyme-Based Biosensors

The glucose biosensor is the most popular clinical biosensor [32]. The prototype enzyme biosensor and its invention paved the way for other enzyme-based biosensors specific for detecting urea, creatinine, and lactate [33].

The glucose biosensor is an amperometric PO_2 sensor coated with a membrane with immobilized glucose oxidase. This outer membrane allows glucose and O_2 to pass to the electrode but blocks the entry of proteins and other molecules into plasma [34].

The reaction between glucose and glucose oxidase proceeds as follows:

$$\text{Glucose} + O_2 \text{ glucose oxidase gluconic acid} + H_2O_2$$

The transducers read glucose concentrations in two main ways.

2.12.1 Mechanism of First-Generation Instruments

First-generation devices made use of the rate of consumption of O_2, which is measured amperometrically by its reduction at the electrode. Another approach was to measure the rate of production of H_2O_2 at the electrode. The generation rate of gluconic acid can be measured using a pH electrode to detect the decrease in pH [35]. The dependence of this method on O_2 concentration introduces challenges due to the non-stoichiometric relationship between O_2 concentration and the glucose oxidase reaction. This nonlinearity is particularly pronounced in diabetic blood samples with significantly elevated glucose levels.

To circumvent this problem, some devices dilute samples and calibrators significantly with a buffer to correct the O_2 concentration in the sample. However, newer generation devices take a different approach to estimate glucose concentration using the glucose oxidase method.

2.12.2 Mechanism of Second-Generation Instruments

This method incorporates compounds on the surface of the electrode capable of capturing electrons in the redox reaction. These compounds include quinones, conductive organic salts, ferrocene, and redox osmium polymers. In these devices, the rate of glucose oxidation is measured by the generation of electrons from oxidized glucose at the surface of the electrode. This method not only eliminated the dependence on glucose estimation of O_2 concentrations but also reduced interference from substances such as uric acid, ascorbic acid, and acetaminophen, which are oxidized by the enzyme. Modern glucometers used for self-blood glucose monitoring make use of this method [36].

2.13 Cell-Based Biosensors

These biosensors incorporate whole cells or tissues into their analytical process [30]. These cells contain the enzyme biocatalysts, thus eliminating the cumbersome process of enzyme extraction and purification. This system is more economical compared to the system that incorporates only enzymes. Cell-based biosensors come in various forms, including single-cell type, multicellular type, and mixed cell and enzyme type; simple systems typically incorporate single-cell microorganisms [30]. An example is the using cholesterol oxidase in microorganisms as a biocatalyst for a cholesterol biosensor [37].

2.14 Enzyme Immunosensors

Enzyme immunosensors make use of the enzymes as the biocatalyst and incorporate antigen-antibody systems for detection [38]. Immunosensors may be labeled or non-labeled, with transducers typically potentiometric; antibodies can be incorporated on the membrane or electrode [39]. Some analytes that use enzyme immunosensors include human chorionic gonadotropin (hCG), serum albumin, and alpha-fetoprotein (AFP) [40].

Antibodies may also be labeled with enzymes, such as IgG coupled to catalase, and the pattern of reaction may be non-competitive or competitive [41].

2.15 DNA Biosensors

DNA biosensors recognize nucleic acids and offer a rapid and simple method for detecting genetic material in infectious diseases and cancers and rare in-born errors of metabolism. The advantage of DNA biosensors is that it is target specific compared to enzymes and immunoglobulins which are subject to cross-reactivity [42]. Sequencer-specific hybridization biosensors are often coupled to either optical, electrochemical, mass-spectrometry, or microarray chips as transducers or detectable methods [43].

2.16 Future Applications of Biosensors

The development of biosensors has accelerated these so-called "nanodevices" in clinical use [44]. Biosensors offer the advantage of miniaturization, which can be incorporated into nanometer scale devices in clinical diagnosis [45]. The advent of diagnostic biochips, an application of biosensor nanotechnology, enables the simultaneous analysis of hundreds of genes [46]. Gene primers and probes bonded to chip surfaces specifically bind to complementary copies in the patient's sample, allowing for the detection of infectious microbes using this method [47].

REFERENCES

1. Stork JT. Potentiometry. *Anal Chem.* 1993;65(13):344A–51A.
2. Walker NL, Roshkolaeva AB, Chapoval AI, Dick JE. Recent advances in potentiometric biosensing. *Curr Opin Electrochem.* 2021 Aug;28:100735. Available from: https://linkinghub.elsevier.com/retrieve/pii/S2451910321000491
3. Ahluwalia VK. Flame photometry. *Instrum Methods Chem Anal.* 2023;505–17. Available from: https://link.springer.com/chapter/10.1007/978-3-031-38355-7_35
4. Bobacka J, Ivaska A, Lewenstam A. Potentiometric ion sensors. *Chemical Reviews* 2008; 13;108(2):329–51.
5. Gandhi K, Sharma N, Gautam PB, Sharma R, Mann B, Pandey V. Atomic absorption spectroscopy and flame photometry. In: *Springer protocols handbooks.* New York, NY: Springer; 2022. p. 219–47. Available from: https://link.springer.com/protocol/10.1007/978-1-0716-1940-7_11
6. Ramírez-Muñoz J, Carrillo-García A, Díaz-Hernández Y, HT-B. A study of the sources of errors in the application of the ponderal ratios method in flame photometry. *Appl Spectrosc.* 1964;18:69–71.
7. Belyustin A, Shultz MM. *To the centenary of glass electrode: prehistory and history of the development: theoretical and practical aspects.* Moscow: Saint-Petersburg State University; 2006.
8. Halley S, Ramaiyan KP, Tsui LK, Garzon F. A review of zirconia oxygen, NOx, and mixed potential gas sensors–History and current trends. *Sensors and Actuators B: Chemical.* 2022 Nov 1;370:132363.
9. Houghton Mifflin. *American heritage dictionary of the English language.* 3rd ed. Houghton Mifflin; Boston, USA, 1992.
10. Garche J, Dyer CK, Moseley PT. Self-discharge. In: Garche J, Dyer CK, Moseley PT, Ogumi Z, Rand DA, Scrosati B, editors. *Encyclopedia of electrochemical power sources.* Amsterdam: Elsevier; 2013. p. 134.
11. Schüring J, Schulz HD, Fischer WR. *Redox: fundamentals, processes and applications.* Berlin: Springer; 2013.
12. Perez N. *Electrochemistry and corrosion of metals.* Springer, New York, USA; 2007; p. 27–70.
13. Albery WJ, Hitchman ML. *Dynamics of ring-disc electrodes.* Clarendon Press, Oxford, England,1971.
14. Yun M-H, Yeon J-W, Hwang J, Hong C, Song K. Applied electrochemistry. *J Appl Electrochem.* 2009;39:2587–92 .
15. Buck RP, Lindner E. Recommendations for nomenclature of ion-selective electrodes (IUPAC Recommendations 1994). *Pure Appl Chem.* 1994 Jan 1;66(12):2527–36. Available from: https://www.degruyter.com/document/doi/10.1351/pac199466122527/html
16. Shanker RM, Nashed NE, Lindenbaum S. An air-gap enzyme electrode: development and applications. *Pharm Res.* 1992 Apr;9(4):485–91. Available from: http://www.ncbi.nlm.nih.gov/pubmed/1495893
17. Jasielec JJ, Mousavi Z, Granholm K, Sokalski T, Lewenstam A. Sensitivity and selectivity of ion-selective electrodes interpreted using the nernst-planck-poisson model. *Anal Chem.* 2018 Aug 7;90(15):9644–9. Available from: https://pubs.acs.org/doi/10.1021/acs.analchem.8b02659
18. Neher E. *Correction for liquid junction potentials in patch clamp experiments.* 1992. p. 123–31. Available from: https://linkinghub.elsevier.com/retrieve/pii/007668799207008C

19. Cammann K. *Working with ion-selective electrodes: chemical laboratory practice:* Springer, Heidelberg, Germany;2012: p. 11–14.
20. Otnes S, Fogh-Andersen N, Rømsing J, Thomsen HS. Analytical interference by contrast agents in biochemical assays. *Contrast Media Mol Imaging.* 2017;2017:1–8. Available from: https://www.hindawi.com/journals/cmmi/2017/1323802/
21. Dimeski G, Badrick T, John AS. Ion Selective Electrodes (ISEs) and interferences—A review. *Clin Chim Acta.* 2010 Mar;411(5–6):309–17. Available from: https://linkinghub.elsevier.com/retrieve/pii/S0009898109006287
22. Burtis CA, Ashwood ER, BDE. *Tietz textbook of clinical chemistry.* Elsevier, Edinburgh, UK, 2012.
23. Zelmat MS. Direct and indirect ion selective electrodes methods: the differences specified through a case of Waldenström's macroglobulinemia. *Ann Biol Clin (Paris).* 2015 May;73(3):345–52. Available from: http://www.john-libbey-eurotext.fr/medline.md?doi=10.1684/abc.2015.1046
24. Mariani F, Gualandi I, Schuhmann W, Scavetta E. Micro- and nano-devices for electrochemical sensing. *Microchim Acta.* 2022 Dec 22;189(12):459. Available from: https://link.springer.com/10.1007/s00604-022-05548-3
25. Krzyczmonik P, Socha E, Skrzypek S. Electrochemical detection of glucose in beverage samples using poly(3,4-ethylenedioxythiophene)-modified electrodes with immobilized glucose oxidase. *Electrocatalysis.* 2018 May 28;9(3):380–7. Available from: http://link.springer.com/10.1007/s12678-017-0442-2
26. Correia R, James S, Lee S-W, Morgan SP, Korposh S. Biomedical application of optical fibre sensors. *J Opt.* 2018 Jul 1;20(7):073003. Available from: https://iopscience.iop.org/article/10.1088/2040-8986/aac68d
27. Kim S, Malik J, Seo JM, Cho YM, Bien F. Subcutaneously implantable electromagnetic biosensor system for continuous glucose monitoring. *Sci Rep.* 2022 Oct 17;12(1):17395. Available from: https://www.nature.com/articles/s41598-022-22128-w
28. Chalklen T, Jing Q, Kar-Narayan S. Biosensors based on mechanical and electrical detection techniques. *Sensors.* 2020 Sep 30;20(19):5605. Available from: https://www.mdpi.com/1424-8220/20/19/5605
29. Robinson PK. Enzymes: principles and biotechnological applications. *Essays Biochem.* 2015 Nov 15;59:1–41. Available from: https://portlandpress.com/essaysbiochem/article/doi/10.1042/bse0590001/88345/Enzymes-principles-and-biotechnological
30. Murugaiyan S, Ramasamy R, Gopal N, Kuzhandaivelu V. Biosensors in clinical chemistry: an overview. *Adv Biomed Res.* 2014;3(1):67. Available from: https://journals.lww.com/10.4103/2277-9175.125848
31. Piroozmand F, Mohammadipanah F, Faridbod F. Emerging biosensors in detection of natural products. *Synth Syst Biotechnol.* 2020 Dec;5(4):293–303. Available from: https://linkinghub.elsevier.com/retrieve/pii/S2405805X20300612
32. Mehrotra P. Biosensors and their applications – A review. *J Oral Biol Craniofacial Res.* 2016 May;6(2):153–9. Available from: https://linkinghub.elsevier.com/retrieve/pii/S2212426815001323
33. Senf B, Yeo W-H, Kim J-H. Recent advances in portable biosensors for biomarker detection in body fluids. *Biosensors.* 2020 Sep 18;10(9):127. Available from: https://www.mdpi.com/2079-6374/10/9/127
34. Li Y-Y, Ma X-X, Song X-Y, Ma L-L, Li Y-Y, Meng X, et al. Glucose biosensor based on glucose oxidase immobilized on BSA cross-linked nanocomposite modified glassy carbon electrode. *Sensors.* 2023 Mar 17;23(6):3209. Available from: https://www.mdpi.com/1424-8220/23/6/3209
35. Yang S, Atanasov P, Wilkins E. A glucose biosensor based on an oxygen electrode: in-vitro performances in model buffer solution and in blood plasma. *Biomed Instrum Technol.* 1996;30(1):55–61. Available from: http://www.ncbi.nlm.nih.gov/pubmed/8850596
36. Ikeda T, Kano K. An electrochemical approach to the studies of biological redox reactions and their applications to biosensors, bioreactors, and biofuel cells. *J Biosci Bioeng.* 2001 Jan;92(1):9–18. Available from: https://linkinghub.elsevier.com/retrieve/pii/S1389172301801912
37. Gui Q, Lawson T, Shan S, Yan L, Liu Y. The application of whole cell-based biosensors for use in environmental analysis and in medical diagnostics. *Sensors.* 2017 Jul 13;17(7):1623. Available from: http://www.mdpi.com/1424-8220/17/7/1623
38. Chen H, Zhang J, Huang R, Wang D, Deng D, Zhang Q, et al. The applications of electrochemical immunosensors in the detection of disease biomarkers: a review. *Molecules.* 2023 Apr 20;28(8):3605. Available from: https://www.mdpi.com/1420-3049/28/8/3605

39. Lim SA, Ahmed MU. Introduction to immunosensors. In: *Immunosensors*. The Royal Society of Chemistry; 2019. p. 1–20. Available from: https://books.rsc.org/books/book/1900/chapter/2494036/Introduction-to-Immunosensors
40. Immunosensors. *Philos Trans R Soc London B, Biol Sci*. 1987 Aug 28;316(1176):121–34. Available from: https://royalsocietypublishing.org/doi/10.1098/rstb.1987.0022
41. Nakane PK, Pierce GB. Enzyme-labeled antibodies for the light and electron microscopic localization of tissue antigens. *J Cell Biol*. 1967 May 1;33(2):307–18. Available from: https://rupress.org/jcb/article/33/2/307/16938/ENZYME-LABELED-ANTIBODIES-FOR-THE-LIGHT-AND
42. Sohrabi N, Valizadeh A, Farkhani SM, Akbarzadeh A. Basics of DNA biosensors and cancer diagnosis. *Artif Cells, Nanomedicine, Biotechnol*. 2016 Feb 17;44(2):654–63. Available from: https://www.tandfonline.com/doi/full/10.3109/21691401.2014.976707
43. Weile J, Knabbe C. Current applications and future trends of molecular diagnostics in clinical bacteriology. *Anal Bioanal Chem*. 2009 Jun 18;394(3):731–42. Available from: http://link.springer.com/10.1007/s00216-009-2779-8
44. Naresh V, Lee N. A review on biosensors and recent development of nanostructured materials-enabled biosensors. *Sensors*. 2021 Feb 5;21(4):1109. Available from: https://www.mdpi.com/1424-8220/21/4/1109
45. Derkus B. Applying the miniaturization technologies for biosensor design. *Biosens Bioelectron*. 2016 May;79:901–13. Available from: https://linkinghub.elsevier.com/retrieve/pii/S0956566316300343
46. Ramesh M, Janani R, Deepa C, Rajeshkumar L. Nanotechnology-enabled biosensors: a review of fundamentals, design principles, materials, and applications. *Biosensors*. 2022 Dec 27;13(1):40. Available from: https://www.mdpi.com/2079-6374/13/1/40
47. Castillo-Henríquez L, Brenes-Acuña M, Castro-Rojas A, Cordero-Salmerón R, Lopretti-Correa M, Vega-Baudrit JR. Biosensors for the detection of bacterial and viral clinical pathogens. *Sensors*. 2020 Dec 4;20(23):6926. Available from: https://www.mdpi.com/1424-8220/20/23/6926

3

Mass Spectrometry-Based Proteomics in Precision Medicine

Refat M. Nimer and Anas M. Abdel Rahman

3.1 Introduction

3.1.1 Mass Spectrometry

Mass spectrometry (MS) is a powerful analytical tool used to identify and measure the molecular mass of macromolecules and small molecules. MS measures the mass-to-charge ratio (m/z) of the ionized molecules in the gas phase under low pressure (high vacuum) [1]. The ionization process is developed in an ion source, separated inside the mass analyzer based on m/z, and then detected for better signal quantification. Biological molecules are often analyzed using MS after ionization using electrospray ionization (ESI) or matrix-assisted laser desorption/ionization (MALDI) [2, 3]. These ionization methods are considered soft ionization techniques that do not significantly fragment the analyzed compounds. The electrospray process involves the generation of a fine mist of charged droplets from a liquid sample, which subsequently undergoes desolvation and ion formation, ultimately allowing for the introduction of the analytes into the mass spectrometer [4]. At the same time, the underlying principle of MALDI-MS involves using a matrix material that absorbs energy from a laser, facilitating the desorption and ionization of the sample. The MALDI process relies on the co-crystallization of the analyte with an energy-absorbing matrix compound, which is then irradiated by a pulsed laser. The matrix absorbs the laser energy, leading to the desorption and ionization of the sample, which are subsequently detected by a mass spectrometer [5]. MALDI-MS is often used to analyze peptide mixtures in less complicated matrices. However, ESI-MS is favored for the analysis of intricate samples.

The MS analyzers are the most critical component for separating the ions based on their m/z. The resolving power of these analyzers is varied, such as quadrupole and conventional ion trap, and high resolution, such as time-of-flight (TOF), orbitrap, and Fourier-transform ion cyclotron resonance (FT-ICR) analyzers. They exhibit significant dissimilarities in structure and efficiency, which are two distinct aspects, each with advantages and disadvantages. These analyzers may function independently or, in some instances, be used in tandem to leverage each other's respective benefits [6]. The performance of the mass analyzers may be assessed by considering factors like resolution, mass accuracy, and acquisition speed [7]. One of the most active areas of mass spectrometric development in recent years has been the improvement of resolution. Resolution in MS refers to the capacity to differentiate between two peaks with slightly varying mass-to-charge ratios ΔM in a mass spectrum [8]. Mass accuracy refers to the difference between the theoretical and measured mass, indicating the deviation of the instrument's response. The measurement is often denoted in parts per million (ppm) [9]. Acquisition speed in mass spectrometry refers to the velocity at which the instrument collects data, specifically how rapidly it can scan over a range of m/z values and capture the quantity of ions at each point.

Another important characteristic of MS is the dynamic range. This refers to the capacity to determine proteins with low abundance in extremely abundant proteins [10].

DOI: 10.1201/9781003486909-3

MS is a prominent technology that facilitates translating research into clinical practice. It is often used in many settings for therapeutic drug monitoring (TDM), toxicology, and conducting newborn screening for genetic abnormalities [11, 12]. Utilizing clinical MS approaches contributes to advancing our comprehension and skills to improve therapy by investigating individual-level chemical pathology in greater depth [13]. MS is an effective tool for integrating precision medicine into practice.

3.1.2 Proteomics

Proteins are organic compounds composed of amino acids, serving as life's fundamental units. The genetic code of the genome is translated into different proteins to encode cell functionality and diversity. While mRNA expression may provide insights into protein expression, mRNA expression levels do not consistently correlate with protein abundance [14]. In addition, the examination of mRNA fails to consider protein post-translational modifications, cleavage, complex formation, and localization, as well as the many alternative mRNA transcripts that might be generated. Several post-transcriptional modifications prevent a direct correlation between gene expression and the final product.

Furthermore, the resulting proteins frequently exhibit variations compared to the initial gene [15]. These factors are crucial for protein functionality [16]. Unlike mRNA, proteins are characterized by greater stability. They are often found in far larger amounts inside the cell, reducing the likelihood of fluctuations in their levels. Proteins are more immediate and essential in preserving cellular activities than transcripts [17]. Furthermore, proteome expression is more sensitively associated with physiological and environmental stresses, such as phenotype, than the genome or the transcriptome [18, 19].

The study of proteins and their collective effects on the structure and function of cells is a part of modern proteomics. Thus, proteomics is an emerging branch of science, categorized within the broader topic of "omics", that investigates the connections, functions, compositions, and architectures of proteins and their activities inside cells [20]. The expression "proteome" was first coined by Mark Wilkins in 1994 to describe the range of proteins from a genome to an organism in proteomics [21]. Proteomics thus involves the identification of the proteins present to understand the complexity of a biological system.

Proteomics is inherently multidisciplinary, made possible by the synchronized integration of several scientific disciplines. Some important areas of study in this field include genome sequencing, protein separation science, MS technique, and bioinformatics [22].

MS was the revolutionized technique in proteomics, especially for protein identification and quantification [23]. The progression of MS-based proteomics technology has enhanced our comprehension of proteomes' intricate and ever-changing characteristics. In addition to MS, the field of proteomics has dramatically profited from advancements in genomics, particularly by completing the Human Genome Project [24]. This landmark achievement provided a comprehensive reference of the human genetic code, enabling researchers to understand the relationship between genes and proteins better. By accessing the complete genome, scientists can accurately identify and quantify proteins, study their functions, and understand how genetic variations influence protein expression and modifications. This synergy between genomics and proteomics has enhanced our ability to explore complex biological systems and diseases at a molecular level.

MS-based proteomics can be categorized into untargeted ("discovery") and targeted proteomics. Untargeted proteomics aims to determine and measure the maximum number of proteins feasible. In contrast, target proteomics seeks to identify and measure a particular group of proteins in a complex biological sample [25]. Targeted proteomics methods enable the establishment of efficient and accurate assays that can test and validate potential biomarkers with high sensitivity, reproducibility, and quantification [26, 27]. In the targeted approach, methods like selective reaction monitoring (SRM), multiple reaction monitoring (MRM), and parallel reaction monitoring (PRM) utilize proteotypic peptides that represent target proteins [28]. These methods are employed to create efficient and sensitive tests for individual proteins or groups of proteins [29]. Bottom-up and top-down proteomics are the two main methods in MS-based proteomics. "Bottom-up" protein analysis involves characterizing proteins by analyzing peptides that arise from the protein through proteolysis [30]. In contrast, "top-down" involves the analysis of intact protein without prior proteolysis [31].

Two commonly used MS data acquisition strategies are data-dependent acquisition (DDA) and data-independent acquisition (DIA). In DDA modes, the mass spectrometer fragments the peptide peaks that are most abundant automatically in every scan [32]. In particular, sequential window acquisition of all theoretical mass spectra (SWATH-MS) fragment peptides in DIA mode falls within a certain mass-to-charge (m/z) range [33].

Success in MS-based proteomics hinges on three key aspects: sample preparation, measurement, and data analysis. Prior to MS analysis, two-dimensional gel electrophoresis (2-DE) and sodium dodecyl sulfate-polyacrylamide gel electrophoresis (SDS-PAGE) were the main techniques used for sample separation with more than 10,000 proteoforms [34].

Since 2011, proteomics has substantially evolved, introducing the age of "next-generation proteomics". The progress has been propelled by the simultaneous utilization of the Orbitrap mass analyzer, upgraded LC technology, and better MS parameters [35, 36].

In medicine, the most immediate benefits of applying proteomics methods include identifying novel disease-specific markers from differential protein profiling, elucidating protein function, understanding the basic mechanisms of many disorders and treatments, and discovering therapeutic targets and treatments [37–40].

Due to the position between genetic and epigenetic inputs, biochemical outputs, and the integration of environmental signals, proteomics is well-suited to contribute substantially to health discovery and management.

3.1.3 Precision Medicine

Clinical decision-making formerly used a "one-size-fits-all" strategy, which depended on pathophysiology knowledge and clinical experience [41].

The inter-individual heterogeneity in many illnesses indicates that approaches for treating, monitoring, and preventing a disease must be diverse or "personalized" to each individual's unique biochemical, physiological, environmental exposure, and behavioral profile [42].

A notable change in how diseases are treated, monitored, and prevented is known as personalized medicine. In this context, personalized medicine tailors individual treatments to achieve maximum efficacy and minimal toxicity [43]. According to the US National Human Genome Research Institute, personalized medicine is "an emerging practice that uses an individual's genetic profile to guide disease prevention, diagnosis, and treatment decisions".

Personalized medicine is not new; it has been around for more than two millennia, as stated in The Yellow Emperor's Canon of Internal Medicine. However, the concept of personalized medicine has gained significant traction recently due to two key factors. First, the realization is that most drugs have limitations in effectiveness and safety. Second, advancements like the Human Genome Project have allowed tailoring treatments based on individual genetic profiles [44].

Precision medicine (PM) and personalized medicine are frequently used interchangeably in practical applications. The White House introduced the PM Initiative in 2016 (https://obamawhitehouse.archives.gov). Since then, it has garnered interest from the worldwide community. PM aims to better "fit" therapy to an individual patient by considering the patient's genetics, epigenetics, proteomics, and other patient variables. Personalized medicine is a fairly old concept considering the patient's genetic composition, beliefs, interests, knowledge, and social circumstances [45]. The phrase "personalized" was first taken with skepticism since some thought it might suggest that preventative and treatment plans are specifically tailored to each person. Due to this, "precision medicine" was chosen above "personalized medicine" by the US National Research Council [46].

PM seeks to stratify patient groups for more efficient and tailored therapy to improve human health while reducing the risk of side effects [47]. Innovations in diagnosis and tailored treatments made possible by integrating massive amounts of data with state-of-the-art computer analysis further benefit the healthcare sector. Technological advancements in patient characterization utilizing "omics" such as proteomics, metabolomics, and genomics, coupled with the recent finishing of the Human Genome Project, open the door for PM to impact clinical decision-making significantly [48]. PM enables anticipating treatment responses and potential negative outcomes by identifying and studying novel prognostic, diagnostic, and therapeutic biomarkers. This helps fill the gap between fundamental research and patient clinical management.

One of the mainstreams of PM is "pharmacoproteomics". The term "pharmacoproteomics" came in parallel with "pharmacogenomics" and was first mentioned in the literature in the early 2000s [49, 50], corresponding with the initial stages of rapid expansion in the broader field of proteomics and its associated technologies. Pharmacoproteomics enables the examination of drug mechanisms at the proteome level, allowing for the exploration of toxicity, resistance, and the identification of possible new therapeutic targets at the early stages of drug development [51].

In addition to biomarkers for diseases and pharmacoproteomics, prototype creation and refining are key to individualized treatment in precision medicine. Cancer diagnostic prototypes such as liquid biopsy tests are being developed to identify circulating tumor DNA (ctDNA) in blood samples. These prototypes provide real-time insights into a patient's tumor biology by monitoring cancer development and therapy response non-invasively. These early-stage diagnostic technologies may discover genetic mutations and modifications to guide targeted medicines, increasing treatment success and reducing adverse effects [52]. As prototypes are evaluated and adjusted, they enable more accurate and tailored cancer therapy, demonstrating precision medicine's transformational potential. While the integration of omics-generated data and clinical data is driving the growth of PM, covering detailed discussions of various omics technologies is beyond the scope of this chapter. Therefore, our focus in this chapter will be only on proteomics.

3.2 Applications of Mass Spectrometry-Based Proteomics in Precision Medicine

Since 2001, the announcement of the human genome draft has resulted in the availability of a significant quantity of knowledge about gene products via genomic sequencing [53]. The advancements in genomics and transcriptomics have contributed significantly to the development of precision medicine [10]. These areas have revolutionized our comprehension of the molecular components of illnesses, resulting in the development of tailored therapies. Genomics thoroughly analyzes the genetic code, whereas transcriptomics specifically studies gene expression in a cell or organism [54]. These technologies have enabled the discovery of many mutations that have spread across various diseases.

Nevertheless, the two issues of indicating the shift from superfluous mutations into "real" disease drivers and the question of managing disease heterogeneity, such as in cancer and its resilient clonal populations, remain challenging. The heterogeneity in the wider population challenges the implementation of precision treatment and customized medicine. This heterogeneity has resulted in limitations in the performance of biomarkers and the effectiveness of therapeutic interventions [55]. Furthermore, these various mutations alone are inadequate indicators of the disease phenotype. The phenotype influences the environment, lifestyle choices, social factors, and epigenetic effects. One method of seeing how those mutations translate to the functional level is by analyzing proteins in cells and tissues affected by diseases like cancer, which can reveal information about disease pathways and potential treatment targets for medical interventions [56]. Drugs that specifically target mitogen-activated protein kinase 1 (MAPK), Phosphoinositide 3-kinases (PI3K), serine/threonine-protein kinase B-raf (BRAF), vascular endothelial growth factor (VEGF), anaplastic lymphoma kinase (ALK), and epidermal growth factor receptor (EGFR) directly inhibit these targets at the protein level, instead of at the level of individual genes [57].

Immunoassays have been the primary method used in medical diagnostics for more than five decades. Although immunoassays have benefits in terms of sensitivity and dynamic range, their inability to conclusively identify the target molecule is a substantial constraint.

On the other hand, MS is becoming a very attractive option since it has high sensitivity, accuracy, and speed, relies less on reagents, does not rely on protein epitopes, and has greater multiplexing capabilities for particular analyses [58]. Advancement in MS technology is positioned to overcome the inherent limits of immunoassays. In this regard, MS-based proteomics offers an emerging tool for comprehensively identifying and quantifying biomolecules in samples like blood and urine. Through this technology, we can understand the relationships among biological elements relevant to various diseases [58]. In addition, this approach has played a role in advancing precision medicine by allowing for tailored treatment and diagnostic strategies for patients [59]. In particular, quantitative proteomics offers a cutting-edge strategy as a vital method in PM since it uncovers physiological distinctions across biological samples by examining protein abundance levels [60].

The main goal is to integrate proteomics data with genetics and clinical information to provide an individualized proteomics profile for every patient, improving the treatment process [61]. For example, by using proteomic and genomic data, it is becoming more feasible to anticipate the medicine or antibody that is most probable to result in effective therapy for a certain patient's cancer [62, 63]. Platinum-based antineoplastic treatments are necessary for advanced ovarian carcinoma. Platinum drugs have different effects on different persons, making it difficult to predict their effects before prescribing. Yu et al. analyzed 130 ovarian carcinoma patients' proteomic profiles and clinical features and established novel models to predict platinum-based chemotherapy response in ovarian carcinoma patients [63].

In contrast to those found in adults, pediatric tumors often show poor mutations in their DNA that can pose a challenge when pinpointing treatment targets using genomics approaches. For instance, medulloblastomas, a type of brain cancer, revealed distinctions that were identified by MS-based proteomics, not by genomics [64]. With such a study, Archer et al. classified the medulloblastoma patients into subgroups with respect to outcomes according to proteomics data. This study indicated that utilizing MS-based proteomics to study protein modifications could be promising for uncovering diagnostic and therapeutic targets in pediatric tumors with limited genetic mutations.

Moreover, MS-based proteomics is considered a powerful approach in identifying a target for future immunotherapies such as in ovarian cancer [65].

In cancer proteomics, Metamark Genetics first identified 12 biomarkers for formalin-fixed paraffin-embedded tissue samples. These biomarkers were subsequently reduced to an 8-marker test. This protein profile has shown the ability to accurately predict outcomes in prostate cancer patients, differentiating between "favorable" and "unfavorable" disease [66, 67]. Furthermore, it enhances the precision of conclusions and therapeutic interventions made after a biopsy by the ability of this test to detect unfavorable pathology during radical prostatectomy and predict risk more accurately.

Another example of the complex nature of cancer is urothelial carcinoma (UC), which may manifest in non-invasive or aggressive forms, each with its own set of distinctive molecular and clinical characteristics [68]. Because of this heterogeneity, the treatments' efficacy varies in UC with tumor stage and molecular profile [69]. Several studies utilizing mass proteomics approaches have found biomarkers like Cyclin D3 and aquaporin-1 [70–72].

Nedjadi et al. found that haptoglobin demonstrated notable sensitivity and specificity in differentiating low-grade bladder cancer patients from controls [73]. Overexpression of aquaporin-1 has been seen in high-grade invasive UC and is linked to worse survival outcomes.

Thus, these biomarkers hold promise for advancing treatment approaches and improving precision treatment outcomes.

MS-based proteomic was utilized to analyze more than 130 clinical breast samples and classify them based on protein expression [74]. Various proteins, such as serotransferrin, alpha-1 antitrypsin, hemopexin, CRP, and albumin, have been found to be expressed differently in ovarian cancer [75]. These results indicate that they might be useful as a combination of many markers for the purpose of screening and detecting the illness.

Lung cancer is a complex disease that often presents with symptoms that complicate early diagnosis and prognosis prediction. In a research conducted by Davies et al., a set of blood proteins was discovered that may be associated with an early risk for lung cancer [76]. Sung et al. showed that quiescin sulfhydryl oxidase 1 (QSOX1) protein was expressed in lung cancer tissue much more than in normal tissues in the area, which could be useful as a potential therapeutic target [77].

A proteomics study by Tang et al. showed that proteins like olfactomedin 4, kininogen-1, and Sec-24 were differently expressed in colon cancer patients [78]. Moreover, Yu et al. found that serine/threonine kinase 4 is downregulated in colorectal cancer and may be utilized as a biomarker for early diagnosis of the disease [79]. Milighetti et al. conducted a study on 36 FFPE samples of several forms of sarcoma in a confined illness context utilizing MS-proteomics. Their study demonstrated that each subtype of sarcoma may have distinct traits that emphasize the importance of proteomics in classifying illnesses

[80]. Regarding chronic illnesses, Yang et al. identified urine proteins that are specifically associated with proliferative diabetic retinopathy in a group of 210 individuals diagnosed with type 2 diabetes [81].

Moreover, proteomic studies have been utilized to predict the susceptibility of drugs and uncover possible protein players that contribute to drug resistance [82, 83]. The successful use of precision medicine to date has been in the use of molecularly targeted therapies, such as Imatinib in Chronic Myelogenous Leukemia (CML), Trastuzumab in HER2-positive breast cancer, EGFR and ALK inhibitors in lung cancer, and B-Raf inhibitors in melanoma [84].

Proteomics analyses were performed on 116 stage IV melanoma patients receiving tumor-infiltrating lymphocytes (TILs) or anti-PD treatments. Patients were categorized as responders or non-responders and their protein composition was examined using high-resolution mass spectrometry. The study found substantial lipid and oxidative metabolism differences between individuals who responded well to both treatments and those who did not. Lipid and ketone metabolisms most negatively impact tumor immunogenicity and cancer cell antigen presentation [85]. Akkour et al. examined tissues collected from patients diagnosed with hyperplasia and endometrial cancer (EC). They found 32 proteins differing between EC and hyperplasia, such as desmin, peptidyl-prolyl cis-trans isomerase A, and zinc finger protein [86].

MS-based proteomics, a rapidly evolving omic technology in PM, is not restricted only to cancer but is seen in complex metabolic, genetics, and inflammatory diseases [87–90].

Ferrannini et al. employed proteomics to identify proteins linked to coronary artery disease (CAD) risk. Multiple proteins linked to either elevated or reduced CAD risk were discovered, aiding in the stratification of patient risk, such as protein shisa-3 homolog (PS-3) and myosin regulatory light chain 2 (MYO) [91].

Multidimensional data, including proteomics, further refine subgroups of neurodegenerative diseases such as Parkinson's, which may benefit from finding novel biomarkers and more tailored treatments [92]. Multi biomarkers could distinguish between early stage of PD and healthy individuals such as Granulin precursor, Mannan-binding-lectin-serine-peptidase-2, Endoplasmatic-reticulum-chaperone-BiP, Prostaglaindin-H2-D-isomaerase, Interceullular-adhesion-molecule-1, Complement C3, Dickkopf-WNT-signaling pathway-inhibitor-3, and Plasma-protease-C1-inhibitor [93].

Neuroinflammation markers, including Transforming growth factor beta (TGF-β), Tumor necrosis factor alpha (TNF-α), Interleukin 1 beta (IL-1β), and Triggering receptor expressed on myeloid cells 2 (TREM2), can be utilized to identify certain subgroups of Alzheimer's disease and to create customized therapeutic approaches that focus on targeting neuroinflammation within the framework of aging-related diseases [94, 95].

MS-based proteomics is also essential in precision medicine for the management of cystic fibrosis (CF), a hereditary condition resulting from mutations in the Cystic Fibrosis Transmembrane Conductance Regulator (CFTR) gene. It has a major impact on the advancement and refinement of CFTR modulators, which are specialized treatments aimed at reinstating or improving the function of CFTR proteins [96]. Both Kalydeco (VX-770) and Orkambi (VX-770 plus VX-809) are medications for CF that were developed via the use of small-molecular compounds that modify the CFTR, ivacaftor/VX-770 and lumacaftor/VX-809 [97, 98].

These examples of studies showed that MS-based proteomics is becoming an additional tool in the precision medicine toolbox as technology has progressed. However, several challenges still need to be overcome before they can be widely used in clinical settings.

3.3 Challenges and Future Directions

Many current developments in the MS-based proteomics field, such as sensitive and robust bioinformatics software, improved sample preparation, including protein digestion and fractionation, high-resolution orthogonal strategies for quantification, alternative protease cleavage to improve sequence coverage, together with new ionization approaches and novel MS instruments which provide rapid serial sampling of large clinical cohorts, have poised the modern MS-based proteomics to move on from research to clinics.

Nevertheless, the development of precision medicine toward integration and implementation into clinical settings represents technological and conceptual obstacles. One of the significant obstacles in using MS-based proteomics in clinical settings is the high cost and the need for specialized skills due to the complexity of these approaches. The complexity inherent in the heterogeneity of diseases, particularly cancer, plays a significant role in slowing down shifting to precision medicine. Advancements in MS-based proteomics, particularly the advent of single-cell proteomics, offer a powerful tool to overcome the challenge of cellular heterogeneity within tumors [99]. In addition, there is a lack of reproducibility and technical standardization. In order to completely verify these potential biomarkers, it is imperative to conduct extensive, prospective multi-center clinical studies in the near future, using standardized methodologies. Moreover, a complete quality control (QC) analysis is required to overcome next-generation proteomics' standardization and reproducibility issues. This framework should include standard reference materials, standard operating procedures (SOPs), and well-defined reference datasets.

Integrated omics datasets with clinical data are essential to complete the picture of our understanding of disease heterogeneity and find potential biomarkers to aid in the development of precision medicine. However, large omics datasets often have limited overlap in the information they capture and poor correlation [100]. Additionally, large-scale data generates computational and statistical challenges.

Future research efforts should focus on overcoming these obstacles in order to provide extensive multiomics data necessary for understanding the intricate biological pathways that control tumor development and progression, resistance to therapy, and the likelihood of recurrence. In order to make significant progress in precision medicine and precision oncology via the use of multiomics techniques, it is necessary to redirect attention away from the limited number of potential diagnostic biomarkers now being promoted to physicians, and instead prioritize the study of comprehensive multiomics signatures and processes. More robust instrumentation, broad training, and standardization are still needed to advance precision medicine. Although there are constraints, MALDI has made progress in identifying bacteria, opening doors for MS use in clinical settings, and the development of precision medicine [62]. Additionally, thanks to advancements in sequencing technology, it is now possible to achieve a proteome that covers over 80% of the transcriptome in just 6 hours [101]. This efficient and cost-effective workflow has made proteomics more accessible than ever before. Currently, precision medicine often depends on funding provided for short periods of time and specific projects. These financing strategies usually have a restricted scope and do not consider long-term viability [102]. In order to effectively achieve precision medicine's future promise, it is essential to transition to finance structures that prioritize long-term viability and expandability.

REFERENCES

1. Kaklamanos G, Aprea E, Theodoridis G. Mass spectrometry: principles and instrumentation. In: Pico Y; *Chemical analysis of food: Techniques and applications.* Elsevier, New York, USA; 2020. p. 525–52.
2. Fenn JB, Mann M, Meng CK, Wong SF, Whitehouse CM. Electrospray ionization for mass spectrometry of large biomolecules. *Science.* 1989;246(4926):64–71.
3. Karas M, Hillenkamp F. Laser desorption ionization of proteins with molecular masses exceeding 10,000 daltons. *Anal Chem.* 1988;60(20):2299–301.
4. Ho CS, Lam CW, Chan MH, Cheung RC, Law LK, Lit LC, Ng KF, Suen MW, Tai HL. Electrospray ionisation mass spectrometry: principles and clinical applications. *Clin Biochem Rev.* 2003;24(1):3–12.
5. Hillenkamp F, Jaskolla TW, Karas M. The MALDI process and method. In: Hillenkamp F, Peter-Katalinic J, editors. *MALDI MS A practical guide to instrumentation, methods, and applications.* 2nd ed. Weinheim, Germany: Wiley Blackwell; 2014.
6. Aebersold R, Mann M. Mass spectrometry-based proteomics. *Nature.* 2003;422(6928):198–207.
7. Abdel Rahman AM. The advanced technology and clinical application in metabolomics. In: Abdel Rahman AM (eds) *Clinical metabolomics applications in genetic diseases.* Springer, Singapore; 2023. p. 1–15.
8. Tamara S, den Boer MA, Heck AJ. High-resolution native mass spectrometry. *Chem Rev.* 2021;122(8):7269–326.

9. De Hoffmann E, Stroobant V. *Mass spectrometry: principles and applications*. John Wiley & Sons, Hoboken, New Jersey; 2007.
10. Doll S, Gnad F, Mann M. The case for proteomics and phospho-proteomics in personalized cancer medicine. *PROTEOMICS–Clin Appl.* 2019;13(2):1800113.
11. Clarke NJ. Mass spectrometry in precision medicine: phenotypic measurements alongside pharmacogenomics. *Clin Chem.* 2016;62(1):70–6.
12. Gelb MH, Basheeruddin K, Burlina A, Chen HJ, Chien YH, Dizikes G, et al. Liquid chromatography-tandem mass spectrometry in newborn screening laboratories. *Int J Neonatal Screen.* 2022;8(4):62.
13. Hristova J, Svinarov D. Enhancing precision medicine through clinical mass spectrometry platform. *Biotechnol Biotechnol Equip.* 2022;36(1):107–17.
14. Liu Y, Beyer A, Aebersold R. On the dependency of cellular protein levels on mRNA abundance. *Cell.* 2016;165(3):535–50.
15. Valenti F, Falcone I, Ungania S, Desiderio F, Giacomini P, Bazzichetto C, et al. Precision medicine and melanoma: multi-omics approaches to monitoring the immunotherapy response. *Int J Mol Sci.* 2021;22(8):3837.
16. Upadhya SR, Ryan CJ. Experimental reproducibility limits the correlation between mRNA and protein abundances in tumor proteomic profiles. *Cell Rep Methods.* 2022;2(9):100288.
17. Reimegård J, Tarbier M, Danielsson M, Schuster J, Baskaran S, Panagiotou S, et al. A combined approach for single-cell mRNA and intracellular protein expression analysis. *Commun Biol.* 2021;4(1):624.
18. Ferkingstad E, Sulem P, Atlason BA, Sveinbjornsson G, Magnusson MI, Styrmisdottir EL, et al. Large-scale integration of the plasma proteome with genetics and disease. *Nat Genet.* 2021;53(12):1712–21.
19. Jacob M, Gu X, Luo X, Al-Mousa H, Arnaout R, Al-Saud B, et al. Metabolomics distinguishes DOCK8 deficiency from atopic dermatitis: towards a biomarker discovery. *Metabolites.* 2019;9(11):274.
20. Wilkins MR, Sanchez J-C, Gooley AA, Appel RD, Humphery-Smith I, Hochstrasser DF, et al. Progress with proteome projects: why all proteins expressed by a genome should be identified and how to do it. *Biotechnol Genet Eng Rev.* 1996;13(1):19–50.
21. Wilkins MR, Pasquali C, Appel RD, Ou K, Golaz O, Sanchez JC, et al. From proteins to proteomes: large scale protein identification by two-dimensional electrophoresis and amino acid analysis. *Biotechnol (NY).* 1996;14(1):61–5.
22. Tyers M, Mann M. From genomics to proteomics. *Nature.* 2003;422(6928):193–7.
23. Domon B, Aebersold R. Options and considerations when selecting a quantitative proteomics strategy. *Nat Biotechnol.* 2010;28(7):710–21.
24. Venter JC, Adams MD, Myers EW, Li PW, Mural RJ, Sutton GG, et al. The sequence of the human genome. *Science.* 2001;291(5507):1304–51.
25. Sobsey CA, Ibrahim S, Richard VR, Gaspar V, Mitsa G, Lacasse V, et al. Targeted and untargeted proteomics approaches in biomarker development. *Proteomics.* 2020;20(9):1900029.
26. Su M, Zhang Z, Zhou L, Han C, Huang C, Nice EC. Proteomics, personalized medicine and cancer. *Cancers (Basel).* 2021;13(11):2512.
27. Malkawi AK, Nimer RM, Almogren M, Masood A, Alarfaj AS, Benabdelkamel H, et al. Quantitative analysis of soluble costimulatory molecules as potential diagnostic biomarkers for rheumatoid arthritis using LC-MS/MS in MRM mode. *Clin Chim Acta.* 2023;548:117501.
28. Borràs E, Sabidó E. What is targeted proteomics? A concise revision of targeted acquisition and targeted data analysis in mass spectrometry. *Proteomics.* 2017;17(17–18):1700180.
29. Sumaily KM, Nimer R, Alzahrani M, Jabar MA, Alodib A, Sabi EM, et al. CFTR protein quantification as a cystic fibrosis diagnostic biomarker in dried blood spots using multiple reaction monitoring tandem mass spectrometry. *J Pharm Biomed Anal.* 2022;216:114801.
30. Zhang Y, Fonslow BR, Shan B, Baek M-C, Yates JR III. Protein analysis by shotgun/bottom-up proteomics. *Chem Rev.* 2013;113(4):2343–94.
31. Kelleher NL, Lin HY, Valaskovic GA, Aaserud DJ, Fridriksson EK, McLafferty FW. Top down versus bottom up protein characterization by tandem high-resolution mass spectrometry. *J Am Chem Soc.* 1999;121(4):806–12.
32. Krasny L, Huang PH. Data-independent acquisition mass spectrometry (DIA-MS) for proteomic applications in oncology. *Mol Omics.* 2021;17(1):29–42.
33. Ludwig C, Gillet L, Rosenberger G, Amon S, Collins BC, Aebersold R. Data-independent acquisition-based SWATH-MS for quantitative proteomics: a tutorial. *Mol Syst Biol.* 2018;14(8):e8126.

34. Nice EC. The separation sciences, the front end to proteomics: An historical perspective. *Biomed Chromatogr.* 2021;35(1):e4995.
35. Köcher T, Pichler P, Swart R, Mechtler K. Analysis of protein mixtures from whole-cell extracts by single-run nanoLC-MS/MS using ultralong gradients. *Nat Protoc.* 2012;7(5):882–90.
36. Thakur SS, Geiger T, Chatterjee B, Bandilla P, Fröhlich F, Cox J, et al. Deep and highly sensitive proteome coverage by LC-MS/MS without prefractionation. *Mol Cell Proteomics.* 2011;10(8).
37. Meissner F, Geddes-McAlister J, Mann M, Bantscheff M. The emerging role of mass spectrometry-based proteomics in drug discovery. *Nat Rev Drug Discov.* 2022;21(9):637–54.
38. Sobsey CA, Ibrahim S, Richard VR, Gaspar V, Mitsa G, Lacasse V, et al. Targeted and untargeted proteomics approaches in biomarker development. *Proteomics.* 2020;20(9):e1900029.
39. Nimer RM, Alfaqih MA, Shehabat ER, Mujammami M, Abdel Rahman AM. Label-free quantitative proteomics analysis for type 2 diabetes mellitus early diagnostic marker discovery using data-independent acquisition mass spectrometry (DIA-MS). *Sci Rep.* 2023;13(1):20880.
40. Nimer RM, Sumaily KM, Almuslat A, Abdel Jabar M, Sabi EM, Al-Muhaizea MA, et al. Dystrophin protein quantification as a Duchenne muscular dystrophy diagnostic biomarker in dried blood spots using multiple reaction monitoring tandem mass spectrometry: a preliminary study. *Molecules.* 2022;27(12):3662.
41. Akhoon N. Precision medicine: a new paradigm in therapeutics. *Int J Prev Med.* 2021;12(1):12.
42. Goetz LH, Schork NJ. Personalized medicine: motivation, challenges, and progress. *Fertil Steril.* 2018;109(6):952–63.
43. Jacob M, Abdel Rahman AM. Metabolomic role in personalized medicine: an update. In: Anas M, Abdel Rahman AM *Clinical metabolomics applications in genetic diseases.* Springer, Singapore; 2023. p. 207–24.
44. Mura S, Couvreur P. Nanotheranostics for personalized medicine. *Adv Drug Deliv Rev.* 2012;64(13):1394–416.
45. Marques L, Costa B, Pereira M, Silva A, Santos J, Saldanha L, et al. Advancing precision medicine: a review of innovative in Silico approaches for drug development, clinical pharmacology and personalized healthcare. *Pharmaceutics.* 2024;16(3):332.
46. Delpierre C, Lefèvre T. Precision and personalized medicine: What their current definition says and silences about the model of health they promote. Implication for the development of personalized health. *Front Sociol.* 2023;8:1112159.
47. König IR, Fuchs O, Hansen G, von Mutius E, Kopp MV. What is precision medicine? *Eur Respir J.* 2017;50(4):1700391.
48. Akhoon N. Precision medicine: a new paradigm in therapeutics. *Int J Prev Med.* 2021;12:12.
49. Witzmann FA, Grant RA. Pharmacoproteomics in drug development. *Pharmacogenomics J.* 2003;3(2):69–76.
50. Chapal N, Molina L, Molina F, Laplanche M, Pau B, Petit P. Pharmacoproteomic approach to the study of drug mode of action, toxicity, and resistance: applications in diabetes and cancer. *Fundam Clin Pharmacol.* 2004;18(4):413–22.
51. Chambliss AB, Chan DW. Precision medicine: from pharmacogenomics to pharmacoproteomics. *Clin Proteomics.* 2016;13:25.
52. Caputo V, Ciardiello F, Corte CMD, Martini G, Troiani T, Napolitano S. Diagnostic value of liquid biopsy in the era of precision medicine: 10 years of clinical evidence in cancer. *Explor Target Antitumor Ther.* 2023;4(1):102–38.
53. Ding C, Qin Z, Li Y, Shi W, Li L, Zhan D, et al. Proteomics and precision medicine. *Small Methods.* 2019;3(7):1900075.
54. Kalisky T, Oriel S, Bar-Lev TH, Ben-Haim N, Trink A, Wineberg Y, et al. A brief review of single-cell transcriptomic technologies. *Brief Funct Genomics.* 2018;17(1):64–76.
55. Uzozie AC, Aebersold R. Advancing translational research and precision medicine with targeted proteomics. *J Proteomics.* 2018;189:1–10.
56. Chutipongtanate S, Dwivedi P. Proteomics: moving toward precision medicine. In: Chutipongtanate S, Hongeng S, editors. *Recent advances in molecular and translational medicine: updates in precision medicine.*Sharjah, UAE, 2021. p. 93–117.
57. Yaffe MB. The scientific drunk and the lamppost: massive sequencing efforts in cancer discovery and treatment. *Sci Signal.* 2013;6(269):pe13.

58. Aebersold R, Mann M. Mass-spectrometric exploration of proteome structure and function. *Nature*. 2016;537(7620):347–55.
59. Clarke NJ. Mass Spectrometry in Precision Medicine: Phenotypic Measurements Alongside Pharmacogenomics. *Clin Chem*. 2016;62(1):70–6.
60. Correa Rojo A, Heylen D, Aerts J, Thas O, Hooyberghs J, Ertaylan G, et al. Towards building a quantitative proteomics toolbox in precision medicine: a mini-review. *Front Physiol*. 2021;12:723510.
61. Sandhu C, Qureshi A, Emili A. Panomics for precision medicine. *Trends Mol Med*. 2018;24(1):85–101.
62. Parker CE, Borchers CH. The special issue: clinical proteomics for precision medicine. *Wiley Online Library*. 2018. p. 1600144.
63. Yu K-H, Levine DA, Zhang H, Chan DW, Zhang Z, Snyder M. Predicting ovarian cancer patients' clinical response to platinum-based chemotherapy by their tumor proteomic signatures. *J Proteome Res*. 2016;15(8):2455–65.
64. Archer TC, Ehrenberger T, Mundt F, Gold MP, Krug K, Mah CK, et al. Proteomics, post-translational modifications, and integrative analyses reveal molecular heterogeneity within medulloblastoma subgroups. *Cancer Cell*. 2018;34(3):396–410. e8.
65. Coscia F, Lengyel E, Duraiswamy J, Ashcroft B, Bassani-Sternberg M, Wierer M, et al. Multi-level proteomics identifies CT45 as a chemosensitivity mediator and immunotherapy target in ovarian cancer. *Cell*. 2018;175(1):159–70. e16.
66. Blume-Jensen P, Berman DM, Rimm DL, Shipitsin M, Putzi M, Nifong TP, et al. Development and clinical validation of an in situ biopsy-based multimarker assay for risk stratification in prostate cancer. *Clin Cancer Res*. 2015;21(11):2591–600.
67. Shipitsin M, Small C, Choudhury S, Giladi E, Friedlander S, Nardone J, et al. Identification of proteomic biomarkers predicting prostate cancer aggressiveness and lethality despite biopsy-sampling error. *Br J Cancer*. 2014;111(6):1201–12.
68. Minoli M, Kiener M, Thalmann GN, Kruithof-de Julio M, Seiler R. Evolution of urothelial bladder cancer in the context of molecular classifications. *Int J Mol Sci*. 2020;21(16):5670.
69. Patel VG, Oh WK, Galsky MD. Treatment of muscle-invasive and advanced bladder cancer in 2020. *CA Cancer J Clin*. 2020;70(5):404–23.
70. Lemańska-Perek A, Lis-Kuberka J, Lepczyński A, Dratwa-Chałupnik A, Tupikowski K, Kątnik-Prastowska I, et al. Potential plasma biomarkers of bladder cancer identified by proteomic analysis: A pilot study. *Adv Clin Exp Med*. 2019;28(3):339–46.
71. Blanca A, Requena MJ, Alvarez J, Cheng L, Montironi R, Raspollini MR, et al. FGFR3 and Cyclin D3 as urine biomarkers of bladder cancer recurrence. *Biomark Med*. 2016;10(3):243–53.
72. Morrissey JJ, Mellnick VM, Luo J, Siegel MJ, Figenshau RS, Bhayani S, et al. Evaluation of urine aquaporin-1 and perilipin-2 concentrations as biomarkers to screen for renal cell carcinoma: a prospective cohort study. *JAMA Oncol*. 2015;1(2):204–12.
73. Nedjadi T, Benabdelkamal H, Albarakati N, Masood A, Al-Sayyad A, Alfadda AA, et al. Circulating proteomic signature for detection of biomarkers in bladder cancer patients. *Sci Rep*. 2020;10(1):10999.
74. Yanovich G, Agmon H, Harel M, Sonnenblick A, Peretz T, Geiger T. Clinical proteomics of breast cancer reveals a novel layer of breast cancer classification. *Cancer Res*. 2018;78(20):6001–10.
75. Swiatly A, Horala A, Matysiak J, Hajduk J, Nowak-Markwitz E, Kokot ZJ. Understanding ovarian cancer: iTRAQ-based proteomics for biomarker discovery. *Int J Mol Sci*. 2018;19(8):2240.
76. Davies MP, Sato T, Ashoor H, Hou L, Liloglou T, Yang R, et al. Plasma protein biomarkers for early prediction of lung cancer. *EBioMedicine*. 2023;93.
77. Sung H-J, Ahn J-M, Yoon Y-H, Na S-S, Choi Y-J, Kim Y-I, et al. Quiescin sulfhydryl oxidase 1 (QSOX1) secreted by lung cancer cells promotes cancer metastasis. *Int J Mol Sci*. 2018;19(10):3213.
78. Quesada-Calvo F, Massot C, Bertrand V, Longuespée R, Blétard N, Somja J, et al. OLFM4, KNG1 and Sec24C identified by proteomics and immunohistochemistry as potential markers of early colorectal cancer stages. *Clin Proteomics*. 2017;14:9.
79. Yu J, Zhai X, Li X, Zhong C, Guo C, Yang F, et al. Identification of MST1 as a potential early detection biomarker for colorectal cancer through a proteomic approach. *Sci Rep*. 2017;7(1):14265.
80. Milighetti M, Krasny L, Lee ATJ, Morani G, Szecsei C, Chen Y, et al. Proteomic profiling of soft tissue sarcomas with SWATH mass spectrometry. *J Proteomics*. 2021;241:104236.

81. Yang J-K, Wang Y-Y, Liu C, Shi T-T, Lu J, Cao X, et al. Urine proteome specific for eye damage can predict kidney damage in patients with type 2 diabetes: a case-control and a 5.3-year prospective cohort study. *Diabetes Care.* 2017;40(2):253–60.
82. Ali M, Khan SA, Wennerberg K, Aittokallio T. Global proteomics profiling improves drug sensitivity prediction: results from a multi-omics, pan-cancer modeling approach. *Bioinformatics.* 2018;34(8):1353–62.
83. Cruz IN, Coley HM, Kramer HB, Madhuri TK, Safuwan NA, Angelino AR, et al. Proteomics analysis of ovarian cancer cell lines and tissues reveals drug resistance-associated proteins. *Cancer Genomics Proteomics.* 2017;14(1):35–51.
84. Duan X-P, Qin B-D, Jiao X-D, Liu K, Wang Z, Zang Y-S. New clinical trial design in precision medicine: discovery, development and direction. *Signal Transduct Target Ther.* 2024;9(1):57.
85. Harel M, Ortenberg R, Varanasi SK, Mangalhara KC, Mardamshina M, Markovits E, et al. Proteomics of melanoma response to immunotherapy reveals mitochondrial dependence. *Cell.* 2019;179(1):236–50.e18.
86. Akkour K, Alanazi IO, Alfadda AA, Alhalal H, Masood A, Musambil M, et al. Tissue-based proteomic profiling in patients with hyperplasia and endometrial cancer. *Cells.* 2022;11(13):2119.
87. Kurgan N, Kjærgaard Larsen J, Deshmukh AS. Harnessing the power of proteomics in precision diabetes medicine. *Diabetologia.* 2024;67(5):783–97.
88. Åkesson J, Hojjati S, Hellberg S, Raffetseder J, Khademi M, Rynkowski R, et al. Proteomics reveal biomarkers for diagnosis, disease activity and long-term disability outcomes in multiple sclerosis. *Nat Commun.* 2023;14(1):6903.
89. Nimer RM, Abdel Rahman AM. Recent advances in proteomic-based diagnostics of cystic fibrosis. *Expert Rev Proteomics.* 2023;20(7–9):151–69.
90. Jacob M, Masood A, Shinwari Z, Abdel Jabbar M, Al-Mousa H, Arnaout R, et al. Proteomics profiling to distinguish DOCK8 deficiency from atopic dermatitis. *Front Allergy.* 2021;2:774902.
91. Ferrannini E, Manca ML, Ferrannini G, Andreotti F, Andreini D, Latini R, et al. Differential proteomics of cardiovascular risk and coronary artery disease in humans. *Front Cardiovasc Med.* 2022;8:790289.
92. Frasier M, Fiske BK, Sherer TB. Precision medicine for Parkinson's disease: the subtyping challenge. *Front Aging Neurosci.* 2022;14:1064057.
93. Hällqvist J, Bartl M, Dakna M, Schade S, Garagnani P, Bacalini M-G, et al. Plasma proteomics identify biomarkers predicting Parkinson's disease up to 7 years before symptom onset. *Nat Commun.* 2024;15(1):4759.
94. Hampel H, Caraci F, Cuello AC, Caruso G, Nisticò R, Corbo M, et al. A path toward precision medicine for neuroinflammatory mechanisms in Alzheimer's disease. *Front Immunol.* 2020;11:456.
95. Arafah A, Khatoon S, Rasool I, Khan A, Rather MA, Abujabal KA, et al. The future of precision medicine in the cure of Alzheimer's disease. *Biomedicines.* 2023;11(2):335.
96. Cholon DM, Gentzsch M. Recent progress in translational cystic fibrosis research using precision medicine strategies. *J Cyst Fibros.* 2018;17(2):S52–S60.
97. Accurso FJ, Rowe SM, Clancy J, Boyle MP, Dunitz JM, Durie PR, et al. Effect of VX-770 in persons with cystic fibrosis and the G551D-CFTR mutation. *N Engl J Med.* 2010;363(21):1991–2003.
98. Boyle MP, Bell SC, Konstan MW, McColley SA, Rowe SM, Rietschel E, et al. A CFTR corrector (lumacaftor) and a CFTR potentiator (ivacaftor) for treatment of patients with cystic fibrosis who have a phe-508del CFTR mutation: a phase 2 randomised controlled trial. *Lancet Respir Med.* 2014;2(7):527–38.
99. Zhu Y, Piehowski PD, Zhao R, Chen J, Shen Y, Moore RJ, et al. Nanodroplet processing platform for deep and quantitative proteome profiling of 10–100 mammalian cells. *Nat Commun.* 2018;9(1):882.
100. Olivier M, Asmis R, Hawkins GA, Howard TD, Cox LA. The need for multi-omics biomarker signatures in precision medicine. *Int J Mol Sci.* 2019;20(19):4781.
101. Ge S, Xia X, Ding C, Zhen B, Zhou Q, Feng J, et al. A proteomic landscape of diffuse-type gastric cancer. *Nat Commun.* 2018;9(1):1012.
102. Lu CY, Terry V, Thomas DM. Precision medicine: affording the successes of science. *NPJ Precis Oncol.* 2023;7(1):3.

4

High-Performance Liquid Chromatography: Usefulness in Medicine and Therapeutics

Sajeeda Shaik, Ruchi Verma, Lalit Kumar, and Rupesh K. Shirodkar

4.1 Introduction

High-performance liquid chromatography (HPLC) is an important analytical tool in medicine and therapeutics. HPLC, known for its precision, versatility, and dependability, separates, identifies, and quantifies components in complicated mixtures. It is a vital instrument in contemporary analytical chemistry, with applications spanning drug discovery, clinical diagnostics, therapeutic monitoring, and pharmaceutical research. This chapter delves into HPLC's numerous utility in medicine and therapeutics, covering its principles, applications, and prospective future use.

Essential components of an HPLC system are:

1. *Mobile Phase:* A solvent or solvent combination that propels the sample across the column.
2. *Pump:* Maintains a constant flow rate by delivering the mobile phase at a consistent pressure.
3. *Injector:* Introduces the sample into the liquid stream of the mobile phase.
4. *Column:* Packed with stationary phase material, wherein separation occurs.
5. *Detector:* Identifies and measures separated items as they exit the column. Common detectors include mass spectrometers, ultraviolet-visible spectroscopy (UV-vis) detectors, mass spectrometry (MS), and fluorescence detectors.
6. *Data System:* Collects, sorts, and assesses data, typically resulting in chromatograms.

The use of HPLC is primarily to separate components between two phases: a mobile phase and a stationary phase. While the mobile phase passes through the stationary phase in a column, different components of a sample mixture separate according to their chemical and physical properties. The choice of a stationary phase, the composition of the mobile phase, the flow rate, the temperature, and the characteristics of the sample all influence the separation process.

4.2 Clinical Utility of HPLC in Medicine and Therapeutics

4.2.1 Drug Discovery

Drug discovery often involves extraction, isolation, and purification of active moieties from plant and animal sources. This is a tedious process and requires skill and expertise in the area. Furthermore, drug molecules may be produced by synthetic procedures; however, that also requires some level of skill and

DOI: 10.1201/9781003486909-4

expertise. Often, synthetic molecules may have higher purity with little adulteration. However, to ensure the safety, stability, and efficacy of molecules obtained from both natural and synthetic sources, a series of characterization steps are required. These characterizations may be both qualitative and quantitative, and HPLC plays a major role. There are a number of HPLC methods that have been developed for plant-based and synthetic molecules. A few of them are listed in Table 4.1.

The development of the new HPLC methods and the detection of molecules are based on several parameters such as the pKa value, partition coefficient, hydrophilicity and lipophilicity, ionization, solubility, temperature, and light sensitivity of the molecules. These parameters are mainly studied at the pre-developmental stage or considered as preliminary pre-formulation data.

HPLC in solubility and dissolution studies helps in estimating the presence of molecules in respective media. HPLC is also useful in the stability studies of drugs where it can assist in determining the degradants produced due to exposure to light, temperature, hydrolysis, and oxidation. It can assist in effectively calculating the conversion of parent molecules or drugs to percent degradants. During the drug discovery process, HPLC is helpful in impurities profiling and can be used in taking a decision on suitable methods or materials for the synthesis of new molecules.

Often, HPLC methods developed should be validated, especially for their specificity, sensitivity, accuracy, precision, and robustness. The HPLC methods developed at this stage are most often utilized even at the drug development stage for the estimation of drugs or molecules in formulations.

4.2.2 Drug Development

Another application of HPLC is its use in drug development. During the drug development process, HPLC is important in the determination of drug content, and drug entrapment, among others. Furthermore, HPLC is also used for in vitro drug release studies, where there is the estimation of drug in dissolution aliquots at different time points. Similar to the drug discovery process, HPLC is also useful in the calculation of the shelf-life of formulations by estimating drug concentrations in them. HPLC methods used at the drug discovery stage can also be used at the drug development stage. However, if chromatographic conditions are modified for any reason, then specificity, sensitivity, precision, accuracy, and robustness should be ensured. Therefore, HPLC may be used as an analytical tool for the optimization of the best drug formulation [11]. HPLC can aid in deciding if formulations need further modifications to improve their quality and shelf-life, as well as the fate of formulations at the preclinical and clinical stages. HPLC methods for the estimation of different drug formulations have been listed in the Table 4.2.

4.2.3 Preclinical Studies

Once drug formulations are developed, they undergo preclinical studies, where pharmacokinetic, bioavailability, and pharmacodynamic studies are performed. At this stage, the formulations are tested in suitable animal models. The formulations are given to animals by a suitable route and samples are collected: blood (serum or plasma) or urine or feces or organ tissues, depending on the requirement of the study. For pharmacokinetic, bioavailability, and tissue distribution studies, collected samples are processed: extraction and isolation of drugs or metabolites with appropriate procedures or methods, and the concentration of isolated molecules estimated using HPLC or liquid chromatography-mass spectrometry (LC-MS). The bioanalytical method used may have similar chromatographic conditions as the analytical method. However, the percent relative standard deviation values may be different for the biological samples and may not be the same as those of the analytical method. Thus, even if the same chromatographic conditions are used at this stage, these should be validated with the optimized method or conditions of extraction and isolation of molecules from biological samples. A few bioanalytical methods for the estimation of molecules, drugs, and/or metabolites are shown in Table 4.3.

TABLE 4.1
HPLC methods for qualitative and quantitative drug screening

No.	Molecule(s)	Instrument used	Detector	Method type	Mobile phase	Reference
1	Hesperetin	HPLC	UV-vis	Isocratic	Acetonitrile (ACN) and orthophosphoric acid (OPA) (50:50, % v/v)	1
2	Gallic acid and hesperetin	HPLC	UV-vis	Gradient	Flow rate 1 mL/min with the gradient from 0 to 5 min 100% (A), from 5 to 15 min 30% (B), from 15 to 20 min 70% (B), and from 20 to 25 min 100%	2
3	Quercetin	HPLC	UV-vis	Gradient	[H_2O (0.1% formic acid, A); Methanol (MeOH): ACN, (40:15, %v/v, B); (40:60, %v/v)] with a flow rate of 0.8 mL/min. The solvent A is 0.2% formic acid in deionized milli Q water and solvent B is 100% ACN	3
4	Andrographolide, eugenol, and zingerone	HPLC	UV-vis	Isocratic	ACN and 0.1% ortho phosphoric acid (30:70, % v/v)	4
5	Carotenoid (lutein, zeaxanthin, beta-cryptoxanthin, and beta-carotene)	HPLC	UV-vis/ MS	Isocratic	ACN: MeOH: CH_2Cl_2: n-heptane (75: 20: 2.5: 2.5, %v/v)	5
6	Lutein	HPLC	UV	Isocratic	n-hexane: Isopropyl alcohol (5%)	6
7	Lutein	HPLC	UV	Isocratic	Water: acetonitrile (10:90, %v/v)	7

(Continued)

TABLE 4.1 (CONTINUED)

HPLC methods for qualitative and quantitative drug screening

No.	Molecule(s)	Instrument used	Detector	Method type	Mobile phase	Reference
8	Bergenin, quercetin, isosalipurposide, and quercitrin	HPLC	UV	Gradient	Solvent A: Acetonitrile; solvent B: water containing 0.2% phosphoric acid. Gradient elution from 10:90 to 100:0, %v/v) to a flow rate of 0.8 mL/min	8
9	Quercetin, caffeic acid, gallic acid, Chlorogenic acid, and naringenin	HPLC	UV	Gradient	Solvent A: Water; Solvent B: acetonitrile. Gradient elution: 0–5 min, 80% A; 5–8 min, 40% A; 8–12 min, 50% A; 12–16 min, 80% A	9
10	Quercetin, ascorbic acid, benzoic acid, gallic acid, vanillin, resorcinol, and catechol	HPLC	Photo diode array (PDA)	Gradient	***Method A:*** Solvent A: ACN; solvent B: 0.1% phosphoric acid in water. Gradient elution: 0–35 min, 92% B; 35–45 min, 78% B. ***Method B:*** Solvent A: Methanol; solvent B: 4% acetic acid. Gradient elution: 0–4 min, 100% B; 4–10 min, 50% B; 10–20 min, 20% B; 20–22 min, 50% B	10

TABLE 4.2

HPLC methods used in the drug development process

No.	Drug(s) or molecule(s)	Instrument used	Detector	Method type	Mobile phase	Reference
1	Biocaluamide and Hesperetin	HPLC	UV-vis	Isocratic	ACN and 0.1% acetic acid (45:55, %v/v)	12
2	Cinacalcet hydrochloride	HPLC	UV-vis	Isocratic	Phosphate buffer and ACN (40:60, %v/v) pH adjusted to 3.0	13
3	Picroside I, Plumbagin, and Z-guggulsterone	HPLC	UV-vis	Gradient	Solvent A: ACN and solvent B: 0.1% orthophosphoric acid in water. The following gradient of: 0 to 12 min, 25% A; 12–17 min, 25–80% A; 17–32 min, 80% A; and 32–37 min 80–25% A at a flow rate of 1 mL/min	14
4	Ritonavir	HPLC	UV-vis	Isocratic	Ortho phosphoric acid: water (pH 3.0) (40:60, %v/v)	15
5	Irinotecan	HPLC	UV-vis	Isocratic	ACN: Potassium phosphate buffer (pH 2.5) with 0.1% triethylamine (45:55, %v/v)	16
6	Gefitinib	HPLC	UV-vis	Isocratic	ACN: Ammonium formate buffer pH 2.5 (30:70, %v/v)	17
7	Asenapine maleate	HPLC	UV-vis	Isocratic	ACN: Potassium phosphate solution containing 0.1 %v/v triethylamine (20:80, %v/v)	18
8	Valsartan	HPLC	UV-vis	Isocratic	Ammonium formate (pH 3.0): ACN (57:43, %v/v)	19
9	Lacidipine	HPLC	UV-vis	Isocratic	ACN: 0.1% triethylamine solution (pH 6.5) (90:10)	20
10	Lamotrigine	HPLC	UV-vis	Isocratic	Ammonium formate buffer: ACN (65:35, %v/v)	21
11	Rivastigmine hydrogen tartrate	HPLC	UV-vis	Isocratic	ACN: Potassium phosphate buffer solution (Ph 3.0) (24:76, %v/v)	22
12	Cilinidipine	HPLC	UV-vis	Isocratic	Ammonium formate (pH 4.0): ACN (22:78, %v/v)	23

TABLE 4.3

Estimation of molecules or drug and/or metabolites in biological samples

No.	Drug(s) or Molecule(s)	Biological sample	Instrument used	Detector	Method type	Mobile phase	Reference
1	Hesperetin and naringenin	Urine	HPLC	UV-vis	Isocratic	MeOH: Water: Acetic acid (40: 58: 02 %v/v/v)	24
2	Naringin, hesperetin, hesperidin, neo-hesperidin, meranzin hydrate, and naringenin	Rat Plasma	HPLC	UV-vis	Gradient	Solvent A: ACN, and solvent B: 0.5% acetic acid in water. Gradient elution procedure: 0–2 min, 20 to 20% A; 2–4 min, 20 to 30% A; 4–5 min, 30 to 30% A; 5–7 min, 30 to 40%, 7–8 min, 40 to 40% A; and 8–10 min, 40 to 20% A	25
3	Glibenclamide	Rat Plasma	HPLC	UV-vis	Isocratic	ACN: water (1:1, %v/v)	26
4	Fisetin	Rat Plasma	HPLC	UV-vis	Isocratic	ACN: orthophosphoric acid (30: 70, %v/v)	27
5	Lacidipine	Rat Plasma	HPLC	UV-vis	Isocratic	ACN: Ammonium acetate buffer (pH 4.5) (60: 40, %v/v)	28
6	Irinotecan and quercetin	Brain, colon, lungs, heart, kidney, liver, spleen, stomach, and intestine	HPLC	UV-vis	Gradient	Solvent A: ACN; Solvent B: Water (pH 3.0 adjusted with 20% o-phosphoric acid). Flow rate: 0–16 min, 8.0 mL/min; 16–27 min, 1.0 mL/min; 27–30 min, 0.8 mL/min. Mobile phase: 0–8 min, 70 %v/v B; 8–14 min, 55 %v/v B; 14–16 min, 40 %v/v; 16–27 min, 98 %v/v; and then equilibrated for 3 min for next injection	29
7	Ritonavir and lopinavir	Plasma, brain, heart, kidney, liver, spleen, stomach, colon, and intestine	HPLC	UV-vis	Gradient	Water with pH 3.0: MeOH (15:85 %v/v)	30,31

4.2.3.1 HPLC in Pharmacokinetic Studies – Quantification of Drugs and/or Metabolites in Serum and Plasma

Pharmacokinetic parameters can be estimated when drugs and/or their metabolites in serum or plasma are determined. The quantification of drugs and/or metabolites can be performed with the help of HPLC. Often, pharmacokinetic parameters are calculated with suitable methods or software. Pharmacokinetic parameters estimated may include bioavailability, clearance, distribution, residence time of a dosage form, and half-life. HPLC methods used here should have high sensitivity and should give accurate results. Based on the drug and metabolites, specific detectors may be used in estimating their presence in the biological samples. These HPLC methods may also be used in estimating the unchanged drug and/or metabolites in urine and feces.

The quantification of some anticancer drugs, such as paclitaxel and doxorubicin, in plasma is quite challenging because of the presence of proteins and other plasma constituents that may interfere with the analysis. HPLC-MS has been used with good effect to quantify these drugs in plasma. For example, methods coupled with HPLC-MS have been developed that quantify paclitaxel with a high degree of accuracy in plasma for dose optimization and toxicity minimization [32].

Antiepileptic drugs (AEDs) such as carbamazepine and phenytoin are commonly assayed in serum to prevent toxicity. Clinical laboratories are currently utilizing HPLC with UV detection for the estimation of these drugs for this very purpose. Separation of AEDs from endogenous serum components allows appropriate therapeutic drug-level monitoring [33]. A few case studies are given below:

Case Study 1: Monitoring Tacrolimus Levels for Transplant Patients

Tacrolimus, an immunosuppressant used to prevent organ rejection in transplant patients, has a narrow therapeutic window and requires precise dose monitoring. Jain et al. [34] used HPLC to assess tacrolimus levels in renal transplant patients. Blood samples were taken at various time intervals following administration, and the drug concentration was quantified by HPLC. The data gained from HPLC analysis allowed clinicians to precisely modify dosages, keeping drug levels within the therapeutic range and reducing the risk of organ rejection or toxicity. This instance demonstrates HPLC's crucial role in therapeutic drug monitoring, resulting in effective and safe immunosuppression.

Case Study 2: Pharmacokinetic Study of the Anticancer Drug Imatinib

Imatinib, a tyrosine kinase inhibitor used to treat chronic myeloid leukemia (CML), necessitates rigorous pharmacokinetic profiling to maximize therapeutic efficacy. Bouchet et al. [35], undertook a pharmacokinetic study on CML patients receiving imatinib treatment. HPLC was used to determine imatinib plasma concentrations at various time points after oral dosing. The resulting pharmacokinetic profile demonstrated inter-individual variability in medication absorption and metabolism. These findings, aided by HPLC analysis, helped improve therapeutic outcomes and decreased side effects in CML patients.

Case Study 3: Evaluating the Pharmacokinetics of the Antiretroviral Drug Efavirenz

Efavirenz, a critical component of antiretroviral therapy for human immunodeficiency virus (HIV) patients, has a narrow therapeutic index and unpredictable pharmacokinetics. Yenny et al. [36], investigated the pharmacokinetics of efavirenz in HIV-positive individuals. The researchers used HPLC to quantify plasma levels of efavirenz at various time intervals. The study found significant inter-individual variability in drug metabolism due to genetic variations in the CYP2B6 enzyme. This HPLC-based pharmacokinetic data allowed the identification of patients at risk of sub-therapeutic level or toxicity. This approach guided personalized dose regimens and improved therapeutic outcomes.

4.2.3.2 HPLC in Pharmacokinetic Studies – Quantification of Drugs or Metabolites in the Urine or Feces

Pharmacokinetic parameters can also be determined by estimating drug and/or metabolites in urine. Metabolites can also be estimated in the feces. However, it depends on the type of metabolites: soluble or insoluble. Based on the types of drugs and/or metabolites, chromatographic conditions and detectors are selected for the estimation of drugs in urine and feces. For this purpose, also, methods previously described for the estimation of drugs and/or metabolites in plasma or serum may be used.

Ciprofloxacin is often measured in urine with other antibiotics either for therapeutic level control or renal clearance studies. The assay is usually carried out with an HPLC with UV detection. Prior to being injected onto the HPLC column, there is the need to clean-up the urine samples by solid-phase extraction. This is necessary to enable accurate quantification of drug in the presence of the complex matrix of urine [37].

4.2.3.3 HPLC in Biodistribution Studies

Biodistribution is the movement of drugs or molecules from systemic circulation to different tissues. This distribution is dependent on the physicochemical properties of the drug or molecules and the physiological and pathological conditions of the patient. Thus, biodistribution is always uneven in the body. Hydrophilic molecules or drugs show their long residence time in systemic circulation and interstitial space, whereas the lyophilic molecules concentrate in fatty tissues. Additionally, pH influences the ionization of molecules which invariably can affect the membrane [38]. Biodistribution studies are preferred for targeted drug delivery systems, where confirmation of drug targeting to a specific site is important [30, 31]. These studies also give critical data that helps to understand modifications in dosing regimens, therapeutic efficacy, and potential drug toxicity.

Drug quantification in biological matrices such as blood, plasma, urine, and organ tissues is an important step in pharmacokinetic, pharmacodynamic, toxicological, and therapeutic drug monitoring studies. HPLC is one of the most used analytical techniques for this purpose because of its great sensitivity, precision, and ability to separate molecules from complicated mixtures. HPLC's capacity to precisely quantify pharmaceuticals even in the presence of impurities makes it indispensable in clinical and laboratory research. HPLC is especially suitable for the quantification of drugs in complex matrices. HPLC has a number of merits, some of which include:

a) *Separate drugs from matrix interferences:* In general, biological matrices contain a number of proteins, lipids, salts, and other endogenous molecules which may interfere with analysis. With advanced stationary phases and the possibility for gradient elution, HPLC can be used to separate drugs from such interferences [39].
b) *High sensitivity and specificity:* HPLC has a high degree of sensitivity and specificity, especially when associated with UV, fluorescence, or MS detectors. This makes it an important tool in situations where only low drug concentrations can be encountered, such as during therapeutic drug monitoring or early drug development phase [40]. These investigations are critical for understanding drug behavior in the body, which ultimately influences dosage regimens. By providing precise and reliable measurements of drug concentrations in biological samples, HPLC assists in modeling the pharmacokinetic characteristics of novel medications [41].
c) *Versatility across different drugs:* HPLC is applied for the analysis of a wide variety of drugs, from small molecules to large peptides, in different matrices – a factor that has greatly contributed to it being one of the methods of choice in many clinical laboratories [42].
d) *Quantification of hormones in tissue samples:* HPLC can be used for the quantification of estradiol and testosterone in tissue samples. The preparation of tissue samples involves homogenization, followed by solvent extraction methods to obtain the extract of these hormones. Separation and quantification of these hormones by HPLC assume a significant relevance in endocrinology research [43].

4.2.4 Quality Control

HPLC is also used in pharmaceutical manufacturing for quality control. To ensure patient safety, pharmaceutical products must meet regulatory criteria for purity, potency, and quality. HPLC is frequently used for detecting contaminants, degradation products, as well as ensuring the uniformity of active pharmaceutical ingredients (APIs) in drug products. Its sensitivity enables the detection of impurities at very low levels, preventing health concerns associated with compromised or low-quality drugs [44].

4.2.5 Therapeutic Drug Monitoring

HPLC is utilized in clinical settings to monitor drug levels in biological matrices, especially for drugs with narrow therapeutic indices. By evaluating drug levels in patient blood, physicians can adjust doses to attain the best therapeutic outcomes. This application is especially crucial for drugs such as immunosuppressants, anticonvulsants, and some antibiotics. Maintaining accurate drug concentrations is critical for drug efficacy and safety [45].

Case Study 1: Cyclosporine Monitoring in Organ Transplant Patients
Cyclosporine is an immunosuppressive drug often used to prevent organ rejection in transplant patients. It has a narrow therapeutic window, which means the difference between an effective and toxic dose is minimal. As a result, monitoring of drug levels in the blood is critical to ensuring maximum therapeutic efficacy while minimizing side effects. In a tertiary care hospital, HPLC was used to evaluate cyclosporine levels in patients who had undergone kidney transplants. The study comprised 50 patients, whose cyclosporine levels were evaluated by HPLC at regular intervals after transplantation. The HPLC method used to identify cyclosporine in whole blood samples was tested for accuracy, precision, and sensitivity [46].

The findings showed that HPLC offered accurate and repeatable assessments of cyclosporine levels, which were utilized to alter dosages accordingly. Patients whose cyclosporine levels remained within the therapeutic range experienced considerably fewer acute organ rejection events than those with sub-therapeutic or supra-therapeutic levels. This case study emphasizes the importance of HPLC in therapeutic drug monitoring for cyclosporine.

Case Study 2: Monitoring Vancomycin in Patients at Intensive Care Units
Vancomycin is an antibiotic used to treat serious infections caused by gram-positive bacteria, such as methicillin-resistant *Staphylococcus aureus* (MRSA). Therapeutic drug monitoring is necessary due to its potential nephrotoxic and ototoxic effects, especially in critically ill patients with altered drug pharmacokinetics.

A study included intensive care unit (ICU) patients with serious infections who received vancomycin. HPLC was used to evaluate vancomycin serum levels. The study comprised 30 patients who were given vancomycin. The HPLC method was chosen for its high specificity and sensitivity in identifying vancomycin at low doses [47].

Results showed that HPLC enabled accurate control of vancomycin dose, ensuring that serum levels stayed within the therapeutic range. This was especially significant for ICU patients with fluctuating renal function, as normal dosage could result in suboptimal drug levels. The study found a significant reduction in nephrotoxicity and improved infection control outcomes, which were attributed to accurate monitoring with the use of HPLC. This case study demonstrates the value of HPLC in managing antibiotic therapy in critically ill patients, guaranteeing effective treatment while minimizing adverse effects.

4.2.6 Detection of Biomarkers in Clinical Diagnostics

HPLC is very useful in detecting biomarkers as well as metabolites within biological samples. Biomarkers are physiological and pathological indicators that are critical for disease diagnosis, prognosis, and monitoring. HPLC's ability to separate and precisely measure these indicators makes it an important tool in clinical diagnostics and biomedical research. For example, HPLC detects and quantifies hemoglobin variations in blood, which is useful for detecting hemoglobinopathies [48]. Furthermore, HPLC helps identify counterfeit medications. HPLC provides the essential analytical capabilities to identify and quantify legitimate active components in medications, separating them from counterfeit versions that may contain erroneous or hazardous substances [49].

Case Study 1: Detection of Cardiovascular Biomarkers
The case study involving the quantification of B type natriuretic peptide (BNP) and its metabolites in heart failure patients demonstrates HPLC's value in detecting cardiovascular biomarkers. BNP is an important biomarker for detecting the degree of heart failure. Traditional immunoassays for measuring

BNP frequently lack specificity due to cross-reactivity with similar peptides. In this investigation, HPLC-MS was used to separate and precisely quantify BNP and its metabolites in plasma samples from patients [50]. The HPLC method had great resolution and sensitivity, enabling discrimination between BNP and its breakdown products. This precise measurement enabled a more accurate assessment of biomarker levels, resulting in better diagnosis and management of heart failure. The study showed that HPLC-MS might overcome the limitations of immunoassays, delivering reliable and specific biomarker measures that are important for clinical decision-making.

Case Study 2: Metabolite Profiling in Cancer Research

Another example of HPLC's usage in cancer research is metabolite profiling. This helps to better understand tumor metabolism and discover possible treatment targets. In a study on colorectal cancer, HPLC combined with tandem mass spectrometry (HPLC-MS/MS) was used to analyze metabolic alterations in malignant and non-cancerous tissues [51]. The researchers employed HPLC-MS/MS to separate and identify different metabolites, such as amino acids, nucleotides, and lipids, which are frequently changed in cancer cells. The study discovered significant changes in metabolic patterns between tumor and normal tissues, pointing to possible biomarkers for early diagnosis and therapeutic intervention. The thorough metabolic profiling acquired by HPLC-MS/MS revealed insights on metabolic reprogramming in cancer cells, which is critical for developing targeted therapeutics and improving patient outcomes.

4.2.7 Future Prospects for HPLC in Therapeutics and Medicine

As technology advances, HPLC applications in drug research, personalized medicine, and clinical diagnostics are projected to increase, providing high precision, efficiency, and sensitivity. One promising future application for HPLC is personalized medicine. Personalized medicine seeks to customize treatments to individual patients' genetic, proteomic, and metabolomic characteristics. HPLC, when combined with mass spectrometry, can be an ideal tool for analyzing complicated biological samples and discovering biomarkers that predict patient response to certain medicines. HPLC has the potential to aid more effective and focused treatments, as well as reduce adverse effects [52].

HPLC is expected to play an even larger role in drug research as biopharmaceuticals become more prevalent. Biologic medications, such as monoclonal antibodies and gene treatments, require advanced analytical techniques for characterization due to their complexity. HPLC's capacity to separate and analyze big macromolecules with great precision makes it essential for ensuring the quality, safety, and efficacy of these novel medicines [53].

Furthermore, the integration of HPLC with cutting-edge technologies like artificial intelligence (AI) and machine learning (ML) is predicted to transform data processing and interpretation. AI and ML algorithms can process large volumes of HPLC data, revealing patterns and correlations that older approaches could have overlooked. This integration can improve the speed and accuracy of drug discovery and development procedures [54].

Furthermore, HPLC is expected to see increased application in the field of metabolomics, which is the comprehensive study of metabolites within a biological system. Metabolomics gives information on disease causes and prospective treatment targets. HPLC's excellent resolution and sensitivity make it ideal for metabolite profiling, which can help identify novel biomarkers for early disease detection and surveillance [55].

4.3 Conclusion

HPLC is an important tool in medicine and therapeutics, providing unrivaled precision, sensitivity, and versatility. HPLC plays an essential role in drug research, quality control, and clinical diagnostics, ensuring the safety and efficacy of pharmaceuticals. HPLC's ability to reliably measure biomarkers and metabolites helps in disease diagnosis, personalized treatment, and therapeutic drug monitoring.

Drug quantification in biological matrices such as blood, plasma, urine, and tissues is an important step in pharmacokinetic, pharmacodynamic, toxicological, and therapeutic drug monitoring studies. HPLC is one of the most utilized analytical techniques for this purpose because of its great sensitivity, precision, and ability to separate molecules in complicated mixtures. HPLC's capacity to precisely quantify pharmaceuticals even in the presence of interfering chemicals makes it indispensable in research contexts.

As technology advances, the use of HPLC is expected to grow, enhancing medical research and patient outcomes. Its integration with developing technology promises to transform data analysis and speed up the creation of new medicines. HPLC has a promising future in medicine and therapeutics, with applications expected to expand and change in tandem with technology advancements. Its use in personalized medicine, biopharmaceutical analysis, and integration with AI and ML has the potential to improve the precision and efficacy of medical therapies.

REFERENCES

1. Jitta SR, Chauhan A, Vaz V, Kumar L. Development and validation of high performance liquid chromatography method for quantification of hesperetin in a topical formulation. *Indian J Pharm Sci.* 2023;85(3):678–85.
2. Saifullah M, McCullum R, Vuong Q. Maximising extraction yields of gallic acid and hesperetin from lemon myrtle (*Backhousia citriodora*) leaf using microwave assisted extraction. *Results Chem.* 2020;2:100080.
3. Pandiyan R, Ilango K. Isolation, characterization, and validation of RP-HPLC method for the quantification of quercetin in *Huberantha senjiana* leaf extract. *J Applied Pharm Sci.* 2020;10(5):110–18.
4. Sivagami B, Sailaja B. Determination of phytochemical markers andrographolide, eugenol, and zingerone in niavembu kudineer by RP-HPLC method. *J Applied Pharm Sci.* 2024; 14(10):128–34.
5. Huck CW, Popp M, Scherz H, Bonn GK. Development and evaluation of a new method for the determination of the carotenoid content in selected vegetables by HPLC and HPLC-MS-MS. *J Chromatogr Sci.* 2000;38:441–49.
6. Fratianni A, Mignogna R, Niro S, Panfili G. Determination of lutein from fruit and vegetables through an alkaline hydrolysis extraction method and HPLC analysis. *J Food Sci.* 2015:80(12):C2686–91.
7. Bhavin SE, Anuradha G. Development and validation of an RP-HPLC method for estimating nutraceutical lutein. *Int J Health Sci.* 2022;6(S5):1710–24.
8. Seo JH, Kim JE, Shim JH Yoon G, Bang MA, Bae CS, Lee KJ, Park DH, Cho SS. HPLC analysis, optimization of extraction conditions and biological evaluation of *Corylopsis coreana* uyeki flos. *Molecules.* 2016;21(1):94.
9. Gheraibia S, Belattar N, Abdel-Wahhab MA. HPLC analysis, antioxidant, and cytotoxic activity of different extract of *Costus speciosus* against HePG-2 cell lines. *South African J Botany.* 2020;131:222–28.
10. Gini TG, Jothi GJ. Column chromatography and HPLC analysis of phenolic compounds in the fractions of *Salvinia molesta* mitchell. *Egyptian J Basic Applied Sci.* 2018;5(3):197–203.
11. Swartz, ME. *Analytical techniques in pharmaceutical development. HPLC: a practical guide.* New York: Springer; 2012.
12. Arya A, Khandelwal K, Singh A, Ahmad H, Agrawal S, Khatik R, Mittapelly N, Dwivedi AK. Validation of R-HPLC method for simultaneous quantification of biocalutamide and hesperetin in polycaprolacton e-biocalutamide-hesperetin-chitosan nanoparticles. *J Chromatogr Sci.* 2015;53(9):1485–890.
13. Rao NM, Sankar DG. Development and validation of stability indicating RP-HPLC method for the estimation of cinacalcet hydrochloride in bulk and their formulations. *Biointerface Res Applied Chem.* 2020;10(6):6610–18.
14. Akhade MS, Agrawal PA, Laddha KS. Development and validation of RP-HPLC method for simultaneous estimation of picroside I, plumbagin, and Z-guggulsterone in tablet formulation. *Indian J Pharm Sci.* 2013;75(4):476–82.
15. Jitta SR, Bhaskaran NA, Kumar L, Shirodkar RK. Development and validation of RP-HPLC method for quantification of total, free, and entrapped ritonavir in lipid nanocarriers and drug content of film coated fixed dosed formulation. *Indian J Pharm Edu Res.* 2022;56(3).S547–58.

16. Bhaskaran NA, Kumar L, Reddy MS, Pai KG. An analytical "quality by design" approach in RP-HPLC method development and validation for reliable and rapid estimation of irinotecan in an injectable formulation. *Acta Pharm.* 2021;71:57–79.
17. Sree KSN, Pai KG, Verma R, Ananthakrishna P, Kumar L. Validation of HPLC method for quantitative determination of gefitinib in polymeric nanoformulation. *Pharm Chem J.* 2017;51(2):159–63.
18. Managuli RS, Kumar L, Chonkar AD, Shirodkar RK, Lewis S, Koteshwara KB, Reddy MS, Mutalik S. Development and validation of a stability-indicating RP-HPLC method by a statistical optimization process for the quantification of asenapine maleate in lipidic nanoformulations. *J Chrom Sci.* 2016;54(8):1290–300.
19. Kumar L, Reddy MS, Managuli RS, Pi KG. Full factorial design for optimization, development, and validation of HPLC method to determine valsartan in nanoparticles. *Saudi Pharm J.* 2015;23:549–55.
20. Shirodkar RK, Shetty P, Kumar L, Mutalik S, Lewis SA. Development and validation of reverse phase HPLC method for the estimation of lacidipine in nanoformulations. *Latin Am J Pharm.* 2015;34(6):1162–6.
21. Gangurde PK, Bhaskaran NA, Verma R, Jose J, Kumar L. Analytical method development using central composite design for estimation of lamotrigine in lipid nanoformulation. *Mater Plast.* 2020;57(1):223–35.
22. Salwa, Kumar L. Quality-by-design driven analytical method (AQbD) development and validation of HPLC-UV technique to quantify rivastigmine hydrogen tartrate in lipid nanocarriers: Forced degradation, and assessment of drug content and in vitro release studies. *Microchemical J.* 2023;193:108944.
23. Marques SM, Shirodkar RK, Kumar L. Analytical 'Quality-by-Design' paradigm in development of a RP-HPLC method for the estimation of cilnidipine in nanoformulations: Forced degradation studies and mathematical modelling of in vitro release studies. *Microchemical J.* 2023;193:109124.
24. Kanaze FI, Kokkalou E, Georgarakis M, Niopas I. A validated solid-phase extraction HPLC method for the simultaneous estimation determination of the citrus flavanone aglycones hesperetin and naringenin in urine. *J Pharm Biomd Anal.* 2004;36(1):175–81.
25. Wang W, Zhao L, Huang H, Yao J, Wang D, Qiu X. Development of an ultra-high performance liquid chromatography method for simultaneous estimation of six active compounds in *Fructus aurantia* and rat plasma and its application to a comparative pharmacokinetic study in rats administered with different doses. *J Analytical Method Chem.* 2018;1:7579136.
26. Mir KB, Abrol V, Wani TU, Jan I, Singh N, Khan NA, Dar AA, Sultan RMS, Lone SA, Iesa MAM, Alhag SK, Al-Shuraym LA, Helm N, Al-Farga A. Validation and development of RP-HPLC method for quantification of glibenclamide in rat plasma and its application to pharmacokinetic studies in wistar rats. *Heliyon.* 2023;9(11):e20876.
27. Kumar R, Kumar R, Khursheed R, Awasthi A, Khurana N, Singh SK, Khurana S, Sharma N, Gunjal P, Kaur J, Corrie L. Development and validation of RP-HPLC method for estimation of fisetin in rat plasma. *South African J Botany.* 2021;140:284–9.
28. Shirodkar RK, Kumar L, Misra C, Managuli R, Attari Z, Mutalik S, Lewis SA. Development and validation of a reverse phase HPLC method for the estimation of lacidipine in rat plasma: application to preclinical pharmacokinetics. *Latin Am J Pharm.* 2016;35(1):124–9.
29. Bhaskaran NA, Jitta SR, Salwa, Kumar L, Sharma P, Kulkarni OP, Hari G, Gourishetti K, Verma R, Birangal SR, Bhaskar KV. Folic acid-chitosan functionalized polymeric nanocarriers to treat colon cancer. *Int J Biol Macromol.* 2023;253:127142.
30. Jitta SR, Salwa, Bhaskaran NA, Marques SM, Kumar L, Cheruku SP, Rao V, Sharma P, Kulkarni OP. Enhanced tissue distribution of ritonavir-loaded nanostructured lipid carriers – recommending its dose reduction. *Drug Delivery Translational Res.* 2024;14:116–30.
31. Jitta SR, Bhaskaran NA, Salwa, Kumar L. Anti-oxidant containing nanostructured lipid carriers of ritonavir: Development, optimization, and in vitro and in vivo evaluations. *AAPS PharmSciTech.* 2022;23:88.
32. Sparidans RW, Lagas JS, Schinkel AH, Schellens JH, Beijnen JH. Quantification of paclitaxel and metabolites in mouse plasma by liquid chromatography/tandem mass spectrometry. *J Mass Spectrom.* 2008;43(1):146–54. doi:10.1002/jms.1281.
33. Soldin SJ, Soldin OP. Review: therapeutic drug monitoring in pediatrics: relevance and clinical applications. *Ther Drug Monit.* 2002;24(1):113–21. doi:10.1097/00007691-200202000-00023.
34. Jain AB, Venkataramanan R, Zuckerman S, Todo S, Fung JJ, Starzl TE. Clinical pharmacokinetics of tacrolimus. *Clin Pharmacokinet.* 1995;29(6):404–30.

35. Bouchet S, Chauzit E, Ducint D, Castaing N, Canal-Raffin M, Moore N, Titier K, Molimard M. Simultaneous determination of plasma levels of several tyrosine kinase inhibitors by ultra performance liquid chromatography–tandem mass spectrometry. *J Chromatogr B Analyt Technol Biomed Life Sci.* 2011;879(25):3454–62.
36. Yenny W, Edianto D, Mangunwardoyo W, Yuniasih W, Indrati A. Pharmacokinetics of efavirenz in Indonesian HIV-infected patients. *J Clin Pharm Ther.* 2014;39(3):321–26.
37. Dautzenberg F, Marini R, Souche E, Lecomte T. HPLC method for the determination of ciprofloxacin in human plasma and urine. *J Chromatogr B Biomed Appl.* 1997;703(1–2):265–71. doi:10.1016/s0378-4347(97)00353-4.
38. Wotring VE. Distribution. In: *Space pharmacology: Springer brief's in space development.* Boston, MA: Springer. https://doi.org/10.1007/978-1-4614-3396-5_3.
39. Niessen WM. *Liquid chromatography-mass spectrometry: an introduction.* Weinheim: Wiley-VCH; 2006.
40. Wermuth CG. *The practice of medicinal chemistry.* 4th ed. London: Academic Press; 2015.
41. Aboul-Enein HY, Ali I. Studies on the enantioselective resolution of drugs by HPLC using immobilized human serum albumin column. *Biomed Chromatogr.* 2002;16(6):399–407. doi:10.1002/bmc.180
42. Chen Y, Zhang L, Zhang Y, Wang X. Applications of HPLC-MS in clinical toxicology—A review. *J Chromatogr B Analyt Technol Biomed Life Sci.* 2015;1002:1–9. doi:10.1016/j.jchromb.2015.07.020
43. Stanczyk FZ, Clarke NJ. Measurement of estradiol—challenges ahead. *J Clin Endocrinol Metab.* 2014;99(1):56–8. doi:10.1210/jc.2013-3642.
44. Kazakevich Y, LoBrutto R. *HPLC for Pharmaceutical scientists.* Hoboken: Wiley; 2007.
45. Dasgupta A, Klein K. *Therapeutic drug monitoring: new drugs and biomarkers.* 1st ed. San Diego: Academic Press; 2012.
46. Shaw LM, Yatscoff RW. Therapeutic drug monitoring of cyclosporine, tacrolimus, and sirolimus. *Clin Biochem.* 2000;33(5):331–47.
47. Pai MP, Neely MN, Rodvold KA, and Lodise TP. Innovative approaches tooptimizing delivery of vancomycin in individual patientss. *Adv Drug Deliv Rev.* 2014;77:50–7.
48. Rifai N, Horvath AR, and Wittwer CT. *Tietz textbook of clinical chemistry and molecular diagnostics.* 6th ed. St. Louis: Elsevier; 2018.
49. Deisingh AK. *Pharmaceutical counterfeiting: detection, identification, and analysis.* London: Wiley; 2005.
50. Lam CSP, Rienstra M, Tay WT, Liu LC, Hummel YM, van der Meer P, et al. Atypical response to loading conditions in heart failure with preserved ejection fraction: insights from HPLC-MS quantification of B-type natriuretic peptide and its metabolites. *Eur J Heart Fail.* 2017;19(7):877–85.
51. Qiu Y, Cai G, Su M, Chen T, Zheng X, Xu Y, et al. Serum metabolite profiling of human colorectal cancer using HPLC-MS/MS. *J Proteome Res.* 2009;8(10):4844–50.
52. Collins FS, Varmus H. A new initiative on precision medicine. *N Engl J Med.* 2015;372(9):793–5.
53. Beck A, Wagner-Rousset E, Ayoub D, Van Dorsselaer A, Sanglier-Cianférani S. Characterization of therapeutic antibodies and related products. Anal Chem. 2013;85(2):715–36.
54. Liang Y, Matharu Z, Dai Y, Liu G, Wang X. Emerging technology and applications of artificial intelligence in chromatography. TrAC Trends Anal Chem. 2020;122:115709.
55. Dunn WB, Ellis DI. Metabolomics: Current analytical platforms and methodologies. TrAC Trends Anal Chem. 2005;24(4):285–94.

5

Diagnostic Imaging Techniques: Current Trends and Challenges

Derick Seyram Sule and Rosemary Ampofo

5.1 Introduction

Wilhelm Conrad Roentgen's discovery of X-rays in 1895 was a milestone that revolutionized healthcare and gave birth to diagnostic imaging [1, 2]. In modern healthcare, diagnostic imaging techniques (DITs) serve as the basis for enabling clinicians to visualize and assess anatomical abnormalities, disease processes, and treatment responses with unprecedented precision and accuracy [3]. Following Conrad's clinical use of X-rays, medical imaging as a field has witnessed remarkable progress. Other imaging techniques that have been used clinically over the years include fluoroscopy, computed tomography (CT), mammography, ultrasonography (USG), magnetic resonance imaging (MRI), and radionuclide imaging.

DITs find extensive applications across various medical specialties; radiology, oncology, cardiology, and neurology. In radiology, CT and MRI play pivotal roles in cancer diagnosis and staging, assessment of musculoskeletal injuries, and evaluation of neurological disorders. Similarly, cardiac imaging modalities like echocardiography and cardiac MRI are indispensable tools for diagnosing heart disease and guiding therapeutic interventions. Moreover, the emergence of molecular imaging techniques like single-photon emission (SPECT)-CT, positron emission tomography (PET)-CT, and PET-MRI enables clinicians to visualize biochemical processes at the molecular level, opening new avenues for precision medicine and targeted therapy [4]. DITs thus play a pivotal role in modern healthcare by enabling the description and presentation of anatomical structures and functional processes within the human body.

Traditionally, diagnostic imaging techniques such as conventional radiography, CT, ultrasound, MRI, and nuclear medicine have been the cornerstone of medical imaging. Over the years, DITs have undergone significant advancements, driven by technological innovation, research breakthroughs, and evolving clinical needs [4]. These advancements have revolutionized medical diagnosis, treatment planning, and patient management [5]. In recent years, a surge in novel imaging technologies and methodologies has been propelled by breakthroughs in areas such as artificial intelligence (AI), molecular imaging, functional imaging, and image-guided interventions [6]. AI, in particular, has emerged as a transformative force in diagnostic imaging, offering promise for enhanced accuracy, efficiency, and automation in image interpretation and analysis [6]. Integrating machine learning algorithms with vast medical image datasets has demonstrated remarkable capabilities in lesion detection, segmentation, classification, and quantification [7].

Since medical imaging is witnessing a rapid change in technologies and methodologies, presenting opportunities and challenges for healthcare systems worldwide, there is a pressing need to systematically examine the existing and current landscape of DITs to identify prevailing trends and challenges. Understanding the current trends and challenges in diagnostic imaging is crucial for healthcare

DOI: 10.1201/9781003486909-5

professionals, researchers, and policymakers. This is to help them in decision-making, promoting innovation, and eventually improving patient care outcomes.

5.2 Conventional Radiography

Conventional radiography is a traditional diagnostic imaging technique by which 2D images of patients' anatomical structures are achieved on an image receptor either made of a piece of radiographic film, an imaging plate, or a digital detector, depending on the system being used.

5.2.1 Principles, Advantages, and Challenges of Conventional Radiography

With conventional radiography, the emergent X-ray beam from the X-ray tube goes through the patient and then to an image receptor, which is processed to produce a visible image. The varied tissue density and attenuation coefficient of body tissues account for differences in the X-ray photon attenuation; hence denser tissues (e.g., bones) produce a whiter (more radiopaque) image while less dense tissues (fat) produce a darker (more radiolucent) image [8]. As X-rays are passed through the body, the resultant images are captured on an image receptor defined by the type of conventional radiography system in use. Conventional radiography is the first line of DIT for many clinical conditions since it is noninvasive, inexpensive, easily accessible, and well known among many health professionals. Compared to other DITs, conventional radiography is relatively harmless and presents a quick turnaround time [8].

Unlike traditional film-screen systems, computed radiography (CR) systems utilize a photostimulable phosphor plate to detect X-rays [8]. As the helium-neon laser navigates the uncovered plate, the light is gathered by a photomultiplier tube, which converts it into a simple electrical circuit before digitalization [8]. With the aid of a semiconductor-based sensor, direct digital radiography (DR) systems clear the invisible image on the imaging plate before reuse by simply converting the X-ray photons into electrical transmissions [8].

In comparison, screen-film systems have a larger client base than direct DR and CR, but this advantage is rapidly diminishing with time. The falling pervasiveness of film-screen radiographic systems in recent times is somewhat a result of their restricted capacity for post-processing contrast enhancement, fixed non-direct dim scale reaction, and dose scope [8]. Moreover, the film-screen systems are relatively labor-intensive, requiring the use of dangerous chemicals (developer and fixer solutions) for image processing, as well as the storage and retrieval of radiographs over an extended period. Additionally, the incompatibility of film-screen systems with picture archiving and communication systems (PACS) poses another challenge.

Given the shortfalls of film-screen systems, digital systems (CR and DR) have recently dominated the healthcare system. With DR systems, the computerized sensor associated with video screens allows continuous image intensification, which to a greater degree is useful for screening during vascular imaging. Without increasing the patient's effective dose, digital systems can enhance image resolution and quality up to multiple times [8]. In summary, the multiple advantages of digital CR and DR systems over film-screen systems include: faster image acquisition, wider latitude, post-processing image enhancement. Further, the possibility of multiple functions such as annotations, measurements, cropping, and panning zooming, darkroom processing is not needed. Additionally, there is no need for film storage space and image dissemination is easy.

5.3 Fluoroscopy

Fluoroscopy is a diagnostic imaging technique that employs continuous and pulsed modes to provide real-time images. Despite the advantage of real-time imaging, there is a higher risk that both the staff and patients may be exposed to radiation [9]. This is principally true during radiological or surgical procedures that require continuous and higher-frequency pulsed modes for a long period. Different types of fluoroscopic machines exist: fixed digital fluoroscopy and C-arm fluoroscopy.

5.3.1 Principles, Advantages, and Challenges of Fluoroscopy

Components of a fluoroscopic system include an X-ray tube (source of radiation), collimator, image intensifier, video camera, and display monitor (Figure 5.1).

The collimator limits the radiation to the field of view where its manual adjustment defines the shape of the X-ray beam. Fluoroscopy can be performed with continuous or pulse X-rays with a frame rate ranging between 1 and 30 frames/sec [9]. Among its numerous advantages, pulsed fluoroscopy can reduce motional blurriness within each image, due to its short acquisition time, which has proven useful in examining moving structures. Fluoroscopy units using image intensifiers operate by converting X-rays into light, which a video camera captures, and the resultant image is displayed on a monitor. Fluoroscopy units using flat-panel detectors (solid-state devices) operate by converting the X-rays into digital electronic signals fed into the computer system for display on a monitor [9].

The clinical application of fluoroscopy covers procedures such as gastrointestinal fluoroscopy (barium studies – barium swallow, barium meal, and barium enema), genitourinary fluoroscopy (intravenous pyelography, hysterosalpingography – HSG), intravenous catheterization, cardiac catheterization, arthrography, lumbar puncture, and angiography [9]. Fluoroscopy is still a standard part of modern radiology practice, despite its volume and referral patterns drastically decreasing in recent decades and some once-common examinations are now performed very infrequently [9].

Although the principles of conventional radiography and fluoroscopy are essentially the same, there are however a few identifiable variations in the two diagnostic imaging techniques. While conventional X-rays produce static images, fluoroscopy provides a real-time live image showing body movements [9]. When fluoroscopic procedures are carried out with contrast, it highlights the lumen of the body's hollow organs, which is a limitation of conventional X-rays. One key challenge with fluoroscopy is that it requires serial X-rays, which relatively makes it carry a higher risk of radiation-related risks than conventional X-rays. Although fluoroscopy is an extremely useful imaging technique for the visualization of surgical tool positions and underlying bone during orthopedic procedures, another challenge with this technology is the need for continued radiation exposure for visual alignment and control which is most often cumbersome [9]. Additionally, fluoroscopy, compared with CT and MRI, has a shortfall due to its inability to provide in-depth detail on the emergent 2D single image produced. To overcome the challenge of difficulty in controlling 3D manipulations, this imaging technique requires that imaging be done at varying viewing angles which often is very cumbersome [9].

5.4 Computed Tomography

Computed tomography, popular as CT scan, is an advanced imaging modality invented in 1972 by British engineer Godfrey Hounsfield and Dr. Andrew Cormack [10]. Their groundbreaking research laid the foundation for the first commercial CT scanner, the EMI Mark I, which was introduced in 1972 [11].

Since its inception, CT scanning technology has undergone continuous refinement and innovation, driven by advances in hardware, software, and imaging algorithms. Early CT scanners utilized single-slice detectors and rotational scanning techniques to acquire cross-sectional images of the body [4]. However, the introduction of multi-slice CT scanners in the 1990s enabled rapid volumetric imaging, allowing for faster scan times, improved spatial resolution, and enhanced diagnostic capabilities [4]. Current generations of CT scanners incorporate dual-energy imaging, electron beam, spectral imaging, and iterative reconstruction algorithms, further enhancing image quality, contrast resolution, and radiation dose optimization [4].

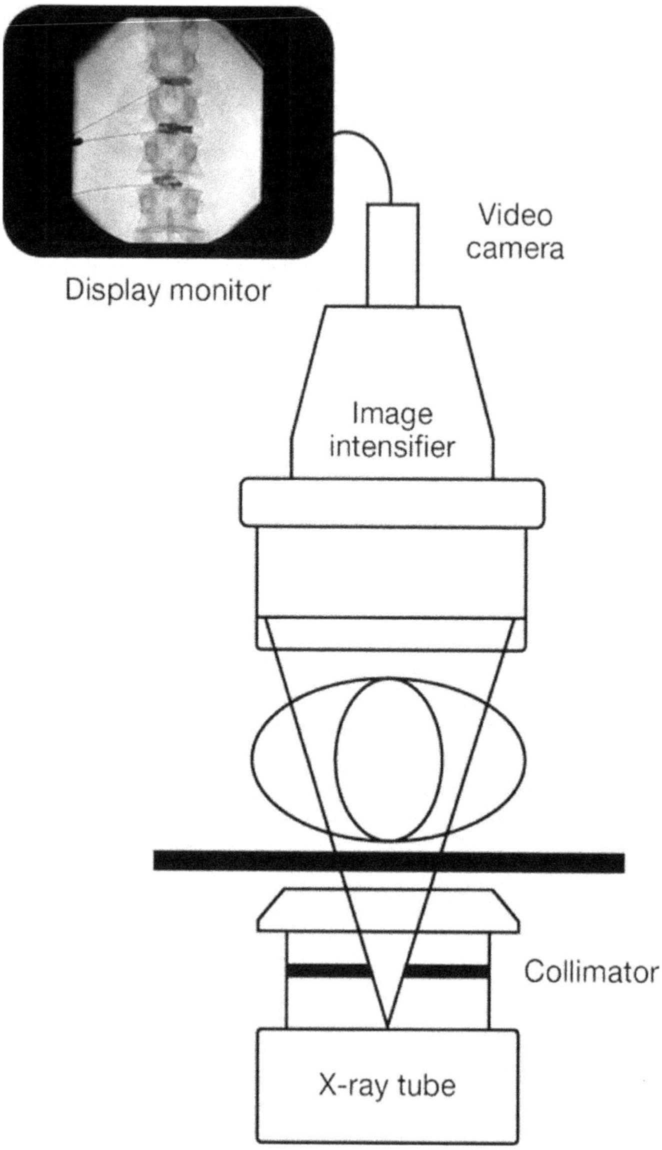

FIGURE 5.1 Components of a fluoroscopic system.

5.4.1 Principles, Advantages, and Challenges of CT Imaging

In CT imaging, cross-sectional images of the body are reconstructed by merging many X-ray projections taken at various angles [4]. A CT image is often made up of a matrix of minuscule squares, or pixels. Every pixel is a 2D depiction of a 3D tissue volume, or voxel [4]. A matrix's spatial resolution improves with the number of pixels it contains and the fewer noticeable transitions between the various pixels. To create a meaningful image, the CT method calculates the linear attenuation coefficient [4]. Since there can be more projections throughout a longer scan period, the image detail is improved; however, there is a chance of motion artifacts and X-ray tube heating [4].

CT imaging is routinely used for the diagnosis and staging of cancer, the evaluation of traumatic injuries, the assessment of vascular diseases, and the detection of neurological disorders [12]. Moreover, CT angiography (CTA) and CT perfusion imaging have emerged as valuable tools for assessing blood flow, tissue perfusion, and treatment response in various clinical scenarios. The versatility of CT imaging has made it an indispensable tool in modern healthcare practice, facilitating timely and accurate diagnoses, treatment planning, and patient management [11, 13]. It is a highly functional tool for keeping track of various forms of cancer, including bladder, kidney, skeletal, neck, and head cancers, as well as for detecting other pathologies [12]. Additionally, CT is instrumental in identifying remote metastases in the lungs, skeleton, liver, and brain, having a remarkable influence on diagnoses.

With tumor detection and tracking changes in tumor mass during treatment, CT scanning surpasses other techniques. For instance, it can reveal a distended abdomen with enlarged lymph nodes in patients with bronchogenic carcinoma, helping with pre-surgical assessments [4]. Furthermore, CT scans play a vital role in detecting heart conditions such as myocardial disease, and congenital heart disease [4]. Again, CT offers numerous benefits compared to other imaging techniques due to its rapidity and widespread availability, enabling physicians to promptly confirm or rule out diagnoses with greater confidence. Its influence on the realm of surgery is profound, as it has significantly reduced the necessity for emergency surgical interventions from 13% to 5% [4]. The number of patients requiring hospitalization has decreased recently due to the widespread use of CT in clinical settings [7, 12]. Likewise, the amalgamation of AI and CT imaging has transformed this imaging modality, allowing automated analysis of images and decision-making [12]. Also, the training of AI algorithms on large data sets of CT images assists radiologists in abnormal pattern recognition, quantifying disease severity, and prognosticating treatment outcomes with high accuracy and efficiency [7, 12]. Furthermore, AI-driven applications such as computer-aided detection (CAD), image segmentation, and radiomics analysis hold promise for advancing personalized medicine, optimizing treatment strategies, and improving patient outcomes. The integration of CT imaging with AI thus has the prospect of transforming healthcare delivery, ushering in an era of precision diagnostics, targeted therapies, and data-driven decision-making [4, 6].

Cone beam computed tomography (CBCT) development is a significant radiologic improvement above conventional CT, owing to the process of tomographic reconstruction which has been found very capable for producing volumetric images [14–16]. This method is being used extensively for invasive radiology diagnosis and treatment, as well as for online image guidance during radiation therapy delivery [17, 18]. CBCT employs an area detector to create a circular or rectangular cone-shaped beam, as opposed to the fan-shaped anode X-ray beam used in typical CT scans [19]. Even with relatively short scan intervals (~1 min), the cone beam technique yields high-quality images with sub-millimeter resolution and remarkable dimensional accuracy [19]. Even though the radiation from a typical CBCT is around ten times less than that of a traditional CT scan, the levels are nonetheless significant and far exceed the background radiation seen in the environment daily [15].

Compared to traditional radiography, CT provides a far higher degree of distinction between particular soft tissue structures. This is because CT can precisely measure the absorption of X-ray beams as they travel through the patient [12]. Using a narrow X-ray beam that revolves around the body, CT scans small slices of the body to avoid the superimposition of underlying tissues on the image that occurs with traditional radiography [12].

On the other hand, CT artifacts are usually a challenge because the actual attenuation coefficient of an object and the reconstructed CT numbers in the image frequently differ. Such artifacts result in erroneous measurements of the transmission of readings by the detectors, resulting in streak and ring artifacts; metal and bone artifacts; beam hardening artifacts; partial volume artifacts; motion artifacts; stair-stepping artifacts; spiral pitch artifacts; and cone beam artifacts.

Despite the widespread use of CT, there are a number of challenges that hinder the modality. One of the primary challenges in CT imaging is radiation dose management. CT scans expose patients to ionizing radiation, which carries inherent risks of radiation-induced malignancies and other adverse effects [12, 20]. Using dose reduction strategies such as tube current modulation, iterative reconstruction, and automatic exposure management in contemporary CT scanners does not make it easy to balance radiation optimization and diagnostic picture quality preservation. Clinicians need to carefully balance the risks of radiation exposure with the advantages of diagnostic information, particularly in vulnerable populations such as children, pregnant women, and individuals undergoing repeated imaging studies [12, 21].

Another challenge is image noise and artifacts, which can degrade image quality and obscure diagnostic information. Common artifacts in CT imaging include beam hardening, metal artifacts, motion artifacts, and partial volume effects. These artifacts may arise from various sources, including patient motion, anatomical heterogeneity, hardware limitations, and reconstruction algorithms. Minimizing artifacts requires meticulous attention to imaging protocols, patient positioning, and scanner calibration, as well as the use of advanced reconstruction techniques and artifact correction algorithms [22].

Clinical interpretation of CT images can be challenging due to the complexity of anatomical structures, overlapping tissue densities, and subtle pathological changes. Radiologists must navigate through vast volumes of image data, differentiate between normal and abnormal findings, and correlate imaging findings with clinical history and laboratory results. Moreover, the subjective nature of image interpretation introduces variability and subjectivity, leading to discrepancies, misdiagnoses, and diagnostic errors. Addressing these challenges requires ongoing training and education for radiologists, interdisciplinary collaboration, and the implementation of standardized imaging protocols and reporting guidelines [20].

Operational challenges in CT imaging include workflow inefficiencies, equipment maintenance, and resource constraints. CT scanners are high-cost, high-maintenance devices that require regular calibration, quality assurance, and downtime for maintenance and upgrades. Additionally, patient throughput and scheduling constraints may lead to long wait times, delayed appointments, and a backlog of imaging studies. To optimize operational efficiency, healthcare institutions must invest in staff training, workflow optimization, and technology upgrades while ensuring adequate staffing levels, equipment availability, and patient-centered care delivery [22].

Addressing the challenges in CT imaging requires a multifaceted approach encompassing technological innovation, clinical practice guidelines, and healthcare policy initiatives [12]. Continued research and development in dose reduction techniques, image reconstruction algorithms, and artifact correction methods will enhance image quality and reduce radiation dose exposure. Furthermore, automating image analysis could be possible with machine learning techniques and AI, improving diagnostic accuracy and streamlining clinical workflows [7]. Moreover, collaborative efforts among healthcare stakeholders, including radiologists, physicists, engineers, and policymakers, are essential for developing standardized protocols, best practices, and quality assurance guidelines to ensure safe, effective, and equitable CT imaging services for all patients [19].

5.5 Magnetic Resonance Imaging

The discovery of nuclear magnetic resonance (NMR) in the 1940s by physicists Felix Bloch and Edward Purcell laid the groundwork for modern MRI. Their efforts established the basis for the advancement of MRI as a medical imaging modality [23]. Raymond Damadian showed that it was possible to use NMR to distinguish between healthy and malignant tissues at the beginning of the 1970s [23]. He found that different tissue emissions had different response lengths with relatively longer signals from malignant tissues. He concluded that these two tissue differentiations had differences in their relaxation times. This led to the invention of the first MRI scanner, known as the "Indomitable", in 1977 [23].

5.5.1 Principles, Advantages, and Challenges of MRI

NMR principles are applied in MRI to produce finely detailed images of the body's interior structures, particularly soft tissue anatomy [7]. This modality relies on hydrogen nuclei in the body due to its abundance in water and fats. Because tissue-resident hydrogen nuclei are composed only of protons, their density in a given region generates a signal that is processed to form an image of the body [7]. Protons in specific compounds are affected by the fields of other atoms to which they are attached, making it possible to separate reactions from hydrogen [24]. To conduct the investigation, the subject is placed within an MRI scanner, which generates a strong magnetic field surrounding the area that has to be investigated [24]. A high magnetic field applied to the body region causes the proton axis to align with the direction of the magnetic field. Initially, the patient is given a brief application of energy at the proper resonance frequency via an oscillating magnetic field. When scanning with X and Y gradient coils, a particular region of the patient is exposed to the exact magnetic field required for the energy to be absorbed [24].

A receiving coil measures the signal produced by a radiofrequency (RF) pulse that excites the atoms. By employing gradient coils to modify the local magnetic field, one may process the RF signal and infer position information by observing changes in RF level and phase [21]. The radio wave introduced exhibits electromagnetic properties and causes the initial magnetic vector to be deflected. The magnitude of deflection depends on the intensity and period at which the radio wave is applied. When particular radio wave frequencies are applied, the proton-absorbed energy changes from a lower energy state to a higher energy level [21].

Due to the windings' slight movement as a result of magnetostriction, these coils, which are quickly switched during the excitation and response to accomplish a moving line scan, provide the distinctive repeating noise of an MRI scan [24]. How quickly stimulated atoms recover to their equilibrium state determines how distinct tissues contrast. The patient may receive exogenous contrast agents to improve the clarity of the image [24]. Subsequent relaxation processes emit RF signals, which are detected by RF coils. MRI can produce images with different contrasts through variations in magnetic field gradients and RF pulse sequences, highlighting various anatomical and pathological features.

MRI is used in medicine for studying the central nervous system (brain and spinal cord), particularly the brain stem and posterior fossa, where abnormalities are more easily seen than with CT scans; lesions (solid and cystic); pathologies of joints (rotator cuff tear, knee meniscus tear); pathologies of intra-abdominal organs (liver, kidneys spleen, gallbladder); origin of pain, unhealthy tissues; and preoperative planning [24]

On one hand, MRI has the advantages of being; extremely sensitive to normal and abnormal patterns of myelination; a painless and noninvasive procedure; and a nonionizing radiation procedure. MRI offers excellent diagnostic information with or without contrast media, is independent of the operator, and has relatively higher spatial resolution and detail [24]. Additionally, its significantly higher soft tissue contrast can be used for treatment planning, follow-up for musculoskeletal neoplasms, and early identification of avascular necrosis of hip and knee injuries [24]. Furthermore, the direct imaging capability of MRI in three orthogonal planes makes it easier to stage and monitor pelvic tumors and other abnormalities [24].

On the other hand, MRI has the challenge of relatively longer scanning and post-processing time; inability to diagnose intra-luminal pathologies; failure to provide real-time information; provides relatively low sensitivity; provides a relatively higher risk of claustrophobic and anxiety-related reactions of patients; and relatively expensive.

5.6 Ultrasonography

High-frequency broadband sound waves in the megahertz range, which are reflected by tissue to variable degrees, are used in ultrasonography, a modern diagnostic imaging technology, to make medical images [25]. On the patient's skin at the desired area, the ultrasonic transducer is positioned. Internal organs are reflected by a stream of high-frequency sound waves that enter the body from the transducer [26]. The transducer picks up sound waves that are reflected off the internal organs and then quantifies this characteristic into an image because various tissues reflect these sound waves in different ways [26]. These waves are received by the ultrasonic device, which transforms them into real-time images. During drainage and biopsy procedures, the obtained real-time moving image might be used as a guide [26]. It is feasible to assess the blood flow in veins and arteries due to the Doppler characteristics of more recent ultrasound scanners. Figure 5.2 (A, B, C, D) shows different types of ultrasound transducers.

5.6.1 Principles, Advantages, and Challenges of Ultrasound Imaging

The application of high-frequency sound to aid in patient diagnosis and treatment forms the basis of medical ultrasonography. Generally speaking, ultrasonic frequencies range from 2 to 15 MHz, while even higher frequencies may be used in some situations [27]. The transducer produces the ultrasonic

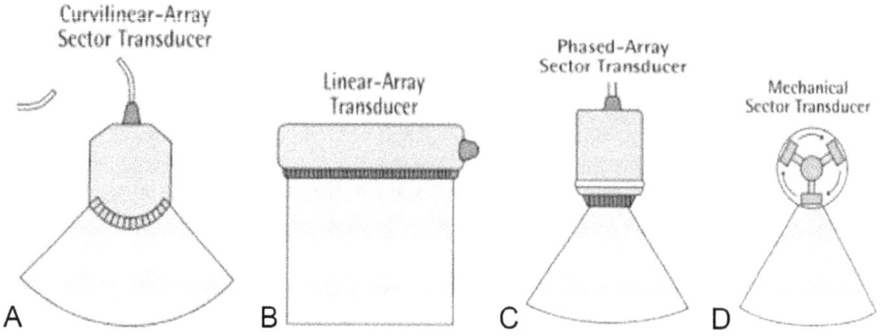

FIGURE 5.2 Types of ultrasound transducers.

beam mechanically, which is driven by electrical pulses (piezoelectric effect) and numerous crystals [27]. A transducer is an apparatus that converts electrical energy into acoustic energy [28]. After leaving the transducer and traveling through various tissues, the ultrasound waves, which are just sound pulses, return to the probe as reflected echoes [28]. The ultrasound image displayed on the screen is created by further processing the returned echoes, which the transducer crystals transform into electrical impulses [25]. Bandwidth is the range of ultrasonic frequencies that are present in ultrasound transducers. As an illustration, 5.0–7.5 MHz is used for imaging superficial structures while 2.5–3.5 MHz is for imaging deeper structures [26].

The reflection of ultrasound waves at the interfaces of denser and thinner tissues is proportionate to the impedance difference. The amount of transmitted sound decreases proportionately with increasing density difference, whereas the amount of reflected sound increases [26]. Complete acoustic shadowing occurs when there is a significant variation in tissue density, which causes all sounds to be reflected. Bones, calculi (kidney stone, gallbladder stone, etc.), and air (bowel gases) exhibit acoustic shadowing [26]. No echoes are generated if there is no variation within or between tissues. Echo-free formations are those that contain homogenous fluids, such as blood, bile, urine, ascites, and the contents of simple cysts [26].

Ultrasound is a useful diagnostic imaging technique for monitoring the development of the fetus during cyesis, examining most head and neck structures, including the glands that control the thyroid and parathyroid hormones, lymph nodes, and salivary glands, examining intra-abdominal organs like the liver, bile ducts, gallbladder, kidneys, pancreas, abdominal aorta, spleen, and inferior vena cava, performing ultrasound-guided biopsies, guiding needles to inject local anesthetic solutions near nerves, and performing echocardiography, which examines the structure and function of the heart [25, 26].

Ultrasound does not only aid in diagnosis but also directs biopsies and therapeutic action. For example, radiologists can evaluate tumors and abnormal findings in the breast or liver using ultrasound-guided biopsy [27]. Physicians who practice pain management also use ultrasound to guide the placement of analgesics in musculoskeletal tissues, which helps patients with both acute and chronic pain [27]. Moreover, recently developed fields of study have brought to light untapped possibilities for high-intensity focused ultrasound in enhanced medication delivery and therapy, such as thrombolysis and drug delivery produced by hyperthermia [27].

Ultrasonography offers several benefits, including being a noninvasive, painless, and nonionizing radiation procedure; it can measure velocity; it can detect changes in flow and extra-luminal abnormalities; it can provide real-time information; and it can be done with high resolution [27]. However, ultrasound has several drawbacks such as the lack of established protocols, reliance on the operator, extended processing times, and limited ability to provide a comprehensive image of the veins, which is frequently impacted by the patient's level of hydration [27].

5.7 Optical Imaging

Optical imaging, first introduced by American physical chemist Britton Chance, is the use of light as an investigative imaging technique for medical uses [28]. Intrinsic optical signal (IOS) imaging, optical microscopy, voltage-sensitive dye imaging (VSD), photoacoustic tomography (PT), optical coherence tomography (OCT), endoscopy, diffuse optical tomography (DOT), scanning laser ophthalmoscopy, spectroscopy, and laser Doppler imaging are a few examples [28, 29]. Similar phenomena occur in X-rays, microwaves, and radio waves since light is an electromagnetic wave [30].

5.7.1 Principles, Advantages, and Challenges of Optical Imaging

Using visible light and the unique characteristics of photons, optical imaging, which is a non-invasive method, is used to obtain fine detailed images of organs, tissues, and even tiny structures like cells and molecules [31]. High-sensitivity charged-coupled device (CCD) cameras are used to capture images. These cameras have a temporal resolution of seconds to minutes and can detect probe concentrations ranging from picomolar to femtomolar.

Low-energy photons, which are highly absorbed and scattered by biological tissues, are detected during optical imaging of living subjects. These photons can only travel a few millimeters. Theoretically, optical imaging systems can be classified into diffusive [27, 32] and ballistic [33]. There exists a model for photon migration in turbid biological mediums. This type of model can be used to create procedures for the therapeutic stimulation of tissue chromophores and to analyze data from laser Doppler blood-flow monitors. The technique of imaging with near-infrared spectroscopy (NIRS) [34] or fluorescence-based techniques [35] is known as diffuse optical imaging (DOI). While 2D imaging techniques are categorized as diffuse optical topography, this type of tomography is used to describe the process of creating 3D volumetric models of the material that has been imaged [34].

Ballistic photons, often referred to as light photons, are used in ballistic optical imaging techniques [33]. These photons go through a turbid or scattering medium in a straight path. The majority of photons in laser pulses that pass through turbid materials like bodily tissue or fog are either randomly scattered or absorbed. On the other hand, some photons travel straight through the scattering medium over short distances. Ballistic photons are the name given to these coherent photons. Snake photons are photons with a small degree of coherence that are somewhat dispersed [33].

Optical imaging technique has applications in many domains, including sports medicine, wound care, neurology, and cancer detection [35]. Usually, DOI methods track variations in hemoglobin concentrations, both oxygenated and deoxygenated. In some cases, the technique could also be referred to as fluorescence diffuse optical tomography (FDOT), near-infrared optical tomography (NIROT), or DOT [35]. Functional measures in neuroscience that employ near-infrared wavelengths and DOI methodologies may be categorized as functional near-infrared spectroscopy (fNIRS) [35].

Due to the fact that ballistic photons in a scattering medium diminish exponentially with distance, image processing techniques are frequently used to recreate high-quality ballistic images from raw, recorded ones [33]. The goal of ballistic imaging modalities is to separate information-carrying ballistic photons from non-ballistic ones [33]. Specific properties of ballistic versus non-ballistic photons are exploited to accomplish this task, including collimation, wavefront propagation, polarization, and time of flight using coherence-gated imaging [36]. Ballistic photons have various uses if they can be detected well, particularly in coherent high-resolution medical imaging systems. Popular optical imaging technologies that use ballistic photon detection to produce images include OCT, which uses the interferometry principle, and ballistic scanners, which use ultrafast time gates [33, 36].

Clinical application of optical imaging is also feasible in the endoscopy setting, detection of tumors, and scanning of the breast, bones, jaws, teeth, gums, and brain [36]. One of the primary benefits of optical imaging, in addition to its affordability and outstanding spatial resolution in the visible and NIR spectrum, is that radiation is not required. Nonetheless, the primary constraints are inadequate tissue penetration and elevated background noise resulting from tissue autofluorescence and light absorption [37]. Therefore, optical imaging has a limited depth of penetration but is generally safe. When compared to other imaging modalities, it is superior because it is very inexpensive, has a high sensitivity of about 10^{-9}–10^{-12} mol/L, does not emit ionizing radiation, can be used in real-time imaging, has a short acquisition time, and can multiplex [37].

This modality is affected by some factors, such as low tissue penetration (0–2 cm), strong tissue scattering of photons in the visible light region (395–600 nm) [38], and a notable background caused by water (above 900 nm), heme groups (maximum absorbance at 560 nm), and protein light absorption (260–280 nm). Several imaging modalities have been studied with the benefits of reduced autofluorescence, reduced tissue scattering, and greater penetration depth for in vivo imaging. These include the NIR window (NIR, 650–900 nm), [39] and the second NIR window (NIR-II, 1000–1700 nm) [40, 41]. Moreover, ballistic imaging, which has a restricted imaging depth, can reach a higher resolution of 1–10 micrometers, which is another benefit of optical imaging over other currently used imaging modalities (such as magnetic resonance imaging and ultrasound). In addition, to boost the signal's "strength" (i.e., signal-to-noise ratio), more dispersed "quasi-ballistic" photons are likewise frequently detected [41].

5.8 Elastography

An organ's stiffness can be determined by using a diagnostic imaging technique called elastography. Stiff spots in the investigated organs may indicate a disease. With stiff patches in the liver indicating scar tissue (fibrosis) brought on by liver disease, elastography can aid in this diagnosis. In other words, elastography is a more recent method that takes into account the fact that pathological conditions can modify a tissue's elastic characteristics [42]. Elastography is a noninvasive diagnostic imaging system that utilizes elasticity as a measure of biological tissues' stiffness in relation to normal tissue [42, 43]. Ultrasonic, magnetic resonance, optical, or tactile elasticity imaging are possible methods for elastography imaging. The first technique to perform elastography was ultrasound elastography, which is now being extensively used for clinical diagnostic applications of soft tissues [44–47].

5.8.1 Principles, Advantages, and Challenges of Elastography

MR elastography uses MRI to image the propagation of shear waves and determine the mechanical characteristics of soft tissues [48–52]. The gradient waveform in the pulse sequence is used by MR elastography to sensitize the MRI scan to shear waves in the tissue. On the skin's surface, an electromechanical transducer produces shear waves. At the same frequency as the motion-sensitizing gradient is the mechanical excitation. Utilizing optical coherence tomography, optical elastography is carried out [53–56]. In order to enable optical coherence elastography on human beings, a simultaneous image can be obtained by designing an annular piezoelectric loading transducer [57]. One medical imaging technology that converts touch perception into a digital image is called tactile imaging [58, 59]. The tactile image is defined by the soft tissue surface pressure under applied deformation. The device's probe, which has a pressure sensor array mounted on its face, acts during the examination like a human finger and slightly distorts soft tissue to detect changes in the pressure pattern. As a result of this, tactile imaging and manual palpation are extremely comparable [59].

Currently, the clinical use of elastography includes the following: measuring the heart muscle's mechanical response at different stages of the cardiac cycle; assessing and diagnosing diseases of the soft tissues, such as breast cancer, age-related changes in material properties, and myofascial trigger points in muscles; examining diseases of the liver, such as liver cirrhosis; assessing the stiffness of the plantar fascia; and using tactile imaging to assess the prostate, vagina, and pelvic floor support structures [59]. The non-invasive and nonionizing radiation character of elastography, the instantaneous nature of the data, the high precision of 2D-time shift-based strain estimate approaches, and the high frame rate that permits the acquisition of a detailed map of the transmural strain in normal conditions are some of its benefits [59]. However, as pressure is increased, elastography is affected by elasticity scores as well as elastography images, which could result in low resolution, incorrect diagnosis, or medical disorders [59].

5.9 Terahertz (THz) Imaging

Terahertz imaging is based on electromagnetic radiation confined to a frequency spectrum from 0.1 to 10 THz referred to as "THz gap" [60], as shown in Figure 5.3.

Terahertz waves, or t-rays, can be used to transport information and produce images, much like visible light. The pronounced absorption of terahertz electromagnetic radiation in water makes reflected terahertz imaging stand out from previous transmission-based techniques [60].

5.9.1 Principles, Advantages, and Challenges of Terahertz Imaging

The measurement of transmitted or reflected ultra-short electromagnetic pulses and a Fourier transform of the recorded waveforms are the fundamental components of terahertz imaging [60]. Probe beams interact with samples in terahertz imaging, and the combination of the terahertz radiation and the probe laser yields the detection signal. The selective absorption of the terahertz radiation allows the image of the subject to be constructed. An image can be created by scanning the sample once the detector receives the signals [60–62].

Owing to its capacity to enable accurate and timely assessment of a material's permeability or permittivity across an extensive bandwidth, the terahertz imaging technique finds its application in the detection of cancers associated with the breast, skin, and colon [63]; imaging the crown of the tooth; both in vivo and in vitro imaging experiments of biological tissues [64].

Advantages of terahertz imaging include its extended wavelength, which allows it to pass through a variety of materials, its unique sensitivity to the vibration modes of water, and its safety and non-ionizing nature. Terahertz radiation is harmless for human health because, unlike X-rays, it does not promote photoionization in biological tissue due to its low photon energy. Moreover, terahertz waves have longer wavelengths than visible and infrared light. The majority of dry dielectric materials, such as plastic, wood, fabric, porcelain, and paper, are transparent to terahertz waves due to this property [63]. To further facilitate their spectroscopic fingerprinting in the terahertz range, a large number of compounds show distinctive absorption and dispersion at terahertz frequencies. Nondestructive inspection utilizing terahertz waves combines this feature with image technology to offer composition information for both target profiles [64].

Terahertz, on the other hand, has drawbacks such as a low signal-to-noise ratio and sluggish processing by detectors; emitters only produce low-brightness, incoherent terahertz radiation [60]; terahertz sources

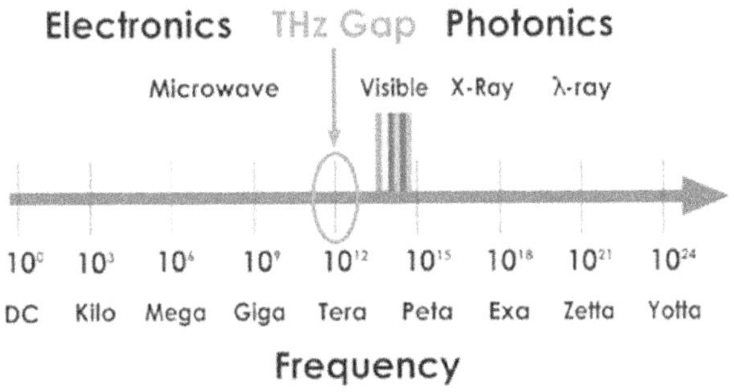

FIGURE 5.3 Frequency spectrum of terahertz imaging.

require cryogenic operating temperatures [65]; and terahertz offers little contrast between healthy and pathological tissues.

5.10 Radionuclide Imaging

A diagnostic imaging method called radionuclide imaging uses trace amounts of radioactive material to create images of the internal structures of the body. Low-level radioactive isotopes in small doses are administered orally or via injection. Particular organs, bones, or tissues are drawn to these isotopes, and these organs or tissues absorb the radioactive substance. After absorbing radioactive material, an organ or tissue releases emissions that can be picked up by specialized radiation detectors. To create an image from the emissions, the scanner collaborates with a computer. Three techniques are used in radionuclide imaging: PET [66–68], SPECT [69–73], and planar scintigraphy [74–76]. Imaging fusion has been applied recently to create unique views for recording data from two distinct exams to be correlated and evaluated on a single image [76]. This includes integrating PET and CT or MRI images. The combination SPECT-CT has also been created by applying image fusion to combine SPECT and CT images [77–79]. A comparison of the radionuclide imaging techniques is summarized in Table 5.1.

The isotopes used in PET imaging decay through positron emission tomography. The released positron doesn't go very far before it experiences an annihilation process that creates two photons that move in opposing directions from one another [66]. Placing two detectors on opposing sides of the patient allows for the localization of the annihilation event. A straight line can be used to determine the position of the positron that was released when the photons were detected simultaneously [67]. Image fusion has been utilized recently to provide unique views for gathering the data from the two separate exams to be correlated and analyzed on one image. This has involved integrating PET scans with CT or MRI images [68]. This provides more precise diagnosis and accurate information. The combinations that are available on the market are PET-MRI [80–82] as well as PET-CT [83–85].

PET-CT, or positron emission tomography-computed tomography, is a nuclear medicine technique that combines a positron emission tomography scanner and an X-ray computed tomography scanner on a single gantry. Sequential images are obtained from both devices during the same session and combined into a single superposed image [86]. As such, anatomic imaging from CT scanning can be more precisely aligned or correlated with functional imaging from PET scanning, which shows the spatial distribution of metabolic or biochemical activity in the body. Reconstructing images in two and three dimensions can be accomplished through the use of a single control system and a set of software [86].

TABLE 5.1

Comparison of radionuclide imaging modalities

	PET	SPECT	Scintigraphy
Methodology	The two photons in two opposite directions produced simultaneously through positron decay are captured in multiple directions	Photons are captured in multiple directions	Only one direction is involved in the capture of the patient's gamma rays (photons)
Source	Positron decay is generated from radioisotope	Gamma decay is generated from radioisotope	One photon is produced randomly at a time during gamma decay, which is produced by radioisotope
Image receptor	Detects two photons in opposite directions simultaneously by using a special coincidence detection circuitry	Captures projection data from multiple angles by using a rotating anger camera	Captures data by using anger scintillation camera

Through the addition of precise anatomic localization to functional imaging, a feature that pure PET imaging was previously lacking, PET-CT has transformed medical diagnosis in numerous disciplines [86]. The emergence of PET-CTs has had a significant impact on several diagnostic imaging processes in oncology, surgical planning, radiation therapy, and cancer staging. As a result, healthcare facilities have been steadily replacing their traditional PET devices with PET-CTs. Despite being significantly more expensive, the hybrid/combined device offers the benefit of doing both tasks as standalone exams because it is two devices in one [86].

The third barrier to a broader application of PET-CT is the expense and difficulty of manufacturing and shipping the radiopharmaceuticals, which are typically very short-lived and needed for PET imaging. For example, radioactive fluorine-18 (18F) used to measure glucose metabolism (with fluorodeoxyglucose, FDG) has a two-hour half-life. An extremely costly cyclotron and a production line for the radiopharmaceuticals are needed for its creation. Ga-68 is created on-site from a gallium-68 generator, which is the source of at least one PET-CT radiopharmaceutical [86].

When using a PET-CT to diagnose, the benefits of the two different approaches are merged, and the outcome significantly outperforms the pictures produced by the two devices used alone [87]. This technique makes it possible to identify any malignant formation in the body, regardless of its size or stage of development. A further benefit of the quick diagnosis process is that it saves the practitioner valuable time while fighting the illness. Even though the material used is radioactive, the risk is extremely low, and the body naturally gets rid of it in less than 24 hours after it is administered [87, 88].

The first demonstration of simultaneous PET/MR detection was made in 1997, but it took another 13 years and new detector technologies for clinical systems to hit the market [89]. At the moment, cancer [90–92], cardiology [93], neurology [94–96], and neuroscience [97] are the primary clinical regions for PET-MRI. The advantages of the novel PET-MRI diagnostic technique are now being investigated through research investigations. Using the sensitivity of PET imaging of metabolism and the ability to track specific cell types or cell receptors, the method combines the excellent structural and functional characterization of tissue offered by MRI with the tracking capabilities of PET imaging. A comparison of PET-CT and PET-MRI is shown in Table 5.2.

Drugs labeled with atoms that decay and release at least one gamma ray are the basis of the imaging method known as SPECT [69–73]. A collimator is required in front of the detector so that only the gamma rays emitted in the detector's direction can be recorded because gamma rays are typically emitted equally in all directions. The collimator defines the direction of the radiation when it is detected in this manner [69–73]. The image is created by using mathematical techniques to track the gamma rays that are released back in the direction in which they were released [69–73].

After a patient receives radioactive materials by injection or mouth, scintigraphy uses a specific organ to temporarily or permanently accumulate these substances [98]. Tc99m and other radioisotopes are utilized no later than 6 hours, but no later than 2 hours after preparation. Tc99m dosage recommendations range from 20 to 25 millicuries [98]. It is recommended that the patient consume four to six glasses of water between the isotope injection and imaging to ensure proper hydration prior to imaging. Imaging is

TABLE 5.2

Comparison of PET-CT with PET-MRI

	PET-CT	PET-MRI
Soft tissue contrast	Lower	Higher
Speed (acquisition time)	Faster	Slower
Total ionizing radiation dose	High	Low (insignificant)
Attenuation maps	Clearly defined	Ill-defined
Atlas technique	Highly applicable	Difficult due to: MR coil attenuation and unusual anatomy

performed two hours after injection in individuals less than twenty years of age, and three to four hours after injection in older patients is advised for higher image quality. It is possible to make some diagnostically helpful inferences about the size of the organ and its normal or pathological location within the body based on the pattern of their distribution [98].

5.10.1 Principles, Advantages, and Challenges of Radionuclide Imaging

The clinical application of radionuclide imaging includes diagnosis of neurological pathologies such as epilepsy, Parkinson's disease, dementia, and Alzheimer's disease; diagnosis of cancers related to the head and neck, thyroid, cervix, lungs, esophagus, breast, pancreas, melanoma, colorectal, lymphoma; diagnosis of cardiovascular pathologies evaluate the effective of treatment [99]. Radionuclide imaging provides precise and accurate functional information with good tissue-specific contrast; useful in staging of cancer and the extent of tissue repair during treatment. Radionuclide imaging is challenging owing to its relatively high cost; use of ionizing radiation which increases radiation risk to patients and personnel; produces images of relatively lower spatial resolution; and sometimes requires the use of sedation for claustrophobic patients [100].

5.11 Conclusion

The book chapter presented an extensive overview of the principles, advantages, and challenges in current applications of diagnostic imaging techniques. The overview included techniques such as conventional radiography, fluoroscopy, CT imaging, MRI, ultrasonography, elastography, optical imaging, terahertz imaging, and radionuclide imaging (PET, SPECT, and scintigraphy). A comparative analysis of these imaging techniques given their safety, image quality, and accessibility is presented in Table 5.3.

TABLE 5.3

Comparison of diagnostic imaging techniques

	Imaging variables					
Diagnostic imaging technologies	**Ionizing radiation effect**	**Heating effect**	**Relative cost**	**Tissue contrast**	**Real-time information**	**Spatial resolution**
Conventional radiography	Yes	Insignificant	Moderate	Soft tissues	No	1 mm
Fluoroscopy	Yes	Insignificant	High	Soft tissues	Yes	1 mm
CT	Yes	insignificant	High	Hard and Soft tissues	No	0.5 mm
Ultrasound	No	Insignificant	Low	Soft tissues	Yes	1 mm
MRI	No	Medium	High	Soft tissues	No	0.5 mm
Optical	No	Medium	Low	Soft tissues	No	100 nm
Elastography	No	Low	Moderate	Soft tissues	Yes	200 μm
Terahertz	No	High	High	Soft tissues	No	40 μm
Radionuclide	Yes	Medium	High	Soft tissues	No	3 mm

REFERENCES

1. Tubiana M. Wilhelm Conrad Röntgen and the discovery of X-rays. *Bull Acad Natl Med.* 1996;180(1):97–108.
2. Panchbhai A. Wilhelm Conrad Röntgen and the discovery of X-rays: revisited after centennial. *J Indian Acad Oral Med Radiol.* 2015;27(1):90.
3. Webb S, Flower MA. *Webb's physics of medical imaging.* CRC Press, Florida, USA; 2016.
4. Hussain S, Mubeen I, Ullah N, Shah SSUD, Khan BA, Zahoor M, et al. Modern diagnostic imaging technique applications and risk factors in the medical field: a review. *BioMed Res Int.* 2022; 2022(1):5164970.
5. Mahara G, Tian C, Xu X, Wang W. Revolutionizing healthcare: exploring the latest advances in medical sciences. *J Glob Health.* 2023;13:03042.
6. Najjar R. Redefining radiology: a review of artificial intelligence integration in medical imaging. *Diagnostics.* 2023;13(17):2760.
7. Pinto-Coelho L. How artificial intelligence is shaping medical imaging technology: a survey of innovations and applications. *Bioengineering.* 2023;10(12):1435.
8. Ansari I, Arfat M, Malik M. Conventional radiography – a comparison with computed radiography (CR). *J Xi'an Shiyou Univ, Nat Sci Ed.* 2022;18(9):338–44.
9. Ballard DH, Sweet DE, Garg T, DiSantis DJ. 21st-century fluoroscopy: what will we be doing? A trainee's perspective. *Radiographics.* 2021;41(6):E166–8.
10. Catalina Imaging. *History of the CT scan – Catalina imaging.* Mobile CT Rental - Mobile Imaging Rental And Lease; 2019. Available from:
11. Bhattacharyya KB. Godfrey Newbold Hounsfield (1919-2004): the man who revolutionized neuroimaging. *Ann Indian Acad Neurol.* 2016;19(4):448.
12. Power SP, Moloney F, Twomey M, James K, O'Connor OJ, Maher MM. Computed tomography and patient risk: facts, perceptions, and uncertainties. *World J Radiol.* 2016;8(12):902.
13. Wesolowski JR, Lev MH. CT: history, technology, and clinical aspects. *Semin Ultrasound CT MRI.* 2005;26(6):376–9.
14. Efird JT, Jindal C, Podder TK, Kang KH, Biswas T. Cone beam computed tomography—the need for future guidance. *J Thorac Dis.* 2022;14:3681-3683.
15. Gingold E. *Modern fluoroscopy imaging systems.* Philadelphia, PA; 2022. Available from: https://www.imagewisely.org/Imaging-Modalities/Fluoroscopy/Modern-Imaging-Systems
16. Schueler BA. The AAPM/RSNA physics tutorial for residents: general overview of fluoroscopic imaging. *Radiographics.* 2020;20:1115–26.
17. Oldham M, Létourneau D, Watt L, et al. Cone-beam CT-guided radiation therapy: a model for online application. *Radiother Oncol.* 2005;75:271–8.
18. Thwaites DI, Tuohy JB. Back to the future: the history and development of the clinical linear accelerator. *Phys Med Biol.* 2006;51:R343–62.
19. Kumar M, Shanavas M, Sidappa A, et al. Cone beam computed tomography - know its secrets. *J Int Oral Health.* 2015;7:64–8.
20. Fred HL. Drawbacks and limitations of computed tomography: views from a medical educator. *Tex Heart Inst J.* 2004;31(4):345–8.
21. McCollough CH, Primak AN, Braun N, Kofler J, Yu L, Christner J. Strategies for reducing radiation dose in CT. *Radiol Clin North Am.* 2019;47(1):27–40.
22. Nowik P, Bujila R, Poludniowski G, Fransson A. Quality control of CT systems by automated monitoring of key performance indicators: a two-year study. *J Appl Clin Med Phys.* 2015;16(4):254–65.
23. Garet L. History of MRIs and the evolution of this life-saving technology. *Ezra.* 2020. Available from: ezra.com
24. McRobbie DW. *MRI from picture to proton.* Cambridge, UK and New York: Cambridge University Press; 2007.
25. Nadrljanski M, Murphy A, Bell D, et al. *Physical principles of ultrasound.* Radiopaedia.org; 2024. Available from: radiopaedia.org
26. Nyland TG, Mattoon JS, Herrgesell EJ, Wisner ER. Physical principles, instrumentation, and safety of diagnostic ultrasound. In: Nyland TG, Mattoon JS, editors. *Small animal diagnostic ultrasound.* 2nd ed. Philadelphia: WB Saunders; 2002. p. 1–18.

27. Phenix CP, Togtema M, Pichardo S, et al. High-intensity focused ultrasound technology, its scope and applications in therapy and drug delivery. *J Pharm Pharm Sci.* 2014;17:136–53.
28. Guevara E, Pouliot P, Dang K, Lesage F. Optical imaging of acute epileptic networks in mice. *J Biomed Opt.* 2023;18.
29. Gibson A, Hebden J, Arridge S. Recent advances in diffuse optical imaging. *Phys Med Biol.* 2015;50(4):R1–R43.
30. Chung SH, Feldman M, Martinez Daniel, et al. Macroscopic optical physiological parameters correlate with microscopic proliferation and vessel area breast cancer signatures. *Breast Cancer Res.* 2015;17:72.
31. Janib SM, Moses AS, MacKay JA. Imaging and drug delivery using theranostic nanoparticles. *Adv Drug Deliv Rev.* 2010;62:1052–63.
32. Durduran T. Diffuse optics for tissue monitoring and tomography. *Rep Prog Phys.* 2010;73(7).
33. Farsiu S, Christofferson J, Eriksson B, Milanfar P, Friedlander B, Shakouri A, Nowak R. Statistical detection and imaging of objects hidden in turbid media using ballistic photons. *Appl Opt.* 2017;46(23):5805–22.
34. Durduran T, et al. Diffuse optics for tissue monitoring and tomography. *Rep Prog Phys.* 2020;75(7):076701.
35. Harvard.edu. Diffuse optical imaging. Archived from the original on June 16, 2012.
36. Lihong VW, Hsin-i Wu. *Biomedical optics: principles and imaging.* John Wiley & Sons, Hoboken, New Jersey, USA; 2012. p. 3.
37. Wang J, Mi P, Lin G, Wang YX, Liu G, Chen X. Imaging-guided delivery of RNAi for anticancer treatment. *Adv Drug Deliv Rev.* 2016;104:44–60.
38. Debbage P, Jaschke W. Molecular imaging with nanoparticles: giant roles for dwarf actors. *Histochem Cell Biol.* 2008;130:845–75.
39. Smith AM, Mancini MC, Nie S. Bioimaging: second window for in vivo imaging. *Nat Nanotechnol.* 2019;4:710–11.
40. Hong G, Zou Y, Antaris AL, et al. Ultrafast fluorescence imaging in vivo with conjugated polymer fluorophores in the second near-infrared window. *Nat Commun.* 2014;5:4206.
41. Robinson JT, Hong G, Liang Y, Zhang B, Yaghi OK, Dai H. In vivo fluorescence imaging in the second near-infrared window with long-circulating carbon nanotubes capable of ultrahigh tumor uptake. *J Am Chem Soc.* 2022;134:10664–9.
42. Tyagi S, Kumar S. Clinical applications of elastography: an overview. *Int J Pharma Bio Sci.* 2010;1:3.
43. Doyley MM, Parker KJ. Elastography: general principles and clinical applications. *Ultrasound Clin.* 2014;9(1):1–11.
44. Ophir J, Alam SK, Garra B, Kallel F, Konofagou E, Krouskop T, Varghese T. Elastography: ultrasonic estimation and imaging of the elastic properties of tissues. *Proc Inst Mech Eng.* 2019;213:203–33.
45. Sarvazyan A, Hall TJ, Urban MW, Fatemi M, Aglyamov SR, Garra BS. An overview of elastography – an emerging branch of medical imaging. *Curr Med Imaging Rev.* 2021;7:255–82.
46. Gennisson JL, Deffieux T, Fink M, Tanter M. Ultrasound elastography: principles and techniques. *Diagn Interv Imaging.* 2013;94(5):487–95.
47. Rivaz H, Boctor EM, Choti MA, Hager GD. Ultrasound elastography using multiple images. *Med Image Anal.* 2014;18(2):314–29.
48. Yin M, Talwalker JA, Glaser KJ, et al. Assessment of hepatic fibrosis with magnetic resonance elastography. *Clin Gastroenterol Hepatol.* 2007;5(10):1207–13.
49. Huwart L, Sempoux C, Vicaut E, et al. Magnetic resonance elastography for the noninvasive staging of liver fibrosis. *Gastroenterology.* 2018;135(1):32–40.
50. Asbach P, Klatt D, Schlosser B, et al. Viscoelasticity-based staging of hepatic fibrosis with multifrequency MR elastography. *Radiology.* 2010;257(1):80–6.
51. Mariappan YK, Glaser KJ, Ehman RL. Magnetic resonance elastography: a review. *Clin Anat.* 2020;23(5):497–511.
52. Schmitt C, Montagnon E, Henni AH, Shijie Q, Cloutier G. Shear wave induced resonance elastography of venous thrombi: a proof-of-concept. *IEEE Trans Med Imaging.* 2013;32(3):565–77.
53. Schmitt G. OCT elastography: Imaging microscopic deformation and strain of tissue. *Opt Express.* 1998;3(6):199–211.
54. Rolland JP, Zvietcovich F, Gary RG, Parker KJ. Perspectives and advances in optical elastography. *Optical Elastography and Tissue Biomechanics VI.* 2019;21;10880:21–32.

55. Pan X, Gao J, Tao S, Liu K, Bai J, Luo J. A two-step optical flow method for strain estimation in elastography: Simulation and phantom study. *Ultrasonics.* 2014; 54(4):990–6.
56. Kennedy BF, Kennedy KM, Sampson DD. A review of optical coherence elastography: Fundamentals, techniques and prospects. *IEEE J Sel Top Quantum Electron.* 2013;20(2):272–88.
57. Kennedy BF, Hillman TR, McLaughlin RA, Quirk BC, Sampson DD. In vivo, dynamic optical coherence elastography using a ring actuator. *Opt Express.* 2009;17(24):21762–72.
58. Hoshi T, Takahashi M, Iwamoto T, Shinoda H. Noncontact tactile display based on radiation pressure of airborne ultrasound. *IEEE Trans Haptics.* 2010;3(3):155–65.
59. Tiwana MI, Redmond SJ, Lovell NH. A review of tactile sensing technologies with applications in biomedical engineering. *Sensors Actuators A Phys.* 2012;179:17–31.
60. Berry E, Walker GC, Fitzgerald AJ, et al. Do in vivo terahertz imaging systems comply with safety guidelines? *J Laser Appl.* 2003;15(3):192–8.
61. Mueller ER. Terahertz radiation: Applications and sources. *Ind Phys.* 2003;9(4):27–9.
62. Parrott E. Terahertz pulsed imaging in vivo: measurements and processing methods. *J Biomed Opt.* 2024; 16(10):106010–10.
63. Taylor ZD, Singh RS, Bennett DB, et al. THz medical imaging: in vivo hydration sensing. *IEEE Trans Terahertz Sci Technol.* 2011;1(1):201–19.
64. Davoudi B. *Comparative study and analysis of THz pulse and continuous-wave imaging towards medical application.* MSc Thesis, University of Waterloo; 2009.
65. Balocco C, Kasjoo SR, Lu X, et al. *Novel terahertz nanodevices and circuits.* IEEE International Conference on Solid-State and Integrated Circuit Technology; 2020. pp. 1176–9, Shanghai.
66. Rahmima A, Zaidib H. PET versus SPECT: strengths, limitations and challenges. *Nucl Med Commun.* 2018;29(3):193–207.
67. Razak HA, Abdul Rahim N, Nordin AJ. Dual time point imaging of FDG PET/CT in a tuberculous spondylodiscitis. *Biomed Imaging Interv J.* 2020;6(2).
68. Bendriem B, Townsend DW. *The theory and practice of 3D PET.* Kluwer,Dordrecht, Netherlands; 1998.
69. Larsson A. *Corrections for improved quantitative accuracy in SPECT and planar scintigraphic imaging.* Print & Media, Umea, Sweden; 2005.
70. Kulkarni S. *Image quality in MAP SPECT reconstructions.* PhD thesis, Electrical and Computer Engineering, Stony Brook University; 2009.
71. DePuey EG. Advances in SPECT camera software and hardware: currently available and new on the horizon. *J Nucl Cardiol.* 2022;19(3):551–81.
72. Madsen MT. Recent advances in SPECT imaging. *J Nucl Med.* 2017;48(4):661–73.
73. Marin T, Kalayeh MM, Parages FM, Brankov JG. Numerical surrogates for human observers in myocardial motion evaluation from SPECT images. *IEEE Trans Med Imaging.* 2014;33(1):38–47.
74. Klutmann S, Bohuslavizki KH, Kroger S, et al. Quantitative salivary gland scintigraphy. *J Nucl Med Technol.* 1999;27:20–6.
75. Lee Z, Ljungberg M, Muzic RF, Berridge MS. Usefulness and pitfalls of planar scintigraphy for measuring aerosol deposition in the lungs: a Monte Carlo investigation. *J Nucl Med.* 2021;42(7):1077–83.
76. Kraft O, Havel M. Sentinel lymph node identification in breast cancer - Comparison of planar scintigraphy and SPECT/CT. *Open Nucl Med J.* 2022;4:5–13.
77. Jacene HA, Goetze S, Patel H, Wahl RL, Ziessman HA. Advantages of hybrid SPECT/CT vs SPECT alone. *Open Med Imaging J.* 2018;2:67–79.
78. International Atomic Energy Agency. *Clinical applications of SPECT/CT: new hybrid nuclear medicine imaging system.* Vienna, Austria: International Atomic Energy Agency; 2018.
79. Carstensen MH, Al-Harbi M, Urbain JL, Belhocine TZ. SPECT/CT imaging of the lumbar spine in chronic low back pain: A case report. *Chiropr Man Ther.* 2011;19(2): 1-5.
80. Catana C, Wu Y, Judenhofer MS, Qi J, Pichler BJ, Cherry SR. Simultaneous acquisition of multislice PET and MR images: Initial results with an MR-compatible PET scanner. *J Nucl Med.* 2016;47:1968–76.
81. Judenhofer MS, Catana C, Swann K, et al. Simultaneous PET/MR images, acquired with a compact MRI compatible PET detector in a 7 Tesla magnet. *Magn Reson Med.* 2021;65(1):269–79.
82. Pichler BJ, Kolb A, Nagele T, Schlemmer HP. PET/MRI: Paving the way for the next generation of clinical multimodality imaging applications. *J Nucl Med.* 2020;51(3):333–6.
83. Omur O, Baran Y, Ora A, Ceylan Y. Fluorine-18 fluorodeoxyglucose PET-CT for extranodal staging of non-Hodgkin and Hodgkin lymphoma. *J Turkish Soc Radiol.* 2014;20(2):185.

84. Straat SJ, Jacobsson H, Noz ME, Andreassen B, Naslund I, Jonsson C. Dynamic PET/CT measurements of induced positron activity in a prostate cancer patient after 50-MV photon radiation therapy. *EJNMMI Res.* 2013;3(6):1–7.
85. Makris NE, Boellaard R, Visser EP, et al. Multicenter harmonization of 89Zr PET/CT performance. *J Nucl Med.* 2014;55(2):264–7.
86. Dureja S, Sen IB, Acharya S. Potential role of F18 FDG PET-CT as an imaging biomarker for the non-invasive evaluation in uncomplicated skeletal tuberculosis: a prospective clinical observational study. *European Spine Journal.* 2014 Nov;23:2449–54.
87. Raylman RR. *Reduction of positron range effects by the application of a magnetic field: For use with positron emission tomography.* Michigan, USA, 1991.
88. Antoch G, Bockisch A. Combined PET/MRI: A new dimension in whole-body oncology imaging? *Eur J Nucl Med Mol Imaging.* 2009;36:113–20.
89. Luna A, Vilanova JC, Hygino da Cruz L, Celso Jr. Rossi SE. *Functional imaging in oncology: biophysical basis and technical approaches.* Springer Science & Business Media, Heidelberg, Germany; 2023. p. 421.
90. Buchbender C, Heusner TA, Lauenstein TC, et al. Oncologic PET/MRI, part 1: Tumours of the brain, head and neck, chest, abdomen, and pelvis. *J Nucl Med.* 2022;53(6):928–38.
91. Buchbender C, Heusner TA, Lauenstein TC, et al. Oncologic PET/MRI, part 2: Bone tumours, soft-tissue tumours, melanoma, and lymphoma. *J Nucl Med.* 2022;53(8):1244–52.
92. Martinez-Möller A, Eiber M, Nekolla SG, et al. Workflow and scan protocol considerations for integrated whole-body PET/MRI in oncology. *J Nucl Med.* 2022;53(9):1415–26.
93. Rischpler C, Nekolla SG, Dregely I, Schwaiger M. Hybrid PET/MR imaging of the heart: potential, initial experiences, and future prospects. *J Nucl Med.* 2023;54(3):402–15.
94. Imaging of traumatic brain injury patients swifter and safer with new technology at NIH. 18 September 2015.
95. Dimou E, Booij J, Rodrigues M, et al. Amyloid PET and MRI in Alzheimer's disease and mild cognitive impairment. *Curr Alzheimer Res.* 2019;6(3):312–19.
96. Bremner JD, Vythilingam M, Vermetten E, et al. MRI and PET study of deficits in hippocampal structure and function in women with childhood sexual abuse and posttraumatic stress disorder. *Am J Psychiatry.* 2023;160(5):924–32.
97. Cho ZH, Son YD, Choi EJ, et al. In-vivo human brain molecular imaging with a brain-dedicated PET/MRI system. *Magn Reson Mater Phys Biol Med.* 2022;26(1):71–79.
98. Nikpoor N. *Scintigraphy of the Musculoskeletal system.* Library of Congress Cataloging-in-Publication Data; 2009.
99. Kasban H, El-Bendary MAM, Salama DH. A comparative study of medical imaging techniques. *Int J Inf Sci Intell Syst.* 2015;4(2):37–58.
100. Nikpoor N. *Scintigraphy of the Musculoskeletal system.* Library of Congress Cataloging-in-Publication Data; 2019.

6

Dual X-Ray Absorptiometry: A Backbone in Bone Mineral Metabolism

Emmanuel Kwaku Ofori and Seth Kwabena Amponsah

6.1 Introduction

Bone health is essential for mobility, quality of life, and overall well-being, particularly as the global population ages. Accurate bone mineral density (BMD) measurement is vital in diagnosing osteoporosis, predicting fracture risk, and assessing treatment effectiveness [1]. Osteoporosis, a public health concern, is characterized by reduced BMD, structural deterioration of bone tissue, increased bone fragility, and the risk of fractures. These fractures can result in significant morbidity, disability, and mortality, particularly in the elderly population [2, 3].

Dual-energy X-ray absorptiometry (DEXA) is a technique for evaluating body composition. Due to its precision and noninvasiveness, DEXA has established itself as the standard for BMD assessment [4]. DEXA also facilitates the evaluation of bone mineral content (BMC) in primary skeletal regions (spine and hip), peripheral areas (heel and forearm), or over the entire body. Although DEXA uses ionizing radiation, an individual's dose is relatively insignificant while getting a DEXA examination. DEXA has been employed in numerous epidemiological studies on bone health and in nearly all pivotal prospective clinical trials that sanctioned medications intended to reduce the occurrence of fragility fractures [5, 6]. Notwithstanding its acknowledged shortcomings, DEXA offers advantages over other technologies. It includes alignment with the World Health Organization (WHO) classification system, proven efficacy in fracture risk assessment, and guidance for medical interventions to reduce fracture risk.

6.1.1 Historical Background

DEXA technology originated in the late 1980s after progress in single-photon absorptiometry (SPA) and dual-photon absorptiometry (DPA) [7]. These foundational techniques established the basis for DEXA's high-resolution and relatively accurate readings.

The advent of DEXA represented a substantial advancement in the precise and reproducible measurement of BMD, paving the way for its extensive clinical application. Subsequent milestones included the first publication of the Fracture Intervention Trial confirming that bisphosphonate therapy prevents bone loss and fractures [8], the issuance of the WHO report defining osteoporosis in postmenopausal Caucasian women as a BMD T-score of ≤–2.5 at the spine, hip, or forearm [9]. The most significant recent development is the Fracture Risk Assessment Tool (FRAX) tool, which enables clinicians to employ a patient's clinical risk factors in conjunction with a hip DEXA scan to assess the ten-year fracture probability for individual patients [10].

DOI: 10.1201/9781003486909-6

6.2 Principles of DEXA

6.2.1 Technical Overview

DEXA is primarily used in clinical settings to evaluate BMD. However, it can also measure or estimate total body mass, lean soft tissue mass, BMC, and fat mass. A DEXA scan is carried out by directing two X-ray beams of various intensities into the body, which allows the scan to penetrate both the bone and other soft tissues, such as adipose and muscle [11]. To differentiate between bone and soft tissues and determine BMD, DEXA uses the differences in the absorption of each beam between the two tissue types. According to the mathematical theory of DEXA, the X-ray transmission through any physical item can be divided into the corresponding areal densities (g/cm^2) of any selected reference materials. Examining how different human tissues absorb specific beams makes determining the body's composition possible. The quantity of soft tissue absorption must be subtracted from the computation to determine the BMD.

A typical DEXA scanner comprises some components, including an X-ray source (tube), X-ray collimators, and X-ray detectors. A C-arm connects the X-ray source, typically beneath the scanner table, to the X-ray detectors located above the table [12]. Depending on the patient, there is a difference in the degree of attenuation that X-ray photons undergo. This difference is partially controlled by the energy of the photons and the density of the tissue they pass through. The dimensions and orientation of the X-ray beam both impact the DEXA densitometers available.

The patient is positioned on a table as part of a DEXA scan. This scan involves the X-ray source and detector moving across the body to obtain the desired results. The process is relatively brief, requiring anywhere from ten to twenty minutes on average, and it results in just a little level of discomfort. During scan acquisition, the C-arm of the scanner moves, but it does not come into contact with the patient. The scan sites most frequently used are the lumbar spine, hip, and forearm. The lumbar spine is the highest-risk area for osteoporotic fractures. A typical DEXA output is shown in Figure 6.1.

6.2.2 Measurement Parameters

DEXA provides various vital measures, including BMC, BMD, T-score, Z-score, and percentage comparisons. Indeed, the output of modern DEXA devices must be more accurate and beneficial to the physician. The findings are presented in a manner that encompasses a variety of distinct regions of interest throughout the display. Consequently, this will make it possible to interpret the data more straightforwardly.

BMC refers to the total mineral content of bone, measured in grams. One method for determining the BMC is to measure the intensity of photons or X-rays transmitted through the entire structure through the measurement process [13]. The computation, which is the responsibility of the machine, is based on the bone's length, width, and density. Children older than five should have their BMC adjusted for height [14].

BMD is the most crucial factor in determining DEXA outcomes. BMD measures the density of minerals in a particular area of bone. It is expressed in grams per centimeter squared (g/cm^2). The calculation of BMD involves dividing the BMC by the area. This outcome is crucial for tracking skeletal alterations and calculating the standardized score (T-score or Z-score). A patient's BMD is evaluated by employing standard deviations for the average BMD of a young and healthy reference group. This allows for a more accurate assessment of the patient's BMD.

The T-score is the number of standard deviations (SD) above or below the mean BMD value of a reference population of young adults. It evaluates the particular patient against the average of individuals aged 20–29 years adjusted for gender and ethnicity. The Z-score represents the standard deviations by which a patient's BMD differs from the mean BMD of an age-matched reference group. The diagnostic criteria for osteoporosis are a T-score of −2.5 or lower [15]. This is the minimum score required to diagnose the condition (Table 6.1). Table 6.2 summarizes the results from a DEXA scan.

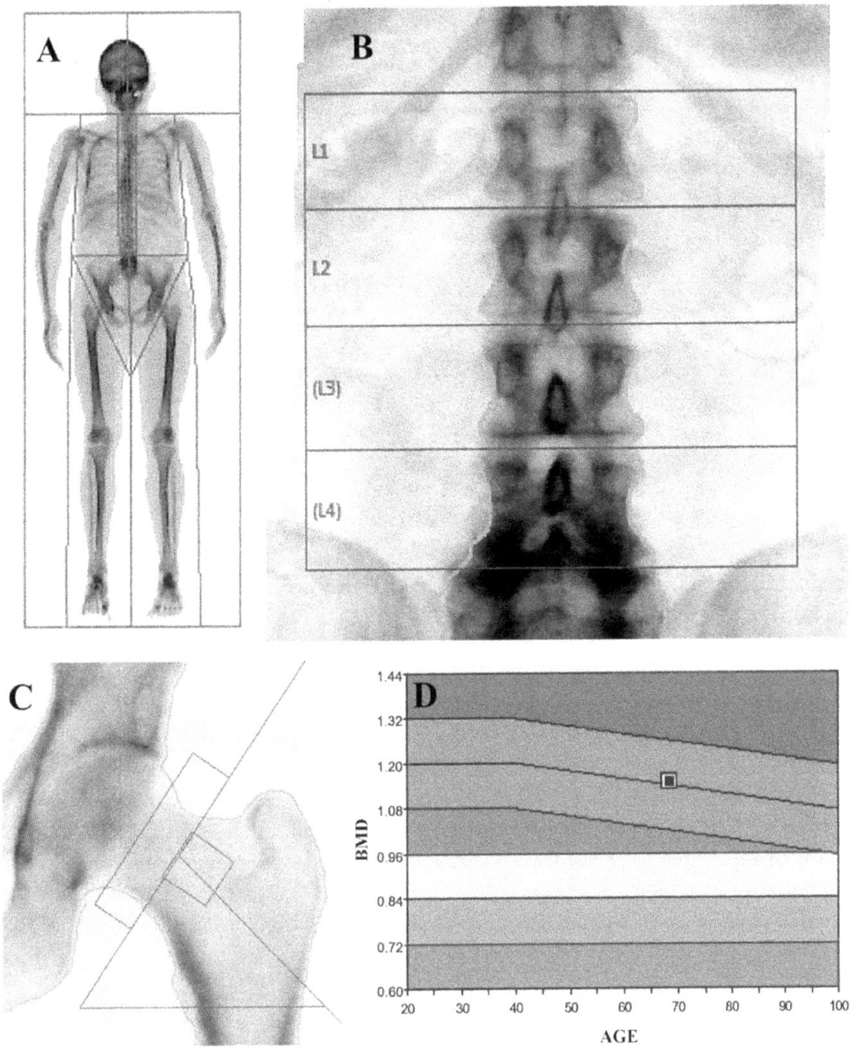

FIGURE 6.1 Components of a DEXA scan.

TABLE 6.1
WHO criteria for diagnosing osteoporosis

Situation	T-score meaning
Normal	T > 1.0
Osteopenia	−2.5 < T < −1.0
Osteoporosis	T ≤ 2.5
Established osteoporosis	T ≤ 2.5 with fractures

6.2.3 Clinical Utility of DEXA

BMD is measured with a DEXA to diagnose osteoporosis or track changes in BMD over time. The correlation between BMD measurement and the probability of a future fracture is the foundation upon which the diagnostic utility of DEXA for osteoporosis is built [16]. This densitometric method also identifies

TABLE 6.2
DEXA results summary

Region	Area (cm²)	BMC (g)	BMD (g/cm²)
Left arm	230.9	228.4	0.986
Right arm	247.2	234.3	0.940
Left ribs	99.8	80.8	0.842
Right ribs	101.7	85.4	0.809
Total spine	117.8	126.2	1.074
Left spine	52.3	61.4	1.173
Pelvis	208.2	286.5	1.376
Left leg	397.4	575.3	1.446
Right leg	380.1	521.4	1.376
	253.8	598.5	2.302
Total	2089.2	2798.2	1.338

T-Score = 1.4 PR (%) = 110 Z-Score = 1.6 AM (%) = 116

people who are at risk before a fragility fracture occurs. One of the critical objectives of osteoporosis treatment is to lessen the likelihood of fractures [17]. Using DXA, one can determine the possibility of a fracture occurring in this scenario. Evaluating fracture risk is also essential to assist the physician in formulating treatment choices. Indeed, the gradient of risk has a relatively substantial predictive capacity and is comparable to the relationship between blood pressure and the risk of cardiovascular disease [18].

Because of the correlation between low DEXA-measured BMD and the risk of fracture, regulatory bodies in both the United States of America and Europe have long advocated including DEXA-measured BMD as a criterion for inclusion in interventional studies. It has been demonstrated that pharmacologic treatment can reduce the risk of fractures among persons selected for trial inclusion based on their low BMD [19]. It is also possible to perform serial DEXA scans to assess changes in BMD over time. It is recommended that a second DEXA scan be performed six months after the first one in individuals who are anticipated to experience rapid bone loss (for instance, beginning glucocorticoid medication) [20].

6.2.4 Whole-Body Composition Analysis

When it comes to acquiring a better understanding of human energy metabolism in physiology and in a variety of clinical diseases, as well as when it comes to evaluating therapies, precise and reliable measures of body composition are helpful. In addition to analyzing BMD, DEXA may also be used to analyze body composition, including fat and lean mass distribution. Bone and soft tissue examinations are regularly performed on infants weighing as little as one kg [21]. DEXA capability is also helpful when it comes to treating illnesses such as sarcopenia and obesity because it provides a holistic perspective on the health of the involved patient. The fact that DEXA offers a comprehensive perspective of body composition is one of the reasons why it is an appealing tool for a wide range of clinical research and practice applications. Whole-body composition analysis can benefit individuals participating in weight control programs. Whole-body composition by DEXA can also assist with nutritional assessments and provide advice regarding activities by athletes.

6.2.5 Advantages of DEXA

Several benefits may be gained from using DEXA, including extensive precision, accuracy, and trustworthy readings essential for diagnosis and monitoring bone disorders (Table 6.3). Precision is frequently evaluated using the coefficient of variation (CV), which usually falls within the range of 1%–1.5% for BMD levels in the spine and the whole hip and within the range of 2%–2.5% for BMD levels in the femoral neck [22]. The amount of radiation exposure caused by a DEXA scan is not high,

TABLE 6.3
Advantages of using DEXA

Advantages: DEXA
Low radiation dose
BMD, T, and Z-score results are very informative in bone health
Stable calibration
Good accuracy and precision
Effective quality control dynamics
Proven ability to predict fracture risk
Used in WHO-FRAX algorithm for predicting ten-year
Proven for effective targeting of anti-fracture treatments
Effective at monitoring response to treatment
Short scan times
Better patient cooperation
Rapid patient setup
It can be used in conjunction with other imaging techniques
Availability of reliable reference ranges

equivalent to the amount consumed regularly. This quantity of radiation exposure is also not considered to be dangerous. DEXA scans are rapid and non-invasive. DEXA can also make correct body composition forecasts, producing accurate predictions. A DEXA scan can be finished in slightly less than five minutes, which is significantly less than the time it takes to obtain data from a whole-body magnetic resonance imaging (MRI) scan, which can take anywhere from 30 to 60 minutes to complete. Patient cooperation is increased because the procedure is performed quickly, and the patient is not uncomfortable. In addition to determining the composition of particular areas of the body, DEXA is also capable of determining the composition of the complete body. DEXA evaluation is also essential to decide on the appropriate treatments to reduce the possibility of fracture. Further, DEXA is applied in pediatric populations to evaluate the bone health of children taking corticosteroid medication for an extended period or who have chronic issues [23]. The utilization of DEXA is advantageous when it comes to the evaluation of secondary causes of osteoporosis. These secondary causes include glucocorticoid-induced osteoporosis, hyperparathyroidism, and other metabolic bone illnesses [24]. This is because DEXA provides a plethora of information. The BMD generated from DEXA is essential to fracture risk assessment devices like FRAX [25]. Based on clinical risk factors and BMD at the femoral neck, this instrument determines the likelihood of osteoporotic fractures occurring over ten years. Because of this integration, medical care can be more individualized with more treatment options.

Indeed, DEXA can comprehensively examine bone health when paired with other diagnostic modalities, such as computed tomography (CT) and MRI. Utilizing multimodal techniques can enhance patient outcomes and further understanding of bone diseases.

6.2.6 Disadvantages or Limitations of DEXA

Ensuring that the appropriate patient demographics are entered into the DEXA information system is paramount when interpreting DEXA examinations. Several things can affect T-scores and Z-scores, including incorrect information on age, gender, and race [26]. The results of a DEXA can be further influenced by several factors, including the patient's positioning, the equipment's calibration, faulty scan capture or analysis, and the operator's experience level [27].

Ensure that the patient is positioned correctly, that the scan is interpreted accurately, and that no artifacts are present. Because DEXA calculates fat mass indirectly by removing the mass of lean soft tissue and the mineral content, it is suggested that DEXA may impact fat mass calculation. The results of the DEXA test also show that the amount of lean soft tissue is an overestimate of the muscle mass. This type of tissue may be responsible for the overestimation because lean tissue comprises different compartments that are not muscle, such as skin, connective tissue, and fat-free adipose tissue [28].

Inaccuracies in BMC measurements can impact the clinical interpretation of DEXA images. In humans, the inhomogeneity of the distribution of adipose tissue can lead to the imaging of bone marrow and other soft tissues placed outside of the bone in the path of the X-ray beam [29]. This can result in an incorrect diagnosis. Furthermore, where an MRI scan can discern between intramuscular and extramuscular lipid levels, a typical DEXA scan cannot provide the added benefit of being able to differentiate between the two [30]. DEXA is a method utilized to determine the BMD present in a specific two-dimensional area. This is different from the accurate three-dimensional volume of the bone evaluated by CT and MRI scans. Thus, DEXA cannot determine the volume of adipose tissue (AT) or differentiate between the numerous AT depots.

Although DEXA employs low-dose radiation, there is still a concern over the possibility of repeated exposure. In particular, this is the case among populations who are more vulnerable to the effects of radiation, such as children and women who are pregnant. Additionally, inter-machine variability is possible, so the same machine ideally should be involved again for follow-up scans whenever feasible. The higher expense of the DEXA equipment and scans may be a barrier to the widespread deployment of this technology, particularly in environments where resources are restricted. Indeed, the results of a DEXA may be challenging to interpret, particularly in people with skeletal dysplasia or osteomalacia, which are disorders that affect bone density in a manner that is unique from osteoporosis [31]. Qualified medical practitioners must consider the clinical situation and any extra diagnostic information to interpret DEXA scans accurately.

The presence of metallic hardware or other artifacts in or overlaying the spine and hip or soft tissue artifacts, such as imaging contrast material, can be some of the additional obstacles that may occur during DEXA measurement [32]. Before beginning the scan, it is necessary to remove any exterior metallic artifacts, such as buttons made of metal, money coins, jewelry, and other items of a similar nature. Specific knowledge and precise attention to detail are essential prerequisites for the acquisition, processing, and subsequent interpretation of DEXA scans. Considering the disadvantages of using DEXA (Table 6.4), it is of the utmost importance to acknowledge the physician and technologist's role in obtaining and interpreting DEXA data to guarantee that the outcomes are consistently high quality.

6.2.7 Alternatives to DEXA

Quantitative computed tomography (QCT) evaluations of the hip and spine, peripheral dual-energy X-ray absorptiometry (pDEXA) systems for evaluating the forearm, heel, or hand, and quantitative ultrasound (QUS) equipment for measuring the heel and other peripheral regions are all examples of the types

TABLE 6.4

Disadvantages of using DEXA

Disadvantages: DEXA
Improper scan capture may invalidate outcome measures
Incorrect information fed into the DEXA machine may affect T- and Z-scores
Inaccurate estimation of fat mass
Potential overestimation of muscle mass
BMC results can be affected by inhomogeneity in adipose tissue distribution
Cannot distinguish between intramuscular and extramuscular lipids
Unable to determine the three-dimensional fat volume
Concerns about repeated radiation exposure
Relatively expensive and unavailable, especially in Africa
Inter-machine variability affecting accuracy and precision
Invalidation with the introduction of a contrast or nuclear material
Expertise required

of diagnostic tools that fall under this category. QCT is a scanner that provides a three-dimensional scanning modality that addresses the two-dimensional limitations of DEXA [33]. This scanning modality allows for evaluating actual physical volumetric BMD (vBMD). Although QCT is typically used for whole-body CT, specialist techniques such as peripheral QCT (pQCT) and high-resolution peripheral QCT (HR-pQCT) can provide focused imaging [34].

These methods can accurately delineate and characterize the trabecular and cortical bone compartments, which DEXA cannot do. pDEXA and QUS devices offer a quick, simple, cost-effective, and straightforward process for evaluating bone health. They are, therefore, enticing for use in a more extensive variety of circumstances. These alternative evaluation methods, however, have a poor relationship with central DEXA of the spine and hip in actual practice. Concerning pediatric patients with spinal abnormalities, contractures, or metallic implants, assessing peripheral regions with pQCT is superior to DEXA scans in terms of its benefits [35].

MRI, a powerful imaging technique that does not ionize, includes noninvasive treatments, and does not cause any patients to experience discomfort, has gained popularity in recent years. The employment of a magnetic field in MRI allows for the development of a comprehensive cross-sectional image of both cortical and trabecular bone, making it easier to perform a study of bone micro-architecture with a high degree of precision. MRI can evaluate soft and hard tissues, making it a valuable clinical tool. The use of MRI is not commonplace because of the high expenses involved and the requirement that general anesthesia be administered to individuals under 18 [36].

Conversely, unlike DEXA and CT, ultrasound is a non-invasive imaging tool that does not use radiation. One of its many benefits is quickly isolating a specific anatomical region. It also offers additional benefits, such as being portable and inexpensive. Although its usefulness depends on the person using it, its benefits make it an effective evaluation tool for determining bone quality in children and adolescents.

6.3 Advancements in DEXA Technology, Artificial Intelligence, and Future Directions

Due to technological breakthroughs, DEXA scans have improved their resolution and accuracy. This has led to the creation of three-dimensional DEXA (3D-DEXA) and high-resolution peripheral quantitative computed tomography (HR-pQCT) [37]. The 3D-DXA is a relatively recent technique that aims to reproduce three-dimensional images from two-dimensional DEXA scans. HR-pQCT is utilized to provide comprehensive insights into the micro-architecture of bones. This technique can produce high-resolution pictures of peripheral regions, such as the wrist and the ankle. These improvements can provide even more comprehensive evaluations of bone micro-architecture and strength, increasing the capacity of DEXA methods to make accurate predictions. Image processing and reconstruction techniques are anticipated to improve the quality of DEXA scans and their application in clinical settings, thereby providing considerable benefits to patients. Indeed, contemporary scanners can discern between cortical and trabecular bone, enabling them to provide more specific insights into bone health. Additionally, new imaging techniques have improved the capability of detecting spinal fractures, which are typically misdiagnosed.

The use of artificial intelligence (AI) in conjunction with DEXA technology has improved the efficiency of data reporting and processing [38]. Furthermore, technologies driven by AI have the potential to aid in risk classification and the development of tailored treatment treatments. These technologies can use massive datasets to recognize patterns and generate predictions regarding the experiment's outcomes. DEXA has the potential to contribute to the development of precision medicine in several ways, one of which is the creation of personalized treatments based on risk profiles and genetic predispositions. Personalized methods of bone health management can boost medication effectiveness while simultaneously minimizing the likelihood of patients experiencing adverse effects [3]. When DEXA data is combined with genetic testing and indications of bone turnover, it is possible to acquire a more comprehensive picture of a person's bone health and the likelihood of bone fracture. Innovative techniques, including optical coherence tomography (OCT), QUS, spatially offset Raman spectroscopy (SORS), and wearable devices, present significant advancements in bone health monitoring [39]. They deliver enhanced-resolution images and more comprehensive molecular-level information. Nonetheless, their application is frequently constrained by elevated expenses and specialized apparatus and training requirements.

Bone health is essential for overall human well-being, and inadequate bone health can result in severe medical diseases, including osteoporosis, fractures, specific skeletal illnesses, and bone malignancies. Consequently, the surveillance and assessment of bone health are crucial for the early detection and intervention of possible abnormalities. Investigations are now being carried out to develop a technology that can be worn or carried around to check the status of bones. This technology would be considered wearable or portable. These devices can provide real-time bone density and quality monitoring. This intervention would significantly improve the accessibility and convenience of bone health care for patients. Progress in sensor technology and data analytics will be an essential component in the design of portable devices that are dependable and easy to operate.

Bone remodeling entails the actions of osteoblasts, which generate new bone tissue, and osteoclasts, which resorb old bone tissue. Osteoblasts, responsible for bone formation, release collagen, the primary constituent of bone, and osteocalcin, which regulates bone development and calcium metabolism. Conversely, enzymes and acids secreted by osteoclasts decompose the mineralized matrix of bone tissue, thereby liberating minerals such as calcium into the bloodstream. The predominant techniques for evaluating bone health comprise QCT, DEXA, and the assessment of bone turnover indicators. Nonetheless, these approaches, particularly the biomarkers, need more accuracy and sensitivity to identify modest changes in bone turnover.

Consequently, there is an immediate necessity for advanced sensing technologies to augment the precision, sensitivity, and ease of bone health evaluation. The integration of technologies, including ultrasound, MRI, and optical imaging, has demonstrated encouraging efficacy in detecting bone disorders and assessing treatment effects. These technologies provide non-invasive, precise, and efficient evaluation of bone health metrics, resulting in enhanced diagnosis, monitoring, and treatment of bone-related disorders.

Progress in nano- and micro-electromechanical systems and AI has demonstrated the capacity to transform bone health evaluation through non-invasive, real-time monitoring [40]. Advanced sensing technologies could profoundly influence clinical practice, improve patient outcomes, and decrease healthcare expenses related to bone illnesses. They also contribute to enhancing specificity, sensitivity, early diagnosis, real-time monitoring, mobility, and cost-effectiveness of treatment. Emerging sensing technologies include wearable devices and biomarker-based sensors. These technologies provide ongoing and individualized monitoring, enabling individuals to actively oversee their bone health, heralding a new epoch of preventative healthcare. Predictive models utilizing machine learning and tissue engineering have the potential to transform bone health evaluation through early diagnosis and ongoing monitoring capabilities.

6.3.1 Portable and Wearable Technologies

Wearable devices (WDs) are becoming popular for collecting biometric data during regular activities, especially in fitness contexts. Although these devices are prevalent and appear cost-effective, their precision in assessing health outcomes needs to be revised, particularly for older folks, as they are designed primarily for younger populations. Most wearable devices have been utilized to monitor cardiometabolic health indicators; however, new devices are being developed to evaluate alterations in mechanical load bearing during regular activities. Wearable devices that assess bone health by delivering real-time input on mechanical loads to avert age-related bone complications have demonstrated promise in the biomedical sector [41, 42]. Nonetheless, the direct correlation between these measurements and tangible bone health outcomes, including fracture risk estimates in older people, has yet to be determined. These devices may assist in selecting exercise programs for elderly individuals, especially those with knee ailments, by providing prompt feedback on the safety and efficacy of the exercises.

Consequently, the existing wearable devices enable clinicians to conduct real-time assessments of bone health; however, there is an urgent necessity for ongoing research advancements and increased collaboration between scientific development and technology-oriented companies to augment the functionality of these devices for broader applications. Due to WDs being a developing technology, its efficiency, specificity, and sensitivity differ among devices and applications; therefore, further study is necessary to achieve consistency among devices. Research on implantable biosensors for detecting bone health biomarkers is at the forefront due to several key advantages, including high sensitivity for specific biomarkers, enabling early diagnosis, real-time monitoring, non-invasive characteristics, enhanced specificity, and long-term stability. Despite their potential, implantable sensors necessitate the evaluation of biocompatibility, long-term reliability, routine calibration and maintenance, and the problem of guaranteeing data confidentiality. Quantum dots, gold nanoparticles, and other nanomaterials enhance the sensitivity and selectivity of biosensors. These developing technologies present significant breakthroughs in bone health monitoring, facilitating more accurate, rapid, and personalized healthcare interventions.

6.3.2 Health Initiatives, Big Data, and Predictive Analytics

To alleviate the burden of osteoporosis and related bone disorders experienced worldwide, efforts must be made to enhance access to DEXA technology in countries with low and intermediate incomes. International partnerships and funding initiatives can assist in disseminating DEXA equipment and training programs, ultimately leading to improved bone health outcomes worldwide. Engaging in advocacy and policy work is essential to elevate bone health to a higher priority and guaranteeing that all individuals have equal access to diagnostic and therapeutic resources. In bone health management, the implementation of big data and predictive analytics has the potential to bring about a complete and total transformation. Constructing prediction models by evaluating big datasets derived from DEXA scans and other sources is possible. This is something that can be taken into consideration. After that, these models can be applied to identify individuals who are at high risk and to optimize the therapy alternatives that are available to them. Through conventional analysis, machine learning algorithms can spot subtle patterns and risk variables that are not immediately visible.

6.4 Conclusion

DEXA is an essential tool for evaluating and managing bone mineral metabolism. It has emerged as a vital instrument for therapeutic practice owing to its precision, noninvasiveness, and capacity to deliver comprehensive insights into bone health. Although DEXA has some disadvantages, the efficacy of DEXA technology is anticipated to increase further, owing to recent innovations and its integration with other diagnostic methods. By perpetually refining and expanding the applications of DEXA and embracing AI approaches, we can enhance bone health outcomes and promote the overarching objective of healthy aging.

REFERENCES

1. Haseltine KN, et al. Bone mineral density: clinical relevance and quantitative assessment. *J Nucl Med.* 2021;62(4):446–54.
2. Palermo A, et al. BMI and BMD: the potential interplay between obesity and bone fragility. *Int J Environ Res Public Health.* 2016;13(6):544.
3. Aibar-Almazán A, et al. Current status of the diagnosis and management of osteoporosis. *Int J Mol Sci.* 2022;23(16):9465.
4. Dimai HP. Use of dual-energy X-ray absorptiometry (DXA) for diagnosis and fracture risk assessment; WHO-criteria, T-and Z-score, and reference databases. *Bone.* 2017;104:39–43.
5. Osuna PM, Ruppe MD, Tabatabai LS. Fracture liaison services: multidisciplinary approaches to secondary fracture prevention. *Endocr Pract.* 2017;23(2):199–206.
6. Khan AA, et al. Osteoporotic fractures: diagnosis, evaluation, and significance from the international working group on DXA best practices. *Mayo Clinic Proceedings.* Elsevier; 2024;99(7):1127–41.
7. Lewiecki EM, Binkley N. DXA: 30 years and counting: Introduction to the 30th anniversary issue. *Bone.* 2017;104:1–3.

8. Hald JD, et al. Bisphosphonates for the prevention of fractures in osteogenesis imperfecta: meta-analysis of placebo-controlled trials. *J Bone Miner Res.* 2015;30(5):929–33.
9. Zhou B, et al. Bone density, microarchitecture and stiffness in Caucasian and Caribbean Hispanic postmenopausal American women. *Bone Res.* 2014;2(1):1–9.
10. Schini M, et al. An overview of the use of the fracture risk assessment tool (FRAX) in osteoporosis. *J Endocrinol Invest.* 2024;47(3):501–11.
11. Silver HJ, et al. Imaging body composition in obesity and weight loss: challenges and opportunities. *Diabetes Metab Syndr Obes.* 2010:337–47.
12. Kang J. Status of DEXA instrumentation using direct and indirect detectors. *Adv X-ray Detector Technol.* 2022; 2022:151–73.
13. Goldstein JI, et al. *X-Rays.* Scanning Electron Microscopy and X-Ray Microanalysis; Heidelberg, Germany, 2018. p. 39–63.
14. Zemel BS, et al. Height adjustment in assessing dual energy x-ray absorptiometry measurements of bone mass and density in children. *J Clin Endocrinol Metab.* 2010;95(3):1265–73.
15. Amarnath S, Kumar V, Das SL. Classification of osteoporosis. *Indian J Orthop.* 2023;57(Suppl 1):49–54.
16. Sangondimath G, Sen RK. DEXA and Imaging in Osteoporosis. *Indian J Orthop.* 2023;57(Suppl 1):82–93.
17. Keen R. Osteoporosis: strategies for prevention and management. *Best Pract Res Clin Rheumatol.* 2007;21(1):109–22.
18. Kanis JA, et al. Assessment of fracture risk. *Eur J Radiol.* 2009;71(3):392–7.
19. Crandall CJ, et al. Comparative effectiveness of pharmacologic treatments to prevent fractures: an updated systematic review. *Ann Intern Med.* 2014;161(10):711–23.
20. Lyu H, et al. Delayed denosumab injections and bone mineral density response: an electronic health record-based study. *J Clin Endocrinol Metab.* 2020;105(5):1435–44.
21. Demerath EW, Fields DA. Body composition assessment in the infant. *Am J Hum Biol.* 2014;26(3):291–304.
22. Elliott ME, Binkley N. Evaluation and measurement of bone mass. *Epilepsy Behav.* 2004;5:16–23.
23. Guss CE, McAllister A, Gordon CM. DXA in children and adolescents. *J Clin Densitom.* 2021;24(1):28–35.
24. Adams JE. Advances in bone imaging for osteoporosis. *Nat Rev Endocrinol.* 2013;9(1):28–42.
25. Schini M, et al. An overview of the use of the fracture risk assessment tool (FRAX) in osteoporosis. *J Endocrinol Invest.* 2024;47(3):501–11.
26. Carey JJ, Delaney MF. T-Scores and Z-Scores. *Clin Rev Bone Miner Metab.* 2010;8(3):113–21.
27. Bazzocchi A, et al. DXA: Technical aspects and application. *Eur J Radiol.* 2016;85(8):1481–92.
28. Rashmi R, Snekhalatha U. Evaluation of body composition parameters using various diagnostic methods: A meta-analysis study. *Obes Med.* 2019;16:100150.
29. Bolotin H, Sievänen H, Grashuis J. Patient-specific DXA bone mineral density inaccuracies: quantitative effects of nonuniform extraosseous fat distributions. *J Bone Miner Res.* 2009;18(6):1020–7.
30. Skalsky AJ, et al. Assessment of regional body composition with dual-energy X-ray absorptiometry in Duchenne muscular dystrophy: Correlation of regional lean mass and quantitative strength. *Muscle Nerve.* 2009;39(5):647–51.
31. Formosa MM, Christou MA, Mäkitie O. Bone fragility and osteoporosis in children and young adults. *J Endocrinol Invest.* 2024;47(2):285–98.
32. Morgan SL, Prater GL. Quality in dual-energy X-ray absorptiometry scans. *Bone.* 2017;104:13–28.
33. Löffler MT, et al. X-ray-based quantitative osteoporosis imaging at the spine. *Osteoporos Int.* 2020;31(2):233–50.
34. Wong AK. A comparison of peripheral imaging technologies for bone and muscle quantification: a technical review of image acquisition. *J Musculoskelet Neuronal Interact.* 2016;16(4):265–82.
35. Binkley T, et al. Bone measurements by Peripheral Quantitative Computed Tomography (pQCT) in children with cerebral palsy. *J Pediatr.* 2005;147(6):791–6.
36. Artunduaga M, et al. Safety challenges related to the use of sedation and general anesthesia in pediatric patients undergoing magnetic resonance imaging examinations. *Pediatr Radiol.* 2021;51(5):724–35.
37. Gazzotti S, et al. High-resolution peripheral quantitative computed tomography: research or clinical practice? *Br J Radiol.* 2023;96(1150):20221016.

38. Dimai HP. New horizons: artificial intelligence tools for managing osteoporosis. *J Clin Endocrinol Metab.* 2022;108(4):775–83.
39. MacRitchie N, et al. Molecular imaging of inflammation - Current and emerging technologies for diagnosis and treatment. *Pharmacol Ther.* 2020;211:107550.
40. Yadav D, et al. Smart diagnostics devices through artificial intelligence and mechanobiological approaches. *3 Biotech.* 2020;10(8):351.
41. Chan M, et al. Smart wearable systems: Current status and future challenges. *Artif Intell Med.* 2012;56(3):137–56.
42. Mirmomeni M, et al. Chapter 12 - From wearables to THINKables: artificial intelligence-enabled sensors for health monitoring. In: Sazonov E, editor. *Wearable sensors*, 2nd ed. Oxford: Academic Press; 2021. p. 339–56.

7

Artificial Intelligence in Diagnostic/ Personalized Medicine

Christian Obirikorang and Hubert Owusu

7.1 Introduction

Artificial intelligence (AI) is one of the fastest-growing fields in computer science. It refers to the design of intelligent machines that could perform tasks with human-like capabilities such as processing thoughts and making decisions. It involves the ability of an intelligent machine to solve problems while also learning to solve new ones [1, 2]. AI could also be thought of as the "artificial thinking power of computers". It is a combination of the terms "artificial", which means man-made, and "intelligence", which indicates the capacity to reason independently. This then requires an AI system to be capable of perceiving its environment, including detecting input data and its parameters, analyzing the data, and making a prediction [3, 4]. Indeed, AI have shown themselves effective at performing these complex tasks at speeds far beyond human ability. This has made the capacity of AI systems to quickly and accurately analyze vast data in many areas of human life. Their impact has been very transformational in industries as widely varied as healthcare, education, banking and finance, retail and e-commerce, manufacturing, information technology, travel, and real estate, among many others.

In recent years, there has been a growing interest in the application of AI in medicine. AI systems have been applied in many areas including clinical decision-making, disease diagnosis, surgery, and rehabilitation [5]. This excitement has also been intensified by the enormous availability of large datasets and advancements in computer processing powers, which have lowered the costs and technical hurdles involved in developing an AI application. Current AI applications are very efficient at diagnosing diseases or providing personalized treatment recommendations. They have also been very successful at improving clinical outcomes, reducing human errors, and streamlining administrative processes. This has freed up time and reduced the toll healthcare professionals experience at work [6].

7.2 Foundations of AI

7.2.1 History and Development of AI

In 1950, Alan Turing proposed the Turing test as a theory for checking a machine's intelligence. The test is used to judge a machine as intelligent if it could fool a person interacting with it into believing that it is also human [7]. At this point, AI was a purely academic research endeavor. Christopher Strachey developed the first AI program and in 1956, a young Dartmouth College associate professor of mathematics, John McCarthy, coined the term "Artificial Intelligence" during the Dartmouth Conference [8]. This signaled a shift in the direction of AI research into mainstream, where many of those who attended the conference anticipated the creation of machine systems with human-level intelligence within a generation or two. After a decade of research, it became apparent that they had grossly misjudged the difficulty

DOI: 10.1201/9781003486909-7

of the enterprise. Their research was limited in many ways, chief among them being the need for large datasets and more computing power [8]. Yet, they also had some success, which included the first real-world AI application to be deployed in healthcare. The MYCIN was a rule-based expert system designed at Stanford University in 1974 to assist clinicians in diagnosing bacterial infections and providing antibiotic recommendations [9]. As a rule-based AI system, the MYCIN system also relied on using rules and logical processes to mimic human reasoning. This limited its capacity to scale and adapt to new changes without manual adjustments being made to its predefined rules. Despite this, the MYCIN system succeeded in demonstrating the potential of AI applications within the medical decision-making process [9].

The 1990s saw AI research shift from a rule-based approach to machine learning algorithms and neural networks. Advancements in computational power and the availability of large datasets also made it possible to perform the complex computations needed to train these algorithms more cheaply and faster. This approach enabled computers to learn from large amounts of data rather than from predefined rules. International Business Machines Corporation (IBM) developed its Deep Blue algorithm during this period. In a highly publicized match in 1997, the Deep Blue algorithm became the first AI system to defeat a world chess champion, Garry Kasparov [8, 10]. A remarkable increase in medical datasets in the 2000s also pushed the applications of AI systems in healthcare to new heights, especially when combined with advancements in deep learning. Deep learning, which involves creating many layers of an artificial neural network to learn and identify complex patterns in a given dataset, made AI systems very much capable of handling intricate tasks such as image recognition and understanding speech. In healthcare, the deployment of AI systems started to show immense promise in areas like medical imaging and predictive analytics [8, 10]. Researchers started to train neural network models on vast datasets of medical images, thereby enabling the automated detection of abnormalities such as cancers.

Another critical area of AI that has made significant strides in healthcare is natural language processing (NLP), which has enabled computers to process and understand human language. This subfield in AI has opened up new possibilities. AI systems are able to provide timely and efficient medical diagnosis by analyzing unstructured medical data including electronic health records (EHRs), physician notes, and medical literature [10, 11]. NLP systems have been useful in extracting insights from medical records, automating clinical documentation, and identifying patients for clinical trials.

7.2.2 Machine Learning

Machine learning is a subfield of AI that focuses on making computers learn without being explicitly programmed to do so. Since the development of computers, scientists have always wondered if computers could learn as humans do. This has allowed researchers to develop new algorithms that enable computers to learn from data to make predictions. To begin with, data is input into the machine learning system, which generalizes the examples in the data to create a mathematical model [12]. This model is then used to make predictions on new examples. In the application of AI systems in medical diagnosis, two of the most widely used machine learning techniques include supervised and unsupervised learning [5].

7.2.2.1 Supervised Learning

Supervised learning is the most widely used AI technique for classification problems. It uses algorithms to learn associations based on a labeled dataset – where a labeled dataset is one in which the output data of an example in the data is correctly matched with its input. An example would be computed tomography (CT) scan images of lung cancer that have been classified by a medical expert; that is, the diagnosis (label) for each example in the data is known. This information is then used to train a machine learning algorithm that creates a model for predicting the outcome of any new input data [5, 13].

In designing a machine learning model, there are two steps in the learning process, which include the training and testing stages. First, the data acquired for the learning process is divided into training and testing data. This begins the training process where the machine learning algorithm takes up the training data as input and uses features from the data to build a mathematical model [13, 14]. The accuracy of the model is then evaluated in the testing phase where it takes up the testing data as input and makes predictions of their outcome [13, 15]. Results from the testing phase would then inform whether the model needs fine-tuning, or is production-ready. The labels provide the ground truth against which values predicted by the model can be compared. This makes evaluating the robustness of the algorithm much easier. However, given the heavy reliance of supervised learning algorithms on these labels, this also makes them very sensitive to the quality of that data [12, 14]. Data that is labeled poorly or incorrectly could lead to a model making biased or faulty predictions [5]. The labels on the data are also important in influencing the type of algorithm architecture to be employed. Depending on whether the label is continuous or discrete, a regressor or classifier algorithm may be used [12].

When the label in a dataset is continuous, a linear regression algorithm is used to train the data. It stands as the most commonly used regression algorithm and the basis for understanding other regression algorithms such as logistics regression for a classification problem. Linear regression aims at plotting a line, or curve, that best fits the given data. To accomplish this, it strives to strike a balance so that the plot does not fit the training data too closely to a point where it can accurately predict results for the training data but fails on the testing or external data. At that point, the model is deemed overfit [12, 13]. In healthcare, linear regression models have been used to predict how long patients may stay at the hospital, and healthcare costs.

Classification algorithms are used to train a machine learning model when the label is a discrete value. It is worth noting that a regression dataset could also be transformed into a classification problem by grouping the continuous values into classes. Classification is a type of pattern recognition algorithm in which the model learns to find patterns in the training data in order to make predictions about the class of a new input [12, 13]. There are many types of classification algorithms that can be used depending on the available data. These include: logistic regression, which is used in predicting a binary outcome; decision tree, which is one of the most humanly understandable classification algorithms that classifies data by splitting them based on features in a hierarchical manner; support vector machine (SVM), which classifies data by finding the optimal hyperplane that separates the classes; and K-nearest neighbors (KNN), which classifies data based on the closest training example in feature space [10]. Over the years, classification algorithms have been used to predict whether a patient has a certain disease based on their symptoms, identifying genetic disorders, or categorizing abnormalities in medical images.

7.2.2.2 Unsupervised Learning

Unsupervised learning algorithms are used for predicting the outcome of datasets with no labels. The aim is to deduce the classes or groups from the dataset without the need for labels. These algorithms are mostly used to identify correlations within a dataset, although they don't have the ability to determine if the observed correlations have any statistical relevance. That is, unsupervised learning algorithms are more likely to identify clusters of little to no relevance to the problem if only such a pattern exists in the data [5, 12, 16]. Given that there are no labels to provide a ground truth basis against which to judge the accuracy of the model, unsupervised learning algorithms are considered to be a less objective method for classification problems than supervised learning algorithms. In view of that, it then becomes necessary for the user to have domain knowledge about the dataset otherwise they may not understand the predictions made by the model [14].

Unsupervised learning algorithms are said to be more difficult to model when compared to supervised learning algorithms. Given that unlabeled data are more abundantly available than labeled ones, the use of this technique has been growing steadily over the years. After all, there are many problems that are uniquely suited to be solved with unsupervised learning algorithms such as: building a recommendation system or classifying the behavior of customers on a website [12, 17].

One of the most popular unsupervised learning techniques is the clustering algorithm, which sorts data into clusters based on their similarities or differences. It is used to identify salient features of the data, form hypotheses, or gain new insights into a given data. Some clustering algorithms group each data point into a single cluster, while others may sort the same data point into one or more overlapping clusters [12]. The number of clusters used in the model is predefined by the user based on domain knowledge of the data. In practice, some methods have been developed to help guide the selection of the "perfect" cluster number. However, it is also generally understood that having domain knowledge about the data could also provide an important perspective in this selection process [17, 18]. That is, faced with the challenge of creating T-shirt sizes for a company based on people's height and weight, one could split the data into three clusters (S, M, and L) or five clusters (S, M, L, XL, and XXL) based on domain knowledge or market dynamics.

Another widely used unsupervised learning algorithm is the *k*-means algorithm, which is also an easier clustering algorithm to understand. It uses a set number of cluster centroids (*k*) to classify data into *k* distinct, non-overlapping clusters. It accomplishes this by assigning each data point to a centroid and then calculating and recalculating their Euclidean distance until each data point is in a cluster with the nearest centroid [18]. In 2020, Singh et al. developed an enhanced *k*-means clustering and improved ensemble learning algorithm that combined data from multiple sources to help clinicians in the early diagnosis of hepatitis disease [19].

7.2.3 Deep Learning and Artificial Neural Networks

Deep learning is a form of AI algorithm where the machine itself performs classification or regression analysis by learning several internal representations from raw data. This differs from classical machine learning algorithms where experts carefully engineer features for the training data [20]. Deep learning algorithms, which are modeled with inspiration from the human brain, are built layer by layer, with each layer learning a set of hidden representations from the data. Each layer is represented as a non-linear composite of representations in the layers before it. As a result, representations learned by the model in the first layer are rather simple, which then combine to create unreasoningly more abstract and complex representations at each additional layer. One illustration of this is when deep learning algorithms are used in image classifications. First, the first layers of the model detect edges and strokes in the images, which combine into simple objects, and then into more complex objects at each other layer. As such, how the model arrives at a prediction is unexplainable due to the high level of abstraction involved, thereby becoming a black box for users [12, 21].

7.2.3.1 Convolutional Neural Networks

A convolutional neural network (CNN) is a type of neural network mainly used for image analysis to find patterns or for object recognition [22]. A CNN algorithm splits an image into small patches with the assumption that each small area can be independently analyzed from the rest of the image in order to obtain basic features in that area. After this, it merges information in each area to create a more abstract representation of the image [21]. This has proved particularly useful in medical imaging diagnosis where CNN algorithms have been used to identify signs of pneumonia in a chest X-ray or malaria diagnosis of plasmodium parasites [23, 24].

7.2.3.2 Recurrent Neural Networks

Recurrent neural network (RNN) is specifically used in analyzing sequential data such as text and time series. In the healthcare environment, such sequential data may include patient health records or their vital signs being monitored over time. In one step at a time, RNNs send data they receive to the hidden layers. However, the neurons in this network have a cyclical connection between them, thereby allowing the network to possess a short-term memory where information previously input into the network could be remembered and acted upon for future predictions [12, 22]. RNN works to predict the next sequence by utilizing information stored in their short-term memory and the current input. At the hospital, RNN systems have been used to predict patient outcomes, such as the likelihood of diabetic patients being readmitted to the hospital or the progression of a chronic disease [25, 26].

7.2.3.3 Generative Adversarial Networks

Generative adversarial networks (GAN), introduced in 2014 by Ian Goodfellow and his colleagues at Google, are based on two artificial neural networks that are competing with each other [27]. It is a generative modeling technique that gives rise to new examples of data such as images, text, or audio by analyzing and identifying patterns in the training data so that the newly generated data is indistinguishable from the training data. It has a generator as the first network to give rise to new data examples, while the discriminator, which is the second network, strives to differentiate between the newly generated examples and those from the original training data [28]. This is often alluded to as a competition between a bank and a scammer who is trying to produce counterfeit money. Anytime the scammer generates counterfeit money, the bank should possess the ability to identify if the money is counterfeit or not. Thus, just as the scammer becomes ever more creative at generating counterfeit money, the bank should also become more competent at identifying them. The hope is to train a GAN to the point where both the generator and discriminator are good at their game and reach a stalemate [12]. GAN have been successfully used to generate images of humans, animals, buildings, and text-to-image generation. In healthcare, some GAN systems have been used to generate synthetic medical images to be used in training CNN, which helps to address the prevailing challenge of having a scarcity of labeled medical images. GAN have also been used in medical imaging to enhance the quality of images by improving the resolution of images or eliminating noises such as artifacts [29, 30].

7.2.3.4 Natural Language Processing

Natural language processing is a field of AI that gives computers the ability to understand human language in the manner in which it is written and spoken – otherwise known as natural language [31]. Computers have long had the ability to understand structured data obtained in the form of spreadsheets and database tables. However, human language, which comes in the form of text or voice, represents a great new challenge as unstructured data. Thus, by combining statistical modeling with deep learning, and computational linguistics, NLP systems are enabling computers to understand and generate text and speech [32]. Computational linguistics deals with analyzing the syntax and semantics of the human language, whereas syntactical analysis deals with the meaning of words, phrases, and sentences by using preprogrammed rules of the language's grammar to parse the syntax of the words. On the other hand, semantical analysis deals with using algorithms to understand the meaning of words based on their syntactic output and using this to interpret their meaning within the sentence structure [33]. There are three different techniques used in NLP, and these include rules-based NLP, statistical NLP, and deep learning NLP.

Rules-based NLP forms the earliest applications of NLPs. It uses handcrafted rules such as a simple if-then decision tree to extract meaning from texts. This system is limited in its ability to offer only answers to specific prompts and as such, unscalable [34]. Some studies have used this method to accurately extract clinically important information from radiology reports to identify stroke patients with cerebral edema or large vessel occlusion [35].

Statistical NLP, which was developed much later, uses machine learning algorithms to automate the extraction, classification, and labeling of text and voice data elements. It then assigns the various possible meanings of each element a statistical probability. Statistical NLP allows a language to be modeled by using mathematical methods to map the various elements of a language (grammatical rules and words) to a vector representation. As such, some statistical NLP models have been successfully deployed in sentiment analysis to determine the emotion expressed in a text [34]. In healthcare, NLP models have been used to gauge the feedback of patients, social media posts, or patient-provider interactions, thereby allowing healthcare providers to assess the sentiments of patients and identify areas for improvements.

Deep learning NLP models are now the predominant method of creating NLP. They are considered as an upgrade of statistical NLP with their algorithms using neural networks. As such, they employ large datasets of raw and unstructured voice and text data to improve their accuracy [36]. There are many different subcategories of deep learning NLPs with the most popular being transformer models. These are large language models trained on vast amounts of text data to perform NLP-related tasks and generate text like humans with high accuracy. Examples of these models include generative pre-trained transformer (GPT), which was developed by OpenAI, and bidirectional encoder representations from transformers (BERT) developed by Google [37, 38].

One area in which NLP systems have been used extensively is in the extraction of information such as diagnosis, medication, and symptoms from EHRs to improve patient care and provide personalized treatment. In 2022, researchers from the University of Waterloo successfully used an NLP model on patient health records to identify patients who were at risk of developing recurrent breast or colorectal cancer [39]. Zheng et al. also used an NLP model to more accurately identify patients at risk of developing an episode of recurrent atrial fibrillation, thereby allowing clinicians to develop more personalized intervention strategies for such patients [40].

Not only that, NLP models have also been used as social media-based surveillance tools to track and predict the outbreak of disease much earlier than traditional methods. In 2009, researchers from the University of Toronto showed that the analysis of tweets with the terms "swine flu" and "H1N1" could be used as a real-time tracking tool to predict the incidence of the pandemic [41]. This was also true during the COVID-19 pandemic where scientists used NLP models to detect and monitor early outbreaks of the disease in Europe [42].

7.3 Importance of AI in Medical Diagnosis

7.3.1 Diagnostic Accuracy

One of the areas where AI systems have had an enormous impact on healthcare delivery is the extent to which they have enhanced the accuracy and speed of medical diagnosis [10]. Traditionally, healthcare professionals have had to rely on their own experience and expertise when making a diagnosis. This has led to diagnostic results that are subjective. On the other hand, AI systems provide a systematic way to quantify diagnostic parameters for a more objective diagnosis. They have the ability to analyze large datasets, which has increased their diagnostic accuracy [43]. Not only that, AI systems have also been used to provide highly consistent diagnoses regardless of the environment in which they are deployed, thereby assisting healthcare professionals to provide good medical diagnoses regardless of their own inefficiencies.

In 2020, McKinney et al. developed an AI algorithm that, when tested on a large dataset of mammograms for the diagnosis of breast cancer, was able to show a better diagnostic performance than radiologists. Not only that, it was also able to bring down the level of false negatives and false positives by 9.4% and 5.7%, respectively [44]. Over the years, other researchers have also demonstrated the superior capabilities of some AI systems to humans, such as one that could quickly predict the onset of electrocardiogram abnormalities in patients, or identify people at risk of developing atrial fibrillation-related strokes [45]. Not only that, studies show that assisting healthcare professionals with AI systems significantly increases their overall performance in disease diagnoses.

7.3.2 Decision Support

In recent years, many AI systems deployed in the healthcare space have been marketed as diagnostic decision support systems (DDSS). These systems are meant to assist healthcare professionals in their decision-making process [46]. Traditionally, clinicians have had to rely on the second opinion of colleagues when reaching a medical decision on a confounding case. This has been a time-consuming effort that often leads to delays in patient care. Using DDSS provides greater insights into patient data, helping to ensure that critical conditions are not overlooked, or a condition misdiagnosed [46].

7.3.3 Handling Complex Data

With advancements in digital healthcare technologies, there has been a stratospheric rise in complex medical data obtained from such varied sources as medical imaging, genomic sequencing, electronic health records, and wearable devices. AI systems excel at integrating and analyzing data obtained from these varied different sources, giving researchers a more holistic understanding of a medical condition. This has helped identify patterns and correlations in these complex data, allowing clinicians to identify unique diagnostic biomarkers to inform personalized treatment strategies [47]. Batras et al. recently developed an AI-based predictive system (AIPS) for lung cancer diagnosis that could predict somatic epidermal growth factor receptor (EGFR) gene mutations by analyzing lung nodules detected in CT images [48]. Whereas earlier studies have focused only on detecting lung nodules from CT images, the AIPS was able to accomplish this feat by being trained on a large dataset of EGFR gene sequencing and CT images, thereby providing a non-invasive method by which genotype information could be obtained from lung nodules. In resource-limited countries such as India where the general public cannot have access to panel-based next-generation sequencing, the AIPS aims to help oncologists effectively triage patients for targeted therapies by identifying and predicting the type of EGFR gene mutation a patient may have [48].

7.4 Applications of AI in Medical Diagnosis

Medical diagnosis is a process that uses a set of signs, symptoms, and/or test results established by medical professionals to identify specific disease conditions. It is a complicated process that involves gathering a sufficient amount of information about a patient and reasoning through them to identify what is affecting them [49]. The goal is to accurately determine if a patient has a disease or not so that an appropriate treatment plan can be developed. A conceptual framework developed by the Committee on Diagnostic Error in Health Care to help understand the process of disease diagnosis includes: first, a person experiencing symptoms of a condition and contacting a healthcare provider. The clinician would conduct a medical interview, review the patient's clinical history, as well as conduct a physical examination and diagnostic tests. All this information is then gathered, collated, and interpreted to make a single or differential working diagnosis. This process can be repeated several times to gather more detailed information about the condition in order to zero in on a more accurate diagnosis. The working diagnosis is communicated to the patient and a treatment plan initiated [5, 50].

As earlier noted, medical diagnosis is a complex procedure with many opportunities for error depending on the clinician's unique experiences, or their emotional or mental state at the time of assessment. This is also complicated by the need for several specialists from different disciplines to provide their input to reach a diagnosis. This also prolongs the timeline needed to reach a diagnosis, thereby delaying the administration of a treatment regimen [5]. Thus, in order to address some of the challenges inherent in the diagnosis process, many healthcare systems are increasingly relying on AI technologies to improve the process.

7.4.1 Emergency Department

A hospital's emergency department (ED) is a unit that provides medical care for acute non-elective medical conditions such as injuries, illnesses, or life-threatening conditions needing immediate medical attention. It is often a chaotic and complex place operating on a 24-hour basis with a multidisciplinary team of healthcare professionals juggling to diagnose and manage a wide range of medical emergencies [3, 51]. Amid a rise in disease burden and an ever-increasing demand on healthcare providers, especially from patients with public insurance, EDs have become overcrowded. This has also led to EDs often functioning as primary care providers even though they are not designed for that purpose [52]. At the ED, any wrongful diagnosis can be both expensive and fatal, resulting in the worsening of a life-threatening condition, or patients waiting for long hours to receive treatment [3, 51]. Fortunately, AI systems are rapidly being deployed at the ED, to assist healthcare providers in their duties.

Over the years, one area where AI systems have been widely researched for their application at the ED is in predictive modeling. ED healthcare providers have come to appreciate the positive impact of these AI systems in their workflow, especially in improving accuracy, efficiency, and overall patient outcomes.

With an increasingly high level of accuracy, AI systems have shown a great ability to identify high-risk patients for treatment by analyzing patient data, which helps to improve patient flow and reduce waiting times. At New York University, Klang et al. tested an ED algorithm on a US nationally representative sample and showed it was able to accurately identify emergency cases that would result in hospitalization within a day or death within 30 days [52]. Not only that, AI-powered symptom assessment tools are being used to predict or rule out the likelihood of a disease condition, thereby cutting down on needless visits to the ED. In 2020, Kim et al. developed a machine learning algorithm for screening septic shock at the ED [53].

Decision support systems that are powered by machine learning algorithms have also been employed to assist ED providers with real-time suggestions in diagnosis and treatment. By using demographic, clinical, and unstructured texts obtained from the notes of doctors and nurses, Klang et al. designed an algorithm that was able to predict and identify patients to be admitted to the neurosciences intensive care unit within 30 minutes of arriving at the ED [54]. Another important task being automated at the ED is crowd management [55, 56]. In 2019, Jilani et al. from the University of Nottingham presented a heuristic-based time series algorithm for addressing overcrowding at EDs by predicting patient attendance or better scheduling for staff and elective surgeries [57].

7.4.2 Clinical Microbiology

AI systems have long existed in the clinical microbiology laboratory in the form of rule-based expert systems using a decision tree to automate microbial identification and susceptibility testing. These rule-based expert systems have been used in direct Gram stains for bacterial differentiation on rules such as bacterial stain color and shape [58]. Today, machine learning and deep learning algorithms have increased and expanded the use of AI systems in the clinical microbiology laboratory with more sophisticated tools. Much like the rule-based systems, new ML systems have also been deployed in the detection, identification, or quantification of microorganisms [59]. By using a CNN, Smith, Kang, and Kirby developed a Gram stain classification algorithm that was able to accurately differentiate between blood culture Gram stain images with 94.9% accuracy [60].

In microscopic imaging, other CNN algorithms have also been developed to aid healthcare providers in the detection and classification of malaria parasites in blood smears or intestinal helminths in stool [61, 62]. Some of these algorithms have then been deployed as smartphone-based AI-assisted tools to assist parasitologists in making a more timely and accurate malaria diagnosis [63, 64]. Other researchers have developed a digital in-line holographic microscopy combined with a machine learning algorithm for malaria parasite detection in unstained red blood cells. In low- and middle-income countries with overcrowded hospitals, such a system promises to provide a quick, accurate, and more economical diagnostic tool for malaria. By analyzing genomic data, machine learning algorithms have also been used to identify viral genotypes such as human papillomavirus (HPV), and further classification of the HPV risk type.

In recent years, advancements in AI algorithms and their incorporation into clinical microbiology instruments have also led to substantial improvement in efficiencies in the laboratory workflow, especially with respect to automated blood culture and susceptibility testing instruments, as well as molecular platforms [58]. With many of these procedures being automated, clinical microbiologists can now have rapid diagnostic results for blood culture tests, thereby making it possible for a suitable antibiotic to be administered to the patient [59].

7.4.3 Precision Medicine

Precision medicine, also referred to as personalized treatment or medicine, is a healthcare approach that uses a patient's unique characteristics to customize medical care. This approach considers factors such as genomics, biomarkers, lifestyle, and the environment to enhance patient treatment outcomes [65]. Advancements in precision medicine have been accelerated by AI systems analyzing complex data from varied sources, making a diagnosis, and optimizing treatment strategies to offer a more targeted intervention [3]. They have been used to analyze large genomic datasets to identify patients with a specific genetic mutation and recommend a more specific treatment plan. This approach has become important to preemptively genotype patients in order to have information when the need arises [66].

Genomics is a relatively new and rapidly growing field in medicine where a patient's genetic information is used to help prevent, diagnose, and treat diseases. This rise has been fueled by advancements in sequencing techniques, from low-throughput sequencing technologies (first-generation sequencing) which were only able to process a small number of deoxyribonucleic acid (DNA) sequences at a time, to high-throughput sequencing technologies (next-generation sequencing, NGS) with their ability to sequence millions of nucleotides in a single run [10, 67]. Sequencing entire genomes in a few hours became possible, generating large amounts of data. However, these data became very complex and too big for the human mind to analyze, or to do so with statistical methods. That is why AI algorithms have been used for this purpose [47]. First, AI systems have been applied to the genome sequencing process itself as a means to eliminate errors intrinsic to the sequencing process. Such applications include using machine learning techniques to improve sequencing accuracy by improving base-calling methods for short-read sequencing technologies [65]. After the data has been generated, AI applications are used to analyze them because of their ability to efficiently handle such large datasets. They are also able to perform complex computations that lead to the discovery of valuable insights far beyond our current understanding of genomic mechanisms and pathways. These insights have allowed scientists to expand their understanding of rare diseases and cancers. The use of AI algorithms in genetic analysis has led to promising breakthroughs in disease diagnosis, surveillance, and precision medicine.

7.4.3.1 Variant Calling

One of the significant applications of AI algorithms in genomics is in the identification of genetic variants associated with diseases. In genome-wide association studies, machine learning algorithms have been used to identify genetic variants such as single-nucleotide polymorphisms (SNPs) that are linked to a specific disease or trait [10]. In 2014, researchers using a SVM classification algorithm trained on millions of high-frequency alleles in humans were able to identify both pathogenic and functional genetic variants with high accuracy [68]. Such models have been beneficial in aiding the discovery of new genetic biomarkers for disease conditions such as diabetes, cardiovascular diseases, and cancers. This has been particularly useful in the diagnosis of rare genetic disorders which often involves the identification of many potential genetic variations. Analyzing large genetic databases has also become very important in identifying what genetic variants make a given population more susceptible to a disease condition so that a more targeted screening, preventive, and intervention program could be designed for them [69]. In 2021, researchers from the Harvard Medical School used deep neural network to accurately identify genetic variants associated with autism spectrum disorder [70]. Another widely cited model used for the identification and classification of rare genetic mutations is DeepVariant, a CNN algorithm developed by researchers at Google Brain, that has improved the accuracy of variant calling [71]. Such application of AI technologies which aid in identifying genetic mutations associated with diseases is indistinguishably linked to precision medicine as it allows for the administration of more specific interventions [65].

7.4.3.2 Pathogen Genomics

In pathogen genomics, traditional microbiology assays are increasingly being replaced or being used alongside whole-genome sequences (WGS), which are producing large datasets of microbial genome. Machine learning has been used to classify and characterize virulent pathogens from non-virulent pathogens [72]. Public health professionals have also employed AI systems as disease surveillance tools to monitor emerging new threats such as the COVID-19 pandemic. As a novel virus, the complete viral genome was sequenced and a machine learning tool was used to define its lineage as a *Betacoronavirus* [73]. After many different SARS-CoV-2 variants were sampled from patients, AI techniques were used to draw a phylogenetic tree that described the evolutionary relationships between these variants, allowing scientists to track the spread and molecular evolution of the virus [74]. A 2022 study used a real-time machine learning application as an infection surveillance tool to analyze a combined dataset of EHRs and WGS that led to the prevention of up to 40% of hospital-borne COVID-19 infections [75].

7.4.3.3 Cancer Genomics

AI applications have also been used to understand how normal cells differ from cancerous ones in both their genetic sequences and expression. This has shed more light on the genetic, metabolic, or systemic factors that contribute toward the formation of tumors and their spread. AI systems provide valuable information for the diagnosis, classification, and management of cancers, especially in the identification of biomarkers. Studies show that the use of AI in genomic cancer diagnosis produces very reliable results [10], and in some instances such as breast cancer [76] and melanoma diagnosis [77], can surpass human experts. In 2017, researchers used deep learning to help identify BRCA1/2 gene mutations, which is a cancer-predisposing gene used in assessing breast cancer risks and selecting treatment [78]. With an ever-increasing availability of large amounts of data in genomics, transcriptomics, proteomics, and metabolomics, machine learning algorithms have made it possible to integrate and analyze these multiomics datasets, thereby allowing for a more comprehensive understanding of biological systems from DNA to metabolites [10, 65]. Multiomics data analysis has enabled scientists to learn more about disease mechanisms that would be impossible with a single omics dataset, thereby allowing for the development of new treatment strategies [79]. By combining transcriptomics and proteomics datasets, Jayaram et al. described the gonadotropin-releasing hormone (GnRH) signaling pathway [80], while Stemke-Hale et al. discovered the altered phosphoinositide 3-kinase (PI3K) pathway by combining genomics and proteomics datasets [81].

7.4.4 Medical Imaging

Medical imaging refers to techniques used to visualize and take images of the body's internal structures for clinical analysis and intervention. These imaging techniques have revolutionized the healthcare environment by providing medical specialists with a non-invasive way to visualize and look for injury, brokenness, or pathology inside the body [82]. Over the years, there has been a lot of advancement in imagining technologies from their use in routine clinical practice to cutting-edge human physiology and pathophysiology. Some of these technologies include X-rays, CT, magnetic resonance imaging (MRI), mammography, and ultrasound [83]. Interpreting images obtained from these techniques, radiologists have long relied on their professional experience and expertise to reach a diagnosis, which is prone to subjectivity and errors. That has led to the adoption of AI applications in medical imaging to help make more accurate diagnoses. Once a very subjective activity, the ability of deep learning techniques to identify complex patterns in images has turned the interpretation of medical images into one that is quantitative and reproducible. It has also improved healthcare decision-making by being able to identify important information in medical images that would have gone unnoticed by humans. Not only that, AI's ability to analyze large amounts of data has made it possible to gather, integrate, and analyze data from diverse sources such as medical imaging, electronic health records, genomics, and pathology to gain a more comprehensive understanding of a disease condition [43]. AI-based systems are used to perform three main tasks when interpreting clinical images: detection, characterization, and disease monitoring.

7.4.4.1 Disease Detection

Computer-aided detection (CAD) tools are AI-based assistant tools used for detecting and localizing objects of clinical importance. CAD tools use pattern recognition algorithms to detect specific characteristics in an image and then highlight them for the radiologist. CADs have become vital tools in reducing screening errors such as missing a diagnostic feature [43]. The usefulness of CAD systems is dependent on whether they can improve the diagnostic ability of a radiologist. In lung cancer screening, low-dose CT is considered a superior screening tool to chest radiography. However, the ability of radiologists to detect subtle lung nodules in numerous CT images is a time-consuming and challenging task [84]. A

CAD system developed by Mingzhu et al. was able to detect about 70% of cancers that radiologists had missed [85]. In breast cancer screening, mammography is considered one of the most reliable tools, with microcalcification clusters (MCC) serving as a biomarker of early breast carcinoma. By detecting MCCs in mammograms, Cheng et al. used a CAD to improve the diagnostic sensitivity of radiographers by 10% [86]. In 2022, Hills et al. designed an AI model that was able to detect pneumothorax in chest radiographs with an accuracy that far exceeded the United States Food and Drug Administration's standard for CADs [87]. Although CAD systems are trained on large datasets annotated by radiologists, the ability of radiologists to provide consistently accurate diagnoses is limited by human bias and a propensity to restrict the region or analysis to a place of most clinical importance. Other CAD systems, such as the Zebra Medical Vision, have also been used as efficient assistant tools for radiologists to improve their diagnoses of osteoporotic vertebral compression fractures (VCF). VCF is frequently an asymptomatic condition yet a risk factor for morbidity and mortality that is often detected during CT scans for unrelated conditions [88].

7.4.4.2 Disease Characterization

Characterization of medical images consists of segmentation, detection, and staging. Segmentation involves defining the extent to which a condition is abnormal. This can include characterizing a condition as benign or malignant, which is important in treatment planning such as calculating the dosage of radiation to be administered in the management of cancer [43]. In clinical practice, defining the extent of a disease condition has been a subjective and qualitative task performed by radiologists, with even expert radiologists unable to consistently reproduce results. In contrast, quantitative features of a condition are processed systematically by CAD systems, making them more reproducible. In diagnosing lung nodules after CT scans, CAD systems have been used to assist radiologists in being more accurate in detecting and differentiating between benign and malignant nodules [89]. Gavrilov et al. developed a web-based CAD system that can be used to detect and classify benign and malignant skin tumors with a high level of accuracy [90]. Diagnoses of prostate lesions from multiparametric MRI have long seen many inconsistent results from expert radiologists. This has led to many studies aiming to design a more capable CAD system to overcome this challenge as current CAD systems have recorded area under the curve (AUC) below 0.90 [91, 92]. Staging is another way to characterize a disease condition such as cancer by categorizing them into predefined groups according to their appearance and spread. Although the commonly used classification system in cancer staging is TNM, most CAD systems are only capable of tumor detection and not staging [43]. Thus, recent CAD applications have extended this by defining other staging methods. A CAD system developed by Paing et al. was not only capable of detecting lung tumors in CT images but also able to extract locational features for cancer staging [93].

7.4.4.3 Disease Monitoring

CAD systems have been used to monitor disease changes over time, either naturally or in response to therapy. By analyzing imaging data from X-rays or CT scans, CAD systems have provided valuable support in assessing and managing patients recovering from fractures or orthopedic surgeries. It accomplishes this by detecting subtle changes in bone density, alignment, and callus formation or by comparing a series of images taken over time. In cancer treatment, the response evaluation criteria in solid tumors (RECIST) has a limited set of predefined metrics for estimating tumor burden and its response to treatment. RECIST also oversimplifies the geometries of tumors, thereby neglecting a lot of useful information that advanced imaging technologies [94]. The aforementioned limitation is particularly relevant in the case of osseous lesions, where chemotherapy improves survival rates for patients with bone metastases, although this benefit is not always evident in radiographic images as measured by RECIST [95]. In contrast, new CAD systems are being developed to offer a more nuanced approach by gathering images over time and identifying a wide range of discriminating features in a manner that surpasses what human readers measure. Despite the promise, this remains an active field of research.

7.4.5 Mental Healthcare

Over the years, AI has seen rapid adoption and integration in physical healthcare, while its influence is only now being felt in the field of mental health [96]. Traditionally, mental health has been a patient-centered enterprise in which mental health practitioners have to heavily rely on interacting directly with patients and observing their behaviors and emotions for their analysis [97]. This often results in clinical data in the form of patient statements and notes that are both qualitative and subjective. Nevertheless, the field is beginning to see some benefits from AI applications, which are helping practitioners detect and diagnose mental health conditions early, as well as offering a more personalized treatment plan [96, 98]. In diagnosing a mental illness, there is still much that is unknown, such as how the biological, psychological, and social systems interact with each other to result in a mental health condition. The capability of AI systems to collate, integrate, and analyze complex data from varied sources offers hope of gaining a more comprehensive understanding of mental illnesses and helps to identify new biomarkers for a more quantitative and objective description of a condition [99]. AI is also being used to design risk assessment models to calculate a patient's risk of developing a mental health condition. These applications are able to help monitor medication adherence and a patient's responsiveness to treatment while also limiting the number of in-person patient consultations [3, 96].

With much of the data from mental health being text-based, many NLP applications have been developed to detect and identify symptoms of severe mental illness [100]. Some other NLP applications have been used to identify and classify patients having suicidal thoughts or have attempted suicide in EHR data [101]. Depression is one of the most studied mental disorders. AI has been used to predict patients who will develop depression from EHR data [102] or those who will remit into depression after a treatment course [103]. AI applications have also been used to identify symptoms of depression using data from people's smartphones, or social media posts [104, 105]. Images from functional MRI scans have also been analyzed with AI to identify patients suffering from schizophrenia with 87% accuracy [106]. Studies have shown that making cognitive-behavioral therapies easily accessible to people, either through chatbots or web-based applications, is an effective way of addressing depression and delivering psychotherapeutic interventions to young adults [107]. Such AI-powered applications include Woebot, which has shown significant promise in alleviating symptoms of depression and improving anxiety and substance abuse [108].

7.5 Future Directions

AI is rapidly evolving and reshaping many areas in healthcare. New advancements in AI promise to further extend these gains in improving patients' outcomes and operational efficiencies. AI adoption in hospitals is expected to increase as more technologies that could easily be integrated into existing electronic infrastructure gain regulatory approval. This would also eliminate high costs associated with institutions seeking to build customized AI applications that would integrate seamlessly into their existing infrastructure [109].

As the accuracy of AI systems continues to improve and even surpass the ability of human experts, a major area in healthcare that is expected to see enormous benefit is in the early detection and diagnosis of diseases. Advancements in NLP models such as ChatGPT are expected to enhance the capabilities of AI systems to analyze and detect clinically important information in EHR data for the early diagnosis of diseases. Advancements in computer vision technologies are also expected to continue to improve, leading to AI systems with abilities surpassing human experts in the diagnosis of diseases. AI applications are also expected to be incorporated directly into medical imaging machines such as the microscope. New studies in AI seek to build intelligent light microscopes that are able to collaborate with human scientists with natural language to acquire and analyze samples. Most of the capabilities of this concept have reached the stage of proof-of-principle [110].

Another area where AI applications are expected to expand in improving patient outcomes is in personalized medicine. As the costs associated with genomic sequencing continue to fall, the adoption of high-throughput sequencing as a routine examination would make personalized care more widely available to patients. The generation of such large datasets is also expected to fuel the training of powerful AI applications, allowing scientists to find new biomarkers, or gain a more comprehensive understanding of disease conditions. In short, there is much to expect in the future of AI applications in healthcare. However, several legal and socioeconomic concerns also need addressing in order to achieve this future.

7.5.1 Data Quality, Sharing, and Privacy

As a digital system, the AI system also operates on the principle of the old adage "garbage in, garbage out". This is especially true given the lack of quality clinical data on which AI systems can be trained; often producing biased or inaccurate predictions [3]. In training supervised learning algorithms, this challenge becomes particularly acute as these applications require good quality data with accurate labels. To address the challenge of obtaining quality data for AI applications, many researchers have resorted to data sharing. Although this solution presents many ethical and economic advantages, it also raises concerns about privacy [10].

With some data obtained from animal research, there's an ethical benefit to reduce the need to repeat such experiments by sharing data among different laboratories. This aligns with the effort to promote health without causing unnecessary harm to animals. It is also more economical to store and share data than to reproduce it in a new experiment. This is particularly important in such fields as medical imaging and genomics, where costs associated with the advanced technologies used in generating data are still relatively high, especially among small laboratories that might be on tight budgets, or those in developing countries that might not have these resources readily available to them. In other words, data sharing could be thought of as a democratic effort to eliminate another barrier to cost that prevents small laboratories from embarking on research relevant to their communities. Not only that, data sharing has allowed for the aggregation and creation of large datasets needed to train and increase the accuracy of AI applications [10, 111].

In order to protect the privacy of individuals, large institutions that indulge in collaborative data sharing projects have invested heavily in software that anonymizes the data and also restricts access to them with well-defined protocols. Such protocols are meant to restrict sensitive and identifiable data such as the raw reads of genomic data to only qualified institutions [112]. As more data with high-dimensionality are being captured for research, the ability to anonymize them has become increasingly difficult with re-identification. Many studies have shown that linking strategies can be used to identify the majority of individuals in a given large dataset [113]. In large international data sharing projects, people can no longer exercise their right to discontinue being part of a research and have their data deleted due to the impracticality of keeping track of the data [10]. With advancements in AI, there have been debates on whether the benefits of these systems are worth the sacrifice of privacy. This has led to an ongoing effort to address the issue of privacy by using methods such as selective data suppression to prevent re-identification [114]. Other methods include k-anonymity, which generalizes certain identifiable attributes of the data so that any given record matches with at least k records on those attributes [115].

7.5.2 Legal, Ethical, and Economic Issues

The use of AI applications in healthcare has been to assist healthcare professionals in detecting and diagnosing diseases. However, these algorithms, especially classification algorithms, are prone to making false positive and false negative errors. Wrongfully classifying a patient as suffering from a condition (false positive) could result in unnecessary distress and costs from unnecessary screening examinations [116]. On the other hand, wrongfully classifying a positive diagnosis as negative (false negative) could result in unnecessary delays in treatment before the correct diagnosis is detected. In conditions such as cancers where the time of diagnosis and commencement of treatment could have a long-term effect on therapy outcome, such an error could be fatal [10]. In healthcare, AI prediction errors are a major source of legal and economic issues. Furthermore, any attempt to quantify the cost penalty based on classification performance has been difficult. While the costs associated with a false positive classification could be reasonably estimated, false negative classifications present a unique challenge akin to placing a price on the value of a human life [117]. Then, there is also the question of who bears legal responsibility for the error: technology companies or the physician? To address the challenge of wrongful classification predictions by AI applications, researchers could define guidelines that require a human expert to re-examine any AI decision concerning a complex case [10]. Another path to addressing these concerns lies in designing an ad hoc AI system to reanalyze samples that have already been analyzed and classified as positive by the main AI application [118].

Another ethical concern affecting the rapid adoption of AI applications is the issue of data fairness with its many reports of AI systems exhibiting discriminatory behaviors against minority groups. The frequency of such reports has been surprisingly high in the healthcare environment where some AI applications have intentionally adjusted for race in a manner that has been harmful to minorities. A well-known example of this is the incidence of an AI system that consistently failed to refer racial minorities for "high risk care management" programs even though they might benefit from such programs [119]. Although the issue of discriminatory behaviors by AI applications abounds, this has been as a result of AI applications being trained on biased datasets that are not a true representation of the population. This is being addressed through large collaborative data sharing projects that collate data from different sources to create a unified, yet diverse, dataset [120].

7.5.3 Will AI Replace Healthcare Professionals?

Technological singularity (TS) is a hypothesis of a point in future where human intelligence would be surpassed by super-intelligent AI technologies. Some scientists predict that this will occur by the year 2040 or 2050. At such a point, it is generally believed that AI applications would replace human healthcare professionals for much faster, accurate, and personalized care [121, 122]. In reality, the debate about this is no longer considered as an unfounded fear given the rapid advancements in AI technologies. However, having a fully autonomous AI system as a primary care provider presents many ethical and legal challenges which require serious public debates [123]. That is, will an AI system be legally liable for making a wrongful diagnosis? Should a less intelligent human expert even be present to second guess the predictions made by the AI? Surely, requiring human experts to second guess predictions made by a more intelligent AI system may seem counterintuitive. However, with healthcare professionals making life and death decisions every day in the course of their duties, the question is to what extent should such decisions be left entirely to an AI system. Given today's social and ethical values, it seems highly unlikely that AI systems would be given such complete autonomy [124].

Another argument against completely replacing human healthcare professionals with AI technologies is the case for empathy. This involves having self-awareness and the ability to understand and share the feelings of another person [125]. Empathy from healthcare providers helps build trust, as well as improve patient satisfaction and their adherence to treatment plans. Thus, it is important for AI systems to exhibit some empathy in order to succeed in replacing human care providers.

REFERENCES

1. Hamet P, Tremblay J. Artificial intelligence in medicine. metabolism. 2017 Apr 1;69:S36–40.
2. Tran BX, Vu GT, Ha GH, Vuong Q-H, Ho M-T, Vuong T-T, et al. Global evolution of research in artificial intelligence in health and medicine: a bibliometric study. *J Clin Med.* 2019;8(3):360.
3. Alowais SA, Alghamdi SS, Alsuhebany N, Alqahtani T, Alshaya AI, Almohareb SN, et al. Revolutionizing healthcare: the role of artificial intelligence in clinical practice. *BMC Med Educ.* 2023;23(1):689.
4. Panch T, Szolovits P, Atun R. Artificial intelligence, machine learning and health systems. *J Glob Health.* 2018;8(2).
5. Mirbabaie M, Stieglitz S, Frick NRJ. Artificial intelligence in disease diagnostics: A critical review and classification on the current state of research guiding future direction. *Health Technol.* 2021;11(4):693–731.
6. Kumar Y, Koul A, Singla R, Ijaz MF. Artificial intelligence in disease diagnosis: a systematic literature review, synthesizing framework and future research agenda. *J Ambient Intell Humaniz Comput.* 2023;14(7):8459–86.

7. Yampolskiy RV. Turing test as a defining feature of AI-completeness. In: Yang XS, editor. *Artificial intelligence, evolutionary computing and metaheuristics: in the footsteps of Alan Turing*. Berlin, Heidelberg: Springer; 2013. p. 3–17.
8. McCorduck P, Cfe C. *Machines who think: a personal inquiry into the history and prospects of artificial intelligence*. AK Peters/CRC Press; Massachusetts, USA, 2004.
9. Sotos JG. MYCIN and NEOMYCIN: two approaches to generating explanations in rule-based expert systems. *Aviat Space Environ Med*. 1990;61(10):950–4.
10. Caudai C, Galizia A, Geraci F, Le Pera L, Morea V, Salerno E, et al. AI applications in functional genomics. *Comput Struct Biotechnol J*. 2021;19:5762–90.
11. Davenport T, Kalakota R. The potential for artificial intelligence in healthcare. *Future Healthc J*. 2019;6(2):94–8.
12. Duarte D, Ståhl N. Machine learning: a concise overview. *Data Sci Practice*. 2019:20:27–58.
13. Nasteski V. An overview of the supervised machine learning methods. *Horizons B*. 2017;4(51–62):56.
14. Krittanawong C, Zhang H, Wang Z, Aydar M, Kitai T. Artificial intelligence in precision cardiovascular medicine. *J Am Coll Cardiol*. 2017;69(21):2657–64.
15. Sandhya N, Charanjeet KR. A review on machine learning techniques. *Int J Recent Innov Trends Comput Commun*. 2016;4(3):451–8.
16. Karpischek S, Michahelles F, Fleisch E. Detecting incorrect product names in online sources for product master data. *Electron Markets*. 2014;24:151–60.
17. Jain AK. Data clustering: 50 years beyond K-means. *Pattern Recogn Lett*. 2010;31(8):651–66.
18. Fujita A, Takahashi DY, Patriota AG. A non-parametric method to estimate the number of clusters. *Comput Stat Data Anal*. 2014;73:27–39.
19. Singh A, Mehta JC, Anand D, Nath P, Pandey B, Khamparia A. An intelligent hybrid approach for hepatitis disease diagnosis: Combining enhanced k-means clustering and improved ensemble learning. *Expert Syst*. 2021;38(1):e12526.
20. Bengio Y, Courville A, Vincent P. Representation learning: a review and new perspectives. *IEEE Trans Pattern Anal Mach Intell*. 2013;35(8):1798–828.
21. Zeiler MD, Fergus R, editors. *Visualizing and understanding convolutional networks*. Springer, Heidelberg, Germany; 2014.
22. LeCun Y, Bengio Y, Hinton G. Deep learning. *Nature*. 2015;521(7553):436–44.
23. Gm H, Gourisaria MK, Rautaray SS, Pandey M. Pneumonia detection using CNN through chest X-ray. *J Eng Sci Technol (JESTEC)*. 2021;16(1):861–76.
24. Turuk M, Sreemathy R, Kadiyala S, Kotecha S, Kulkarni V. CNN based deep learning approach for automatic malaria parasite detection. *IAENG Int J Comput Sci*. 2022;49(3).
25. Suo Q, Ma F, Canino G, Gao J, Zhang A, Veltri P, et al., editors. A multi-task framework for monitoring health conditions via attention-based recurrent neural networks. American Medical Informatics Association; 2017;2017:16665.
26. Chopra C, Sinha S, Jaroli S, Shukla A, Maheshwari S, editors. *Recurrent neural networks with non-sequential data to predict hospital readmission of diabetic patients*. 2017;2017:18–23.
27. Goodfellow I, Pouget-Abadie J, Mirza M, Xu B, Warde-Farley D, Ozair S, et al. Generative adversarial nets. *Adv Neural Inf Process Syst*. 2014;27:1–9.
28. Creswell A, White T, Dumoulin V, Arulkumaran K, Sengupta B, Bharath AA. Generative adversarial networks: An overview. *IEEE Signal Process Mag*. 2018;35(1):53–65.
29. Yi X, Walia E, Babyn P. Generative adversarial network in medical imaging: A review. *Med Image Anal*. 2019;58:101552.
30. Chen Y, Yang X-H, Wei Z, Heidari AA, Zheng N, Li Z, et al. Generative adversarial networks in medical image augmentation: a review. *Comput Biol Med*. 2022;144:105382.
31. Locke S, Bashall A, Al-Adely S, Moore J, Wilson A, Kitchen GB. Natural language processing in medicine: a review. *Trends Anaesth Crit Care*. 2021;38:4–9.
32. Jiang F, Jiang Y, Zhi H, Dong Y, Li H, Ma S, et al. Artificial intelligence in healthcare: past, present and future. *Stroke Vasc Neurol*. 2017;2(4):e000101.
33. Tsujii J. Natural language processing and computational linguistics. *Comput Linguist*. 2021;47(4):707–27.
34. Nadkarni PM, Ohno-Machado L, Chapman WW. Natural language processing: an introduction. *J Am Med Inform Assoc*. 2011;18(5):544–51.

35. Siddiqui Z, Bhatia K, Corbin A, Dhar R. Rules-based natural language processing to extract features of large vessel occlusion and cerebral edema from radiology reports in stroke patients. *Neurosci Informatics.* 2023;3(2):100129.
36. Wu S, Roberts K, Datta S, Du J, Ji Z, Si Y, et al. Deep learning in clinical natural language processing: a methodical review. *J Am Med Inform Assoc.* 2020;27(3):457–70.
37. Kotei E, Thirunavukarasu R. A systematic review of transformer-based pre-trained language models through self-supervised learning. *Inf.* 2023;14(3):187.
38. Gupta R. Bidirectional encoders to state-of-the-art: a review of BERT and its transformative impact on natural language processing. *Informatics Econ Manag.* 2024;3(1):0311–20.
39. Kaka H, Michalopoulos G, Subendran S, Decker K, Lambert P, Pitz M, et al. Pretrained neural networks accurately identify cancer recurrence in medical record. In: Séroussi B, Weber P, Dhombres F, Grouin C, Liebe J, Pelayo S, Pinna A, Rance B, Sacchi L, Ugon A, Benis A, Gallos P. *Challenges of trustable AI and added-value on health.* IOS Press, Amsterdam, Netherlands; 2022. p. 93–7.
40. Zheng C, Lee M-s, Bansal N, Go AS, Chen C, Harrison TN, et al. Identification of recurrent atrial fibrillation using natural language processing applied to electronic health records. *Eur Heart J Qual Care Clin Outcomes.* 2024;10(1):77–88.
41. Chew C, Eysenbach G. Pandemics in the age of Twitter: content analysis of Tweets during the 2009 H1N1 outbreak. *PLoS One.* 2010;5(11):e14118.
42. Lopreite M, Panzarasa P, Puliga M, Riccaboni M. Early warnings of COVID-19 outbreaks across Europe from social media. *Sci Rep.* 2021;11(1):2147.
43. Bi WL, Hosny A, Schabath MB, Giger ML, Birkbak NJ, Mehrtash A, et al. Artificial intelligence in cancer imaging: clinical challenges and applications. *CA Cancer J Clin.* 2019;69(2):127–57.
44. McKinney SM, Sieniek M, Godbole V, Godwin J, Antropova N, Ashrafian H, et al. International evaluation of an AI system for breast cancer screening. *Nature.* 2020;577(7788):89–94.
45. Raghunath S, Pfeifer JM, Ulloa-Cerna AE, Nemani A, Carbonati T, Jing L, et al. Deep neural networks can predict new-onset atrial fibrillation from the 12-lead ECG and help identify those at risk of atrial fibrillation–related stroke. *Circulation.* 2021;143(13):1287–98.
46. Miller RA. Diagnostic decision support systems. *Clin Decis Support Syst: Theory Pract.* 2016:181–208.
47. Dias R, Torkamani A. Artificial intelligence in clinical and genomic diagnostics. *Genome Med.* 2019;11(1):70.
48. Batra U, Nathany S, Nath SK, Jose JT, Sharma T, Preeti P, et al. AI-based pipeline for early screening of lung cancer: integrating radiology, clinical, and genomics data. *Lancet Reg Health Southeast Asia.* 2024; 24:100352.
49. Jutel A. Sociology of diagnosis: a preliminary review. *Sociol Health Illn.* 2009;31(2):278–99.
50. Baerheim A. The diagnostic process in general practice: has it a two-phase structure? *Fam Pract.* 2001;18(3):243–5.
51. Mueller B, Kinoshita T, Peebles A, Graber MA, Lee S. Artificial intelligence and machine learning in emergency medicine: a narrative review. *Acute Med Surg.* 2022;9(1):e740.
52. Gandhi SO, Gandhi S, Sabik L. *Emergency department visit classification using the NYU algorithm. American Journal of Managed Care*, 2014;20(4):315–320.
53. Kim J, Chang H, Kim D, Jang D-H, Park I, Kim K. Machine learning for prediction of septic shock at initial triage in emergency department. *J Crit Care.* 2020;55:163–70.
54. Klang E, Kummer BR, Dangayach NS, Zhong A, Kia MA, Timsina P, et al. Predicting adult neuroscience intensive care unit admission from emergency department triage using a retrospective, tabular-free text machine learning approach. *Sci Rep.* 2021;11(1):1381.
55. Lee S, Lee YH, editors. Improving emergency department efficiency by patient scheduling using deep reinforcement learning. MDPI; 2020;8(2):77.
56. Pak A, Gannon B, Staib A. Predicting waiting time to treatment for emergency department patients. *Int J Med Inform.* 2021;145:104303.
57. Jilani T, Housley G, Figueredo G, Tang P-S, Hatton J, Shaw D. Short and long term predictions of hospital emergency department attendances. *Int J Med Inform.* 2019;129:167–74.
58. Smith KP, Wang H, Durant TJS, Mathison BA, Sharp SE, Kirby JE, et al. Applications of artificial intelligence in clinical microbiology diagnostic testing. *Clin Microbiol Newslett.* 2020;42(8):61–70.

59. Peiffer-Smadja N, Dellière S, Rodriguez C, Birgand G, Lescure FX, Fourati S, et al. Machine learning in the clinical microbiology laboratory: has the time come for routine practice? *Clin Microbiol Infect.* 2020;26(10):1300–9.
60. Smith KP, Kang AD, Kirby JE. Automated interpretation of blood culture gram stains by use of a deep convolutional neural network. *J Clin Microbiol.* 2018;56(3):10–1128.
61. Delahunt CB, Jaiswal MS, Horning MP, Janko S, Thompson CM, Kulhare S, et al., editors. *Fully-automated patient-level malaria assessment on field-prepared thin blood film microscopy images.* IEEE; 2019; 2019:1–8.
62. Viet NQ, ThanhTuyen DT, Hoang TH, . *Parasite worm egg automatic detection in microscopy stool image based on Faster R-CNN.* Association for Computing Machinary 2019; 2019:197–202.
63. Yang F, Poostchi M, Yu H, Zhou Z, Silamut K, Yu J, et al. Deep learning for smartphone-based malaria parasite detection in thick blood smears. *IEEE J Biomed Health Inform.* 2019;24(5):1427–38.
64. Sri NT, Sahithi P, Lavanya P, Amrin SK. Deep learning for smartphone-based malaria parasite detection in thick blood smears. *Turkish J Comput Math Educ (TURCOMAT).* 2023;14(03):672–6.
65. Quazi S. Artificial intelligence and machine learning in precision and genomic medicine. *Med Oncol.* 2022;39(8):120.
66. Johnson KB, Wei WQ, Weeraratne D, Frisse ME, Misulis K, Rhee K, et al. Precision medicine, AI, and the future of personalized health care. *Clin Transl Sci.* 2021;14(1):86–93.
67. Heather JM, Chain B. The sequence of sequencers: The history of sequencing DNA. *Genomics.* 2016;107(1):1–8.
68. Kircher M, Witten DM, Jain P, O'Roak BJ, Cooper GM, Shendure J. A general framework for estimating the relative pathogenicity of human genetic variants. *Nat Genet.* 2014;46(3):310–5.
69. Vilhekar RS, Rawekar A. Artificial intelligence in genetics. *Cureus.* 2024;16(1):e52035.
70. Wang H, Avillach P. Diagnostic classification and prognostic prediction using common genetic variants in autism spectrum disorder: Genotype-based deep learning. *JMIR Med Inform.* 2021;9(4):e24754.
71. Poplin R, Chang P-C, Alexander D, Schwartz S, Colthurst T, Ku A, et al. A universal SNP and small-indel variant caller using deep neural networks. *Nat Biotechnol.* 2018;36(10):983–7.
72. Suster CJE, Pham D, Kok J, Sintchenko V. Emerging applications of artificial intelligence in pathogen genomics. *Front Bacteriol.* 2024;3:1326958.
73. O'Toole Á, Scher E, Underwood A, Jackson B, Hill V, McCrone JT, et al. Assignment of epidemiological lineages in an emerging pandemic using the pangolin tool. *Virus Evol.* 2021;7(2):veab064.
74. Ye C, Thornlow B, Kramer A, McBroome J, Hinrichs A, Corbett-Detig R, et al. Pandemic-scale phylogenetics. *bioRxiv.* 2021;12(3):470766.
75. Sundermann AJ, Chen J, Kumar P, Ayres AM, Cho ST, Ezeonwuka C, et al. Whole-genome sequencing surveillance and machine learning of the electronic health record for enhanced healthcare outbreak detection. *Clin Infect Dis.* 2022;75(3):476–82.
76. Bejnordi BE, Veta M, Van Diest PJ, Van Ginneken B, Karssemeijer N, Litjens G, et al. Diagnostic assessment of deep learning algorithms for detection of lymph node metastases in women with breast cancer. *JAMA.* 2017;318(22):2199–210.
77. Haenssle HA, Fink C, Schneiderbauer R, Toberer F, Buhl T, Blum A, et al. Man against machine: diagnostic performance of a deep learning convolutional neural network for dermoscopic melanoma recognition in comparison to 58 dermatologists. *Ann Oncol.* 2018;29(8):1836–42.
78. Doncescu A, Tauzain B, Kabbaj N,. *Machine learning applied to BRCA1 hereditary breast cancer data.* IEEE; Bradford, UK, 2009; 942–47.
79. Curtis C, Shah SP, Chin S-F, Turashvili G, Rueda OM, Dunning MJ, et al. The genomic and transcriptomic architecture of 2,000 breast tumours reveals novel subgroups. *Nature.* 2012;486(7403):346–52.
80. Jayaram S, Gupta MK, Raju R, Gautam P, Sirdeshmukh R. Multi-omics data integration and mapping of altered kinases to pathways reveal gonadotropin hormone signaling in glioblastoma. *Omics.* 2016;20(12):736–46.
81. Stemke-Hale K, Gonzalez-Angulo AM, Lluch A, Neve RM, Kuo W-L, Davies M, et al. An integrative genomic and proteomic analysis of PIK3CA, PTEN, and AKT mutations in breast cancer. *Cancer Res.* 2008;68(15):6084–91.
82. Bibault J-E, Xing L. Screening for chronic obstructive pulmonary disease with artificial intelligence. *Lancet Digit Health.* 2020;2(5):e216–e7.

83. Panayides AS, Amini A, Filipovic ND, Sharma A, Tsaftaris SA, Young A, et al. AI in medical imaging informatics: current challenges and future directions. *IEEE J Biomed Health Inform.* 2020;24(7):1837–57.
84. Doi K. Current status and future potential of computer-aided diagnosis in medical imaging. *Br J Radiol.* 2005;78(suppl_1):s3–s19.
85. Liang M, Tang W, Xu DM, Jirapatnakul AC, Reeves AP, Henschke CI, et al. Low-dose CT screening for lung cancer: computer-aided detection of missed lung cancers. *Radiology.* 2016;281(1):279–88.
86. Cheng H-D, Cai X, Chen X, Hu L, Lou X. Computer-aided detection and classification of microcalcifications in mammograms: a survey. *Pattern Recognit.* 2003;36(12):2967–91.
87. Hillis JM, Bizzo BC, Mercaldo S, Chin JK, Newbury-Chaet I, Digumarthy SR, et al. Evaluation of an artificial intelligence model for detection of pneumothorax and tension pneumothorax in chest radiographs. *JAMA Netw Open.* 2022;5(12):e2247172.
88. Kolanu N, Silverstone EJ, Ho BH, Pham H, Hansen A, Pauley E, et al. Clinical utility of computer-aided diagnosis of vertebral fractures from computed tomography images. *J Bone Miner Res.* 2020;35(12):2307–12.
89. Nishio M, Nagashima C. Computer-aided diagnosis for lung cancer: usefulness of nodule heterogeneity. *Acad Radiol.* 2017;24(3):328–36.
90. Gavrilov D, Lazarenko L, Zakirov E, editors. *AI recognition in skin pathologies detection.* IEEE; Belgrade, Serbia, 2019.
91. Mehta P, Antonelli M, Ahmed HU, Emberton M, Punwani S, Ourselin S. Computer-aided diagnosis of prostate cancer using multiparametric MRI and clinical features: A patient-level classification framework. *Med Image Anal.* 2021;73:102153.
92. Wang S, Burtt K, Turkbey B, Choyke P, Summers RM. Computer aided-diagnosis of prostate cancer on multiparametric MRI: a technical review of current research. *Biomed Res Int.* 2014;2014(1):789561.
93. Paing MP, Hamamoto K, Tungjitkusolmun S, Pintavirooj C. Automatic detection and staging of lung tumors using locational features and double-staged classifications. *Appl Sci.* 2019;9(11):2329.
94. Jaffe CC. Measures of response: RECIST, WHO, and new alternatives. *J Clin Oncol.* 2006;24(20):3245–51.
95. Guenther LM, Rowe RG, Acharya PT, Swenson DW, Meyer SC, Clinton CM, et al. Response Evaluation Criteria in Solid Tumors (RECIST) following neoadjuvant chemotherapy in osteosarcoma. *Pediatr Blood Cancer.* 2018;65(4):e26896.
96. Graham S, Depp C, Lee EE, Nebeker C, Tu X, Kim H-C, et al. Artificial intelligence for mental health and mental illnesses: an overview. *Curr Psychiatry Rep.* 2019;21:1–18.
97. Gabbard GO, Crisp-Han H. The early career psychiatrist and the psychotherapeutic identity. *Acad Psychiatry.* 2017;41:30–4.
98. Luxton DD. Artificial intelligence in psychological practice: Current and future applications and implications. *Prof Psychol Res Prac.* 2014;45(5):332.
99. Shatte ABR, Hutchinson DM, Teague SJ. Machine learning in mental health: a scoping review of methods and applications. *Psychol Med.* 2019;49(9):1426–48.
100. Jackson RG, Patel R, Jayatilleke N, Kolliakou A, Ball M, Gorrell G, et al. Natural language processing to extract symptoms of severe mental illness from clinical text: the Clinical Record Interactive Search Comprehensive Data Extraction (CRIS-CODE) project. *BMJ Open.* 2017;7(1):e012012.
101. Fernandes AC, Dutta R, Velupillai S, Sanyal J, Stewart R, Chandran D. Identifying suicide ideation and suicidal attempts in a psychiatric clinical research database using natural language processing. *Sci Rep.* 2018;8(1):7426.
102. Arun V, Prajwal V, Krishna M, Arunkumar BV, Padma SK, Shyam V, editors. *A boosted machine learning approach for detection of depression.* IEEE; Bangalore, India, 2018.
103. Chekroud AM, Zotti RJ, Shehzad Z, Gueorguieva R, Johnson MK, Trivedi MH, et al. Cross-trial prediction of treatment outcome in depression: a machine learning approach. *Lancet Psychiatry.* 2016;3(3):243–50.
104. Wahle F, Kowatsch T, Fleisch E, Rufer M, Weidt S. Mobile sensing and support for people with depression: a pilot trial in the wild. *JMIR mHealth uHealth.* 2016;4(3):e5960.
105. Aldarwish MM, Ahmad HF,. *Predicting depression levels using social media posts.* IEEE; Bangkok, Thailand, 2017.
106. Kalmady SV, Greiner R, Agrawal R, Shivakumar V, Narayanaswamy JC, Brown MRG, et al. Towards artificial intelligence in mental health by improving schizophrenia prediction with multiple brain parcellation ensemble-learning. *npj Schizophr.* 2019;5(1):2.

107. Williams AD, Andrews G. The effectiveness of internet cognitive behavioural therapy (iCBT) for depression in primary care: a quality assurance study. *PLoS One*. 2013;8(2):e57447.
108. Prochaska JJ, Vogel EA, Chieng A, Kendra M, Baiocchi M, Pajarito S, et al. A therapeutic relational agent for reducing problematic substance use (Woebot): development and usability study. *J Med Internet Res*. 2021;23(3):e24850.
109. Singh RP, Hom GL, Abramoff MD, Campbell JP, Chiang MF. Current challenges and barriers to real-world artificial intelligence adoption for the healthcare system, provider, and the patient. *Transl Vis Sci Technol*. 2020;9(2):45.
110. Carpenter AE, Cimini BA, Eliceiri KW. Smart microscopes of the future. *Nat Methods*. 2023;20(7):962–4.
111. Halevy A, Norvig P, Pereira F. The unreasonable effectiveness of data. *IEEE Intell Syst*. 2009;24(2):8–12.
112. Kaye J. The tension between data sharing and the protection of privacy in genomics research. *Annu Rev Genomics Hum Genet*. 2012;13(1):415–31.
113. Montjoye Y-Ad, Farzanehfar A, Hendrickx J, Rocher L. Solving artificial intelligence's privacy problem. *Field Actions Sci Rep*. 2017;17:80–3.
114. Azencott CA. Machine learning and genomics: precision medicine versus patient privacy. *Philos Trans R Soc A Math Phys Eng Sci*. 2018;376(2128):20170350.
115. Sweeney L. k-anonymity: A model for protecting privacy. *Int J Uncertainty Fuzziness Knowl Based Syst*. 2002;10(05):557–70.
116. Wolff J, Pauling J, Keck A, Baumbach J. The economic impact of artificial intelligence in health care: systematic review. *J Med Internet Res*. 2020;22(2):e16866.
117. Rao RR, Makkithaya K. Learning from a Class Imbalanced Public Health Dataset: a Cost-based Comparison of Classifier Performance. *Int J Electr Comput Eng*. 2017;7(4).
118. Aboutalib SS, Mohamed AA, Berg WA, Zuley ML, Sumkin JH, Wu S. Deep learning to distinguish recalled but benign mammography images in breast cancer screening. *Clin Cancer Res*. 2018;24(23):5902–9.
119. Hoffman S, Podgurski A. Artificial intelligence and discrimination in health care. *Yale J Health Policy Law Ethics*. 2019;19:1.
120. Nagashima T, Yamaguchi K, Urakami K, Shimoda Y, Ohnami S, Ohshima K, et al. Japanese version of The Cancer Genome Atlas, JCGA, established using fresh frozen tumors obtained from 5143 cancer patients. *Cancer Sci*. 2020;111(2):687–99.
121. Shuaib A, Arian H, Shuaib A. The increasing role of artificial intelligence in health care: will robots replace doctors in the future? *Int J Gen Med*. 2020;19: 891–6.
122. Solez K, Bernier A, Crichton J, Graves H, Kuttikat P, Lockwood R, et al. Bridging the gap between the technological singularity and medicine: Highlighting a course on technology and the future of medicine. *Glob J Health Sci*. 2013;5(6):112.
123. Leenes R, Palmerini E, Koops B-J, Bertolini A, Salvini P, Lucivero F. Regulatory challenges of robotics: some guidelines for addressing legal and ethical issues. *Law Innov Technol*. 2017;9(1):1–44.
124. Braga A, Logan RK. The emperor of strong AI has no clothes: limits to artificial intelligence. *Information*. 2017;8(4):156.
125. Bringsjord S. Ethical robots: the future can heed us. *AI Soc*. 2008;22:539–50.

8

Digital Health Diagnostics: Current Trends and Future Directions

Junaid Tantray, Akhilesh Patel, Hiba Parveen, and Bhupendra G. Prajapati

8.1 Introduction

Digital health is a broad term that includes mobile health, health information technology, wearable devices, and personalized medicine. The supervision of digital health solutions is essentially determined by the level of risk they cause to patients [1]. Digital approaches in healthcare have traditionally been associated with health systems such as electronic health records (EHR), electronic medical records (EMR), laboratory information systems (LIS), hospital information systems (HIS), and middleware [1]. As the digital healthcare revolution continues, artificial intelligence (AI), algorithms, and clinical decision aids are becoming more widely recognized and integrated into the world of healthcare. Laboratory findings and choices based on them are now being made outside of established laboratories, clinics, and hospitals. The COVID-19 pandemic greatly boosted the acceptance of digital healthcare internationally, with a projected annualized growth rate of 15.1% between 2021 and 2028 [2].

Recent years have seen a dramatic revolution in medicine as a result of the thorough incorporation of computer technology and AI. Medical specialities like radiography have evolved tremendously, transitioning from traditional to digital approaches [2]. Furthermore, there is an increase in the clinical utility of AI in healthcare; some of these include invoicing, diagnostic assessment, and workflow improvement. Anatomic pathology has also started this transformation by introducing whole slide imaging (WSI). Several pathology facilities have begun to use digital WSI for tissue examination and evaluation, with some labs substituting this with the typical light microscopes [3, 4]. However, the adoption of WSI in cytopathology has been delayed due to variances in the preparation of samples and technological barriers such as focus problems [5, 6]. Despite these challenges, recent improvements in scanners, infrastructure, and growing experience from surgical pathology have led many cytopathology laboratories to begin adopting WSI [7]. Concurrently, AI applications are being developed for clinical use in cytopathology practices [8].

Digital health has evolved into a phase that encompasses electronically collected data, technological and communication systems, and healthcare-related applications. Significant advances in digital health are transforming medical care and biomedical research by reframing and reengineering devices needed to create a healthier tomorrow. Cloud computing, AI, machine learning (ML), blockchain, digitally assisted diagnostics and therapy, telemedicine, and consumer-facing mobile health applications are now widely used in self-management, healthcare, and biological science fields. These developments are projected to enable quicker diagnoses and therapies, enhance overall health, and inspire greater participation by patients [9].

In the mid-20th century, the newly formed World Health Organization (WHO) defined health as "a state of complete physical, mental, and social well-being, and not merely the absence of disease or infirmity" (WHO, 2006). Even in prosperous nations like the United States, this integrative notion represents

DOI: 10.1201/9781003486909-8

an audacious and ambitious aim. The WHO's concept underlines that health is far greater than just medical care. Since the foundation of the WHO, research has revealed how different factors other than medical care combine to impact health outcomes. According to studies, social and behavioral factors are more important in defining health status and regulating the impacts of genetics and physical settings [10–12].

8.2 Current Trends in Digital Health Diagnostics

Technological advancement can now be found in all aspects of healthcare. Digital health technologies have many applicable areas; some of these are summarized in Figure 8.1.

8.2.1 Digitalization in Healthcare

The integration of technology in the field of healthcare has improved tremendously. Statistics indicate that 66% of persons in the United States who are 65 years and above utilize online platforms. Among this, 42% possess a mobile device and 34% engage with social media [13]. According to a recent survey, 80% of internet users actively search for medical advice online, while 25% watch health information commercials and view care-related videos [14]. A significant number of individuals rely on internet-based tools and information to make informed health decisions, utilizing these resources to choose healthcare providers and treatment options [15]. Access to health information via mobile phones is also rising, with a significant portion of mobile phone users utilizing their devices for this purpose [16].

Many applications and websites currently enable the collection and monitoring of health data, while also offering prescription reminders and instructional resources [17]. These applications are extensively utilized to collect the most up-to-date medical data, providing patients with comprehensive information about their ailments. Employing such technology can decrease expenses associated with therapy, aid in the supervision of dietary habits and nutritional intake, and provide recommendations for nutritious food options. In addition, these technologies assist patients with identifying medicines, verifying drug interactions, and overseeing personal health care. This is especially advantageous for individuals with persistent illnesses who are prescribed many drugs. Several applications provide diagnostic assessments, and detailed knowledge about the indications and symptoms of diseases, serve as medical calculators, measure kidney functionality, and assist in the management of chronic kidney disease. Both consumers and healthcare professionals are increasingly utilizing online resources to remain informed about medical breakthroughs, as evidenced by testimonials that suggest alterations in treatment strategies based on search results [14].

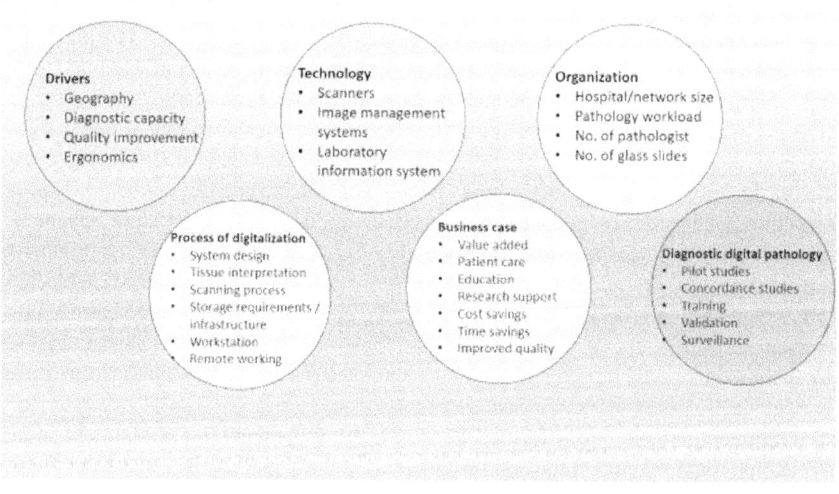

FIGURE 8.1 Use of digital technology in healthcare and health services.

Programs such as SCAN-ECHO provide the delivery of educative sessions by health professionals to primary care physicians in rural or remote regions [18]. Videoconferencing facilitates the connection between primary care physicians and specialists, promoting learning among peers by allowing any practitioner to ask questions or debate clinical situations with an expert. Similarly, the term "digital pathology" is a broad term for computerized methods employed in pathology, specifically in anatomic pathology. This encompasses the utilization of entire slide imaging, algorithms for precise measurement, and analysis of shape and size, as well as sophisticated microscopic procedures that frequently include physical interfaces [19]. Digital pathology enables the real-time sharing of computerized images and video streams, facilitating the connection between local hospitals, educational institutions, and companies, regardless of their physical locations. Furthermore, it enables the spatial integration of pathological observations across several slides and staining techniques [19].

8.2.2 Artificial Intelligence and Machine Learning in Healthcare

The inclusion of AI into the field of mental healthcare signifies a substantial transformation in this aspect of healthcare. Historically, mental health has often been dismissed and sometimes disregarded; however, currently, it is recognized as a fundamental component of general well-being [20, 21]. The WHO has reported that mental health problems greatly add to the total disease burden worldwide [22]. Indeed, the increasing frequency of mental problems has resulted in excessive pressure on healthcare systems, thereby exposing the shortcomings of conventional mental healthcare approaches. The traditional method, which mostly depends on face-to-face consultations and treatments, is inadequate to satisfy the growing need for easily available, reasonably priced, and adaptable health services. This discrepancy in the availability of appropriate mental healthcare services necessitates creative ideas [23].

AI exhibits extraordinary capabilities, such as effectively managing large data and enabling the analysis of intricate designs and relationships. Within the field of mental health, where understanding complicated human emotions and behaviors is vital, AI has the power to transform the sector by generating solutions formerly impossible with traditional approaches [24]. This transforming technology offers virtual therapeutic platforms, tailored treatments, and sophisticated detection techniques. This can expand healthcare access, reduce stress, and enhance treatment outcomes [24].

AI inclusion into mental health care is transforming the sector. Although early intervention, individualized treatments, and broad access are promised with the use of AI, it raises ethical questions, legal difficulties, and the need for constant study and improvement. As the uses of AI in healthcare are investigated, cooperation between human knowledge and AI capacity could start a new age in mental health treatment [25].

AI has also made significant advancements in evaluating speech, words, and glances to identify early mental health issues. Natural language processing (NLP) approaches are employed to derive significant details from either written or spoken words [26]. For example, sentiment analysis can detect shifts in a person's emotional condition by analyzing their online chat or written memoirs. Furthermore, alterations in speech patterns, such as fluctuations in pitch, tone, and timing, could potentially signify the presence of stress, depression, or other forms of mental illness [27–30]. Facial expression analysis, typically employing computer vision techniques, offers valuable insights into one's emotional condition by identifying minute facial movements and small alterations in facial characteristics. This technology facilitates remote psychological monitoring through video chats or mobile applications, allowing for rapid identification and intervention [31].

AI-powered mental health applications such as "Woebot" utilize sentiment analysis to assess user text input, providing advice or professional assistance when signs of depression or despair are identified [32]. The term "Cogito" employed in telemedicine services, tracks and analyses patient speech during treatment sessions, notifying therapists of any alterations that could potentially signify the presence of anxiety or despair. A company called "Affectiva" has created tools for analyzing facial expressions. These technologies have been utilized in mental health research for the timely detection of mental illness [33]. AI also demonstrates potential in examining EHRs for prompt identification of mental health issues.

Furthermore, ML algorithms can analyze patient data and detect patterns that indicate the presence of a mental health disorder. These algorithms can then identify patients who are at risk and require

TABLE 8.1

AI tools used in mental healthcare

AI tool	Function	References
Woebot	Uses sentiment analysis to provide guidance or recommend professional help based on user text input	[44]
Cogito	Monitors speech patterns during therapy sessions to detect anxiety or depression	[45]
Affectiva	Uses facial expressions to detect mental health issues early	[46]
Google Depression Screening Tool	Offers a depression assessment questionnaire	[47]
Ginger	Finds and helps mental health-risk individuals using predictive analytics	[48]
Watson for Drug Discovery	Identifies mental health drug candidates using genetic and chemical data	[49]
Mindstrong	Smartphone usage trends can indicate mental health difficulties	[50]
Koko	Uses AI to offer peer support and analyze text for signs of distress	[51]

more careful monitoring. AI also enables the incorporation of mental health data into patient health profiles, promoting a comprehensive approach to healthcare. The "Google Depression Screening Tool" is designed to prompt users who search for depression-related topics to fill out a questionnaire. The tool then offers suggestions based on the users' responses [34, 35].

Predictive simulation with AI takes individuals into account environmental factors, dietary habits, and genetic and social aspects of health to forecast the likelihood of acquiring mental health disorders [36, 37]. Platforms such as "Ginger" utilize guessing analytics to identify persons who are at risk and provide preventive assistance. Wearable technologies and mobile health applications gather up-to-date information on habits like sleep patterns and physical activity, improving the accuracy of predictive models [38, 39]. AI-driven predictive models help improve treatment outcomes by predicting patient responses to different treatments and ensuring personalized interventions (Table 8.1 and Figure 8.2). Additionally, these models can predict advancement in diseases, which can assist healthcare practitioners in making correct choices about treatment strategies and resources [40–42]. IBM's "Watson for Drug Discovery" uses AI to detect new pharmaceutical candidates for mental health disorders, expediting medication advancement and providing enhanced therapeutic interventions [43].

Recent evidence suggests that ML models outperform traditional cardiovascular disease (CVD) risk prediction tools. In a multi-ethnic study of atherosclerosis (MESA), researchers created an ML model utilizing the same inputs as the American College of Cardiology (ACC)/American Heart Association (AHA) atherosclerotic CVD risk estimator [52]. This ML model predicted CVD occurrences with an area under the receiver operator characteristic curve (AUROC) of 0.94, compared to 0.72 for the classical calculator. Statins were suggested for 46% of study participants by the ACC/AHA estimate, however, 24% of severe CVD events happened to non-statin users [52]. Only 11% of the group was advised statins by the ML model, whereas 14% of severe CVD events occurred in those not prescribed statins. The ML model may prescribe fewer statins and detect fewer events compared to the ACC/AHA estimator, resulting in more tailored treatment and better CVD risk identification. Due to low event frequencies, this ML model's validation cohort was only non-Hispanic whites, underlining the need for more diverse validation [52]. ML may identify complex, non-linear interactions and improve its precision providing more accurate risk estimates than conventional risk estimators.

8.2.3 Wearable Health Devices

Currently, the market for wearable biomedical devices that monitor vital signs is expanding rapidly. Key factors in the development of these wearable devices include low cost, minimal power consumption,

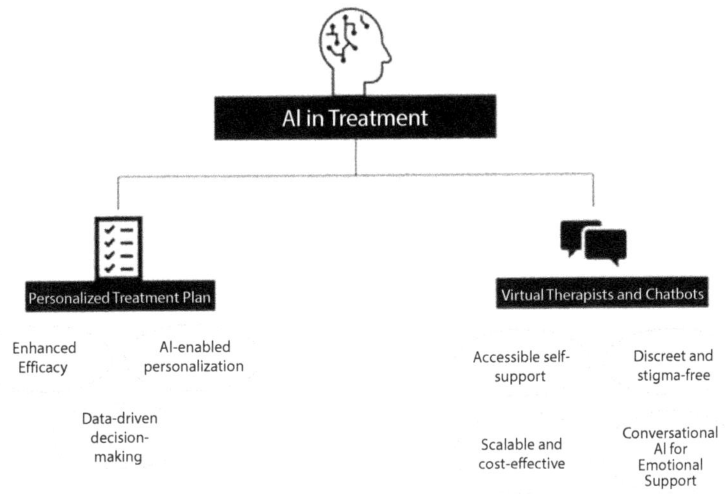

FIGURE 8.2 Application of AI in mental health treatment.

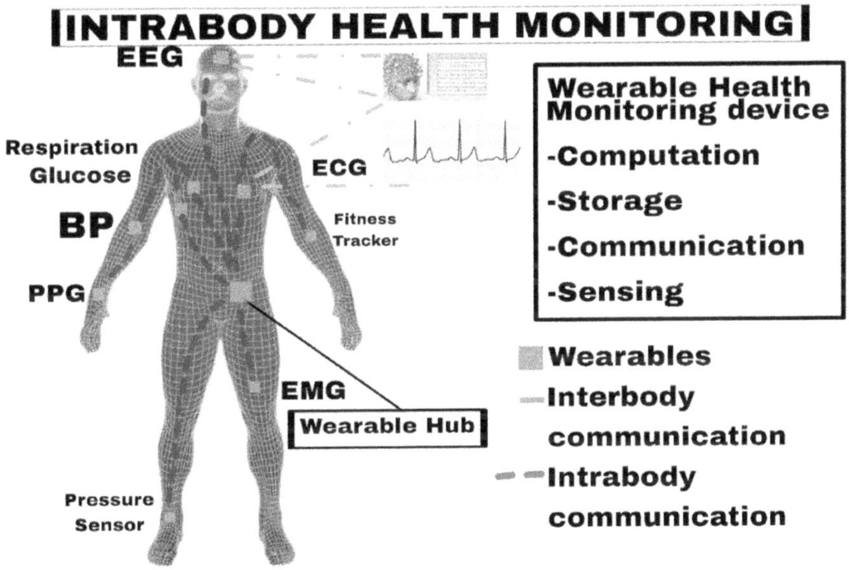

FIGURE 8.3 Wearable telemedicine technology.

compact size, and advanced intelligence. These wearable health devices (WHDs) offer numerous advantages, such as continuous clinical monitoring and real-time access to healthcare information [53]. WHDs are innovative tools that enable continuous monitoring of vital signs in everyday activities such as work, home, and sports (Figure 8.3). These devices reduce discomfort and minimize interference with daily life. Introduced in the late 1990s, WHDs aim to place individuals at the center of the healthcare system, empowering them to manage their health and stay connected with care providers. The objective is to enhance health awareness, improve the quality of care, and leverage the latest technological advancements [54].

Health data is collected by an on-body hub using human body communication (HBC) from various wearable and implantable physiological sensors. Metal electrodes are used to connect the signal to the body, and the wearable hub (WH) receives and transmits this data to a remote station via encrypted wireless media. The WH, equipped with a large battery for extended operation, can also securely store and transfer health data to a terminal using HBC [55]. Remote health tracking faces challenges due to limited energy supply, necessitating ultra-low-power communication solutions like wireless body area networks (WBANs).

WBANs integrate physiological sensors using commercial, scientific, and medical bands, including 2.4 and 5.8 GHz frequencies. Ultra-Wide-Band (UWB) technology, operating in the 3.1–10.6 GHz range, offers fast data speeds (up to 1 Gbps) over short distances (up to 10 meters) with low power consumption. UWB antennas, beneficial for high data rate applications, face design challenges such as size reduction and interference from other applications within the frequency range. Various band-rejection strategies, including notch structures, have been developed to mitigate interference from Wi-Fi, WLAN, and Bluetooth, ensuring efficient WBAN functionality [56, 57].

8.2.4 Telehealth Platforms

According to a study conducted by Goenka and colleagues [58], the Department of Radiation Oncology had a total of seven outpatient radiation treatment sessions and employed 20 faculty members in the metropolitan area of New York. Before March 2020, all patient consultations were conducted in person. Although a telehealth strategy had been in trial for three years, the complete execution commenced in mid-March 2020 due to the COVID-19 crisis. They implemented the HIPAA-compliant Amwell Telehealth System (American Well Corporation, Boston, MA), which had already been acquired for use in all outpatient facilities. The required equipment was promptly obtained, and the physicians were authorized for the 2-way audio-video technology.

Secretarial and billing teams were trained to be involved in the telehealth workflow, scheduling telehealth appointments and assisting patients with platform access. Resident trainees were trained to initiate telehealth encounters and address technical issues before transferring the session to attending physicians [58]. As of March 28, 2020, all providers had obtained credentials for telehealth utilization. Telehealth was utilized for initial consultations, post-treatment meetings, and subsequent appointments, employing 2-way audio-video communication, with telephone-only meetings available as a contingency. On-treatment visits conducted in person proceeded without any changes.

Goenka and colleagues analyzed billable interactions from six radiation oncology locations, utilizing the administrative database complied with HIPAA regulations. The analysis covered a period from January 1 to May 1, 2020. Every interaction was categorized as either face-to-face, over the phone, or through two-way audio-video communication. Patient income was estimated using 2018 census data, and age was calculated based on the encounter date (available for four facilities). From January 1 to May 1, 2020, a total of 2,997 billable assessment and leadership encounters occurred. In short, the amount of billable activity experienced a 35% decline between January and April. In January and February, all visits were conducted in person. This percentage decreased to 90% in March and further dropped to 21% in April. During April, 60% of telehealth visits were carried out using two-way audio-video communication, while the remaining 40% were conducted solely through telephone calls. Substantial growth in telephone-only consultation ($p < 0.01$) was seen after the stabilization of the telehealth program [58].

An analysis was conducted on clinical and demographic factors to ascertain the probability of completing a two-way audio-video session compared to a telephone-only consultation. Univariate analysis revealed a significant association between older patient age ($p < 0.01$; odds ratio, 0.97) and a reduced probability of 2-way audio-video encounters. The physician's effect on the type of telehealth session was statistically significant ($p < 0.01$), with the utilization of 2-way audio-video ranging from 22% to 100% across physicians. The type of telehealth visit was not influenced by patient income. After doing a multivariable analysis, it was shown that the physician providing the visit ($p < 0.01$) and older patient age ($p = 0.01$; odds ratio, 0.97) were factors linked with a decrease in the utilization of 2-way audio-video appointments.

8.3 Application of Digital Health Diagnostics

Case studies and scoping investigations from various global healthcare systems offer extensive insights into the drivers behind digital pathology deployment, its operational requirements, and effective business case planning [59]. These studies, mainly focusing on pathologists' viewpoint, emphasize the requirements of digital pathology, such as necessary hardware and software. In addition, they offer a thorough examination of the digitalization procedure and possible frameworks for clinical execution. Nevertheless, there is uncertainty over the number of pathologists who provide information digitally.

The study by Retamero et al. [60] is the only one that clearly states the adoption of digital pathology. According to their findings, within two weeks of implementation, all pathologists were utilizing digital pathology for initial diagnosis, and the traditional analog processes were discontinued. The precise proportion of pathologists utilizing computerized pathology for diagnostic procedures within individual departments or networks remains uncertain, with estimates ranging from 5% to 28%. Additionally, the long-term viability and widespread implementation of this technology are also unclear [61].

Digital pathology has mostly been implemented in healthcare settings by early adopters, assessment and verification studies, and larger networks like the three UK digital pathology/AI centers of excellence [62]. Diagnostic digital pathology has spread slowly, as is common for healthcare technologies [63]. Van Limburg et al. [64] mentioned financial and legal constraints, scattered innovation installation, and implementation strategies as structural impediments to healthcare innovation uptake. The adoption of telehealth solutions often lacks sustained use. To address these challenges, Greenhalgh et al. [65] have suggested the "Nonadoption, Abandonment, Scale-up, Spread and Sustainability (NASSS)" framework to improve the implementation of health technology innovations.

8.3.1 Personalized Medicine

The use of modern, data-driven biomedical tools like DNA sequencing, the field of proteomics imaging protocols, and cellular monitoring devices have shown large inter-individual variability in the etiology of diseases. This variability has prompted questions about how much these differences should influence decisions regarding the best ways to treat, monitor, or prevent diseases. It is now widely accepted that the inherent heterogeneity of many diseases necessitates strategies that are appropriate to each person's unique profile. Numerous comprehensive reviews and textbooks on personalized medicine, intended for medical students and clinicians, have been published [66, 67].

Drugs like warfarin and imatinib have generated considerable interest due to their effectiveness or reduced adverse effects in patients with specific genetic profiles. This has led to a focus on identifying variations in genes that influence an individual's reaction to different drugs and therapies. The emphasis on developing tailored medications has also expanded to encompass customized disease monitoring approaches, such as early detection and individualized preventive strategies [68].

Rather than following the traditional approach in drug development and then conducting observational studies to find characteristics that influence its effectiveness or adverse effects, as observed with warfarin and imatinib, current efforts focus on identifying genetic patterns in patients and designing therapies specifically targeted to those profiles. For example, ivacaftor was specifically designed for cystic fibrosis (CF) patients with particular pathogenic mutations in the CFTR gene. The CFTR gene influences various functions, including a gate-like structure in its encoded protein that regulates salt movement in and out of cells. When the CFTR gene is dysfunctional, the gate remains closed, leading to mucus buildup in the lungs. Different mutations cause different dysfunctions, such as a complete lack of CFTR production or gate mechanism failure. Ivacaftor targets mutations that result in the gate being closed by prolonging its opening, making it effective only for CF patients with these specific gating issues [69].

There are also a number of new drugs (immunotherapies) that are used in cancer management that have been developed based on genetic characteristics of the patient [70]. One of the approaches involves identifying the special genetic changes in a cancer patient's tumor cells known as neo-antigens which, if correctly identified by the patient's immune cells, can set off an immunological response. Under this immunotherapy, immune cells such as T cells are obtained from the patient, altered to especially target the neo-antigens in the tumor, and subsequently reintroduced into the patient's body to attack the tumor cells (releasing the neo-antigen signals). Although very patient-specific, cytotoxic T-cell treatments and other immunotherapies have demonstrated notable results. This specificity arises because each patient's neo-antigen profile is unique, making targeted T cells effective only for tumors with matching neo-antigens. Additionally, using autologous constructs, where the patient's T cells are modified, limits the therapy's applicability to other patients, although research is ongoing to develop allogeneic constructs, where T cells from one individual are modified for use in another [70].

8.3.2 Early Disease Prevention

Although the scientific community is aware of the need to use genetic details to create customized disease prevention plans, their general clinical acceptance is lacking. Many cases show how genetic information can lower the risk of disease and adverse effects from accepted therapies and screening programs. In 2012, Liao et al. found that patients with a somatic PIK3CA mutation in their colorectal cancers who took postoperative aspirin had improved overall survival and reduced cancer-specific mortality compared to those with the wild-type PIK3CA gene [71]. In 2015, Nan et al. reported that aspirin's effect on colorectal cancer risk varied by genotype, with some genotypes showing decreased risk, increased risk, or no change. Given aspirin's potential adverse effects, such as intestinal and intracranial bleeding, it is ideal to prescribe it only to individuals whose genotypes predict substantial benefit [72].

Jeon et al. (2018) advanced risk prediction models for colorectal cancer screening beyond traditional guidelines based solely on age and family history. Their study demonstrated significant potential by incorporating additional factors such as environmental exposures and genetic profiles, particularly genetic variants associated with colorectal cancer [73]. They found that integrating these factors into the predictive model could lead to substantial changes in screening recommendations: up to 12 years earlier for men and 14 years earlier for women compared to guidelines based only on age and family history. This underscores the impact of personalized medicine in optimizing healthcare decisions. The accuracy of their predictive models was evaluated using the area under the curve (AUC), a metric where 1.0 represents perfect prediction. For models incorporating environmental and genetic factors, the AUC values were 0.63 for men and 0.62 for women. In contrast, models based solely on family history yielded lower AUC values of 0.53 for men and 0.54 for women. While the AUCs around 0.62 indicate room for improvement, the considerable enhancement over models lacking genetic and environmental data justifies their integration into clinical practice. This advancement suggests a promising future for enhancing risk prediction and guiding personalized screening strategies in colorectal cancer [67].

8.4 Challenges in Digital Health Diagnostics

Developing countries frequently have scattered digital health rules, where different parties exert influence without established responsibilities. The lack of structure can impede the efficient deployment of digital health technology, leading to possible health hazards and commercial inefficiencies. Regulatory authorities often struggle to keep up with the rapid speed of technological changes, resulting in obsolete norms and legal uncertainties that add complexity to the regulatory process. In India, various institutions, including the Central Drugs Standard Control Organization (CDSCO), the Ministry of Health and Family Welfare (MoHFW), and the Ministry of Electronics and Information Technology (MeitY), are involved in the regulation of digital health. Nevertheless, the lack of a well-defined system outlining their obligations can lead to perplexity, inefficiency, and regulatory inconsistencies [74]. Telemedicine and digital health services, which could increase access to care, are financially unattainable to many due to the lack of regulatory procedures requiring insurance companies to pay them. Regulation of digital health products including mHealth applications, wearable devices, and EHRs is complicated by their diversity. Indeed, regulatory processes and tool requirements are unclear due to this confusion. Some mHealth applications are regulated as medical devices, while others are not. This creates gaps that could compromise patient safety and data security [75].

Technical incompetence among regulators is another issue in digital health regulation. This weakness affects digital health technology implementation and oversight. Regulatory staff may not comprehend the technologies they oversee, making at-risk and benefit assessments difficult. Thus, laws may be inefficient, misguided, or unduly restrictive, stifling innovation and reducing the health advantages of new technology [76].

8.4.1 Integrity

Every day, digital health companies manage enormous volumes of delicate patient data: personal identities, medical histories, genetic details, and more, all of which need strong security measures to defend the confidentiality of patients. Strong data protection rules help to reduce the possibility of data breaches exposing patient information. Indeed, privacy invasion or identity theft may cause patients to refuse to adopt digital health technology, therefore restricting their advantages. Regulating the gathering, preservation, and use of private health data is sadly lacking in some African nations. For example, one of the most populous countries in Africa, Nigeria only adopted its first thorough data security law in 2019. Generally, it has been challenging to enforce and apply these rules in many jurisdictions [77]. Such regulatory shortcomings reveal sensitive health data and might lead to breaches of privacy, therefore discouraging people from using digital health devices. Similar difficulties confront Southeast Asia. For example, records of HIV patients were unintentionally leaked in 2019 following a hack in a Singaporean health database. This event emphasizes the crucial requirement of strong data security policies since more medical treatments have migrated online [78].

8.4.2 Infrastructure and Maintenance

Inadequate infrastructure poses substantial technical difficulties that restrict the widespread implementation of electronic tools in medical facilities. The absence of reliable services, such as power and secure internet connectivity, restricts the successful adoption and utilization of digital health solutions. This issue has been documented in countries such as India and Brazil [79, 80]. Healthcare institutions located in rural places often have challenges in accessing crucial services, leading to limitations in device operation and disruptions in regular services. Internet connectivity is essential for the transfer of data, conducting online consultations, and viewing medical records. Nevertheless, the utilization of cloud-based applications and real-time telemedicine solutions is hindered in certain places due to sluggish or sporadic connections, resulting in adverse effects on patient care and decision-making procedures [80]. In Ethiopia, a comprehensive analysis revealed that inadequate infrastructure is a major obstacle to the use of electronic medical records [81]. Furthermore, problems in transmitting data might result in delays and errors when exchanging vital healthcare information, which may hinder the process of diagnosing and planning therapy.

Insufficient infrastructure also weakens the effectiveness of telemedicine and remote assistance, making them unreliable or inaccessible in regions with connectivity difficulties [82]. For instance, in rural Nigeria, frequent blackouts impede the functioning of medical equipment, while unreliable internet connection hampers real-time counseling and data retrieval [83]. Moreover, the task of upkeeping and assisting digital health equipment is difficult due to the scarcity of skilled technicians and spare parts, leading to extended periods of inactivity and complications in replacing defective devices [84]. This problem is particularly widespread in sub-Saharan Africa. In Tanzanian hospitals, there were substantial delays in the repair of malfunctioning equipment, such as CT scanners and MRI machines, mostly caused by a scarcity of proficient technicians and essential replacement parts [85].

8.5 Future Directions in Digital Health Diagnostics

A recent research by WHO has identified a minimum of 12 functions that digital technology offers in healthcare. At present, they are in the process of establishing a set of suggestions for global implementation [86]. The functions encompass the dissemination of accurate and concise information to the general public regarding health and disease, provision of immediate assistance to healthcare professionals and supervisors in the diagnosis and treatment of patients, maintenance of reliable and easily accessible records of births, deaths, and healthcare interactions, furnishing health managers at all hierarchical levels with crucial operational and strategic data about medication availability, financial matters, and human resource management. These effects will radically alter the way healthcare is provided in unanticipated ways. The subsequent five components delineate the anticipated impact of technological advances on healthcare delivery and society [87]

8.5.1 Health Workers Will Be Digitally Supported

Today's system of care relies on properly trained health staff to diagnose, treat, and interact with patients. Training alone cannot guarantee high-quality care, but it is essential. Decision support technologies for clinical procedures or pathways are increasingly advocated by the WHO to improve quality. Each medical professional will soon have a computerized tool for evaluation, therapy, and patient communication [88]. Lists for routine treatment like antenatal check-ups, decision support for detecting illnesses, and provider-to-patient video or graphic counseling messages are examples. Numerous research has shown that decision help, video counseling, and digital monitoring increase care quality. These initiatives are still developing, but governments are adopting them as part of their health policies [89, 90]. Technology will also change training. Online instruction tailored to the health worker's counseling interests and work environment will substitute direct instruction and interactions. Health workers will receive ongoing training. Regular education will become the standard, although face-to-face instruction will still be needed for surgery. Instead of memorizing each sign and its meaning, health personnel will learn to traverse the digital world and use decision support technologies to make better clinical decisions. Information will also change, with illustrations, animations, and graphics replacing vocal guidance from healthcare professionals [91].

8.5.2 Data Will Be Central to Health Systems

Data management and utilization will be greatly affected by digital technologies. Presently, despite significant financial commitments toward health information systems, only a limited number of low-income nations have dependable data. The majority of data is still documented on physical paper, consolidated solely at the national scale, and mostly utilized for reporting the occurrence of diseases or the number of patients. There is an imminent change about to occur [92]. Implementing digital data collection tools at the point of care will facilitate faster and more thorough data gathering, enhance data accuracy, and give health planners compelling reasons to employ the data for administration and planning [93]. One important advancement is that the gathering of data, which occurs as a result of tools for decision-making utilized by healthcare professionals, will become prompter and seamlessly incorporated into patient care. Entering data will be integrated into the clinical process, eliminating the need for it to be a distinct task. Data collected throughout the diagnostic process will be documented in a digital patient record, allowing for prompt access and utilization of individual data across all levels of the system. Providers will benefit from getting access to a patient's history since it will simplify the diagnosis procedure. Implementing universal biometric authorization will reduce the necessity of repeatedly gathering demographic data. The collected information can be employed for reporting, monitoring, and planning. For example, sudden increases in complaints can be promptly examined to detect disease outbreaks such as diarrheal disorders or malaria [94].

8.6 Conclusion

The great progress in digital health diagnostics is revolutionizing healthcare. The current change is being driven by the combination of AI and ML, the advancement of wearable health devices, and the use of telehealth platforms. These technologies empower customized medicine, expedite the early identification of diseases, and enhance long-term disease management. Nevertheless, the implementation of digital health diagnostics is not free of obstacles. Addressing the crucial challenges of data privacy and safety, legal compliance, and regulation and interoperability is essential. In order to fully harness the promise of digital health diagnostics, it is imperative to address and overcome these limitations. Eventual success of digital health diagnostics will depend on seamless connectivity with existing healthcare systems, developments in big data analytics, and the spread of services to marginalized areas. By focusing on these specific areas, digital health diagnostics can further develop and offer substantial advantages to healthcare systems globally, boosting the standard of care and better findings for patients.

REFERENCES

1. Hellmann A, Emmons A, Prime MS, Paranjape K, Heaney DL. Digital health: today's solutions and tomorrow's impact. *Clin Lab Med.* 2023;43(1):71–86.
2. Paranjape K, Schinkel M, Hammer RD, Schouten B, Nannan Panday RS, Elbers PW, et al. The value of artificial intelligence in laboratory medicine: current opinions and barriers to implementation. *Am J Clin Pathol.* 2021;155(6):823–31.
3. Yu KH, Beam AL, Kohane IS. Artificial intelligence in healthcare. *Nat Biomed Eng.* 2018;2(10):719–31.
4. Jain E, Patel A, Parwani AV, Shafi S, Brar Z, Sharma S, Mohanty SK. Whole slide imaging technology and its applications: current and emerging perspectives. *Int J Surg Pathol.* 2024;32(3):433–48.
5. Fraggetta F, Garozzo S, Zannoni GF, Pantanowitz L, Rossi ED. Routine digital pathology workflow: the Catania experience. *J Pathol Inform.* 2017;8(1):51.
6. Pinto DG, Bychkov A, Tsuyama N, Fukuoka J, Eloy C. Real-world implementation of digital pathology: results from an intercontinental survey. *Lab Investig.* 2023;103(12):100261.
7. Kumar N, Gupta R, Gupta S. Whole slide imaging (WSI) in pathology: current perspectives and future directions. *J Digit Imaging.* 2020;33(4):1034–40.
8. Li Z, Pantanowitz L. Whole slide imaging in cytopathology. In: Pantanowitz L, editor. *Whole slide imaging: current applications and future directions.* Springer, New York, 2022. p. 179–91.
9. McGinnis JM, Fineberg HV, Dzau VJ. Advancing the learning health system. *N Engl J Med.* 2021;385(1):1–5.
10. Templeton K, Bernstein CA, Sukhera J, Nora LM, Newman C, Burstin H, Busis N. Gender-based differences in burnout: issues faced by women physicians. *NAM Perspectives.* 2019. Available from: https://nam.edu/gender-based-differences-in-burnout-issues-faced-by-women-physicians/
11. McGovern L, Miller G, Hughes-Cromwick P. The relative contribution of multiple determinants to health. *Health Aff Health Policy Brief.* 2014;10(10.1377).
12. McGinnis JM, Williams-Russo P, Knickman JR. The case for more active policy attention to health promotion. *Health Aff.* 2002;21(2):78–93.
13. Mejia C, Libby BA, Bracken ML, Shanley B, Holovatska MM, Wanik J, et al. Interest in digital dietary support among adults with kidney failure receiving hemodialysis. *J Ren Nutr.* 2021;31(3):327–32.
14. Fareed N, Swoboda CM, Jonnalagadda P, Huerta TR. Persistent digital divide in health-related internet use among cancer survivors: findings from the Health Information National Trends Survey, 2003–2018. *J Cancer Survivorship.* 2021;15:87–98.
15. Bhavnani SP, Parakh K, Atreja A, Druz R, Graham GN, Hayek SS, et al. 2017 Roadmap for innovation—ACC health policy statement on healthcare transformation in the era of digital health, big data, and precision health: a report of the American College of Cardiology Task Force on Health Policy Statements and Systems of Care. *J Am Coll Cardiol.* 2017;70(21):2696–718.
16. Krebs P, Duncan DT. Health app use among US mobile phone owners: a national survey. *JMIR Mhealth Uhealth.* 2015 Nov 4;3(4):e101. doi: 10.2196/mhealth.4924. PMID: 26537656; PMCID: PMC4704953.
17. Dubin R, Rubinsky A. A digital modality decision program for patients with advanced chronic kidney disease. *JMIR Form Res.* 2019;3(1):e12528.
18. Mattson CJ. *Grounds for a new normal: integration of telenephrology in rural communities.* Seattle, USA, 2021.
19. Jahn SW, Plass M, Moinfar F. Digital pathology: advantages, limitations and emerging perspectives. *J Clin Med.* 2020;9(11):3697.

20. Lee EE, Torous J, De Choudhury M, Depp CA, Graham SA, Kim HC, et al. Artificial intelligence for mental health care: clinical applications, barriers, facilitators, and artificial wisdom. *Biol Psychiatry Cogn Neurosci Neuroimaging*. 2021;6(9):856–64.
21. Espejo G, Reiner W, Wenzinger M. Exploring the role of artificial intelligence in mental healthcare: progress, pitfalls, and promises. *Cureus*. 2023;15(9):e44748.
22. World Health Organization. Mental disorders. Available from: https://www.who.int/news-room/fact-sheets/detail/mental-disorders. Accessed 11 Oct 2023.
23. Wainberg ML, Scorza P, Shultz JM, Helpman L, Mootz JJ, Johnson KA, et al. Challenges and opportunities in global mental health: a research-to-practice perspective. *Curr Psychiatry Rep*. 2017;19:1–10.
24. Bouhouita-Guermech S, Gogognon P, Bélisle-Pipon JC. Specific challenges posed by artificial intelligence in research ethics. *Front Artif Intell*. 2023; 6:1149082.
25. Gerke S, Minssen T, Cohen G. Ethical and legal challenges of artificial intelligence-driven healthcare. In: Bohr A, Memarzadeh K. *Artificial intelligence in healthcare*. Academic Press, Massachusetts, USA; 2020. p. 295–336.
26. Zhang T, Schoene AM, Ji S, Ananiadou S. *Natural language processing applied to mental illness detection*. 2022; NPJ Digital Medicine 5(1):46.
27. Khurana D, Koli A, Khatter K, Singh S. Natural language processing: state of the art, current trends and challenges. *Multimed Tools Appl*. 2023;82(3):3713–44.
28. Uban AS, Chulvi B, Rosso P. An emotion and cognitive-based analysis of mental health disorders from social media data. *Future Gener Comput Syst*. 2021;124:480–94.
29. Flanagan O, Chan A, Roop P, Sundram F. Using acoustic speech patterns from smartphones to investigate mood disorders: scoping review. *JMIR Mhealth Uhealth*. 2021;9(9):e24352.
30. Fagherazzi G, Fischer A, Ismael M, Despotovic V. Voice for health: the use of vocal biomarkers from research to clinical practice. *Digit Biomarkers*. 2021;5(1):78–88.
31. Haines N, Southward MW, Cheavens JS, Beauchaine T, Ahn WY. Using computer-vision and machine learning to automate facial coding of positive and negative affect intensity. *PLoS One*. 2019;14(2):e0211735.
32. Zhao G, Li X. Automatic micro-expression analysis: open challenges. *Front Psychol*. 2019;10:465651.
33. Kuziemsky C, Maeder AJ, John O, Gogia SB, Basu A, Meher S, et al. Role of artificial intelligence within the telehealth domain. *Yearb Med Inform*. 2019;28(01):035–040.
34. Mittelsteadt M. *Artificial intelligence: an introduction for policymakers*. Mercatus Research Paper; 2023.
35. Catanzariti B. *Seeing affect: knowledge infrastructures in facial expression recognition systems*. Edinburgh University Press, Edinburgh, Scotland, UK; 2023.
36. Krause FC, Linardatos E, Fresco DM, Moore MT. Facial emotion recognition in major depressive disorder: a meta-analytic review. *J Affect Disord*. 2021;293:320–8.
37. Lee YS, Park WH. Diagnosis of depressive disorder model on facial expression based on fast R-CNN. *Diagnostics*. 2022;12(2):317.
38. Iyortsuun NK, Kim SH, Jhon M, Yang HJ, Pant S. A review of machine learning and deep learning approaches on mental health diagnosis. *Healthcare*. 2023 Jan;11(3):285.
39. Chekroud AM, Bondar J, Delgadillo J, Doherty G, Wasil A, Fokkema M, et al. The promise of machine learning in predicting treatment outcomes in psychiatry. *World Psychiatry*. 2021;20(2):154–70.
40. Al Kuwaiti A, Nazer K, Al-Reedy A, Al-Shehri S, Al-Muhanna A, Subbarayalu AV, et al. A review of the role of artificial intelligence in healthcare. *J Pers Med*. 2023;13(6):951.
41. Yu J, Shen N, Conway S, Hiebert M, Lai-Zhao B, McCann M, et al. A holistic approach to integrating patient, family, and lived experience voices in the development of the BrainHealth Databank: a digital learning health system to enable artificial intelligence in the clinic. *Front Health Serv*. 2023;3:1198195.
42. Olawade DB, David-Olawade AC, Wada OZ, Asaolu AJ, Adereni T, Ling J. *J Med Surg Public Health*.
43. Olawade DB, Wada OZ, Odetayo A, David-Olawade AC, Asaolu F, Eberhardt J. Enhancing mental health with artificial intelligence: current trends and future prospects. *J Med Surg Public Health*. 202417:100099.
44. Darcy A, Beaudette A, Chiauzzi E, Daniels J, Goodwin K, Mariano TY, et al. RETRACTED ARTICLE: Anatomy of a Woebot®(WB001): agent-guided CBT for women with postpartum depression. *Expert Rev Med Devices*. 2022;19(4):287–301.

45. Ben-Zeev D, Scherer EA, Wang R, Xie H, Campbell AT. Next-generation psychiatric assessment: using smartphone sensors to monitor behavior and mental health. *Psychiatr Rehabil J.* 2015;38(3):218.
46. D'Mello S, Dieterle E, Duckworth A. Advanced, analytic, automated (AAA) measurement of engagement during learning. *Educ Psychol.* 2017;52(2):104–23.
47. Gathright EC, Vickery KD, Ayenew W, Whited MC, Adkins-Hempel M, Chrastek M, et al. The development and pilot testing of a behavioral activation-based treatment for depressed mood and multiple health behavior change in patients with recent acute coronary syndrome. *PLoS One.* 2022;17(2):e0261490.
48. Hall PS, Morris A. Predictive analytics and population health. In:Sheikh A, Wright A, Cresswell KM, Bates DW. *Key advances in clinical informatics.* Academic Press, Cambridge, Massachusetts, USA. 2017. p. 217–25.
49. Mbatha SZ, Mulaudzi TV, Mbita Z, Adeola HA, Batra J, Blenman KR, et al. Artificial intelligence-enhanced drug discovery and the achievement of next-generation human-centered health system. In: Zodwa Dlamini, *Society 5.0 and next generation healthcare: patient-focused and technology-assisted precision therapies.* Springer Nature Switzerland; 2023. p. 155–77.
50. Onnela JP, Rauch SL. Harnessing smartphone-based digital phenotyping to enhance behavioral and mental health. *Neuropsychopharmacology.* 2016;41(7):1691–6.
51. Mutahi J, Kangwana B, Khasowa D, Muthoni I, Charo O, Muli A, Kumar M. Integrating mental health management into empowerment group sessions for out-of-school adolescents in Kenyan informal settlements: a process paper. *Int J Environ Res Public Health.* 2024;21(2):223.
52. Kakadiaris IA, Vrigkas M, Yen AA, Kuznetsova T, Budoff M, Naghavi M. Machine learning outperforms ACC/AHA CVD risk calculator in MESA. *J Am Heart Assoc.* 2018;7(22):e009476.
53. Raad HK, Al-Rizzo HM, Abbosh A, Hammoodi AI. A compact dual band polyimide-based antenna for wearable and flexible telemedicine devices. *Prog Electromagn Res C.* 2016;63:153–61.
54. Di Rienzo M, Rizzo F, Parati G, Brambilla G, Ferratini M, Castiglioni P. MagIC system: *A new textile-based wearable device for biological signal monitoring. Applicability in daily life and clinical setting.* 2005 IEEE Engineering in Medicine and Biology 27th Annual Conference; 2006 Jan. p. 7167–9.
55. Leander G, Paar C, Poschmann A, Schramm K. *New lightweight DES variants.* Fast Software Encryption: 14th International Workshop, FSE 2007; Luxembourg, Luxembourg, March 26–28, 2007. Revised Selected Papers 14. Springer Berlin Heidelberg; 2007. p. 196–210.
56. De Canniere C, Dunkelman O, Knežević M. *KATAN and KTANTAN—a family of small and efficient hardware-oriented block ciphers.* International Workshop on Cryptographic Hardware and Embedded Systems; 2009 Sep. p. 272–88. Springer Berlin Heidelberg.
57. Tantray J, Kosey S, Prajapati JB, Prajapati B. The future of the healthcare system: a meta-analysis of remote patient. In: *Handbook on augmenting telehealth services.* CRC Press; p. 105–26.
58. Goenka A, Ma D, Teckie S, Alfano C, Bloom B, Hwang J, Potters L. Implementation of telehealth in radiation oncology: rapid integration during COVID-19 and its future role in our practice. *Adv Radiat Oncol.* 2021;6(1):100575.
59. Chen J, Jiao Y, Lu C, Zhou J, Zhang Z, Zhou C. A nationwide telepathology consultation and quality control program in China: implementation and result analysis. *Diagn Pathol.* 2014 Dec;9:1–5.
60. Retamero JA, Aneiros-Fernandez J, Del Moral RG. Complete digital pathology for routine histopathology diagnosis in a multicenter hospital network. *Arch Pathol Lab Med.* 2020;144(2):221–8.
61. Zarella MD, Bowman D, Aeffner F, Farahani N, Xthona A, Absar SF, et al. A practical guide to whole slide imaging: a white paper from the digital pathology association. *Arch Pathol Lab Med.* 2019;143(2):222–34.
62. Alami H, Fortin JP, Gagnon MP, Pollender H, Têtu B, Tanguay F. The challenges of a complex and innovative telehealth project: a qualitative evaluation of the eastern Quebec Telepathology network. *Int J Health Policy Manag.* 2018;7(5):421.
63. Betmouni S. Diagnostic digital pathology implementation: learning from the digital health experience. *Digit Health.* 2021;7:20552076211020240.
64. van Limburg M, van Gemert-Pijnen JE, Nijland N, Ossebaard HC, Hendrix RM, Seydel ER. Why business modeling is crucial in the development of eHealth technologies. *J Med Internet Res.* 2011;13(4):e124.
65. Greenhalgh T, Wherton J, Papoutsi C, Lynch J, Hughes G, A'Court C, Hinder S, Fahy N, Procter R, Shaw S. Beyond adoption: a new framework for theorizing and evaluating nonadoption, abandonment, and challenges to the scale-up, spread, and sustainability of health and care technologies. *J Med Internet Res.* 2017 Nov 1;19(11):e367. doi: 10.2196/jmir.8775. PMID: 29092808; PMCID: PMC5688245.

66. CDC. 2016. Available from: https://blogs.cdc.gov/genomics/2016/04/21/shift/
67. Garrod A. The incidence of alkaptonuria: a study in chemical individuality. *Lancet.* 1902;160(4137):1616–20.
68. Goetz LH, Schork NJ. Personalized medicine: motivation, challenges, and progress. *Fertil Steril.* 2018 Jun;109(6):952–63. doi: 10.1016/j.fertnstert.2018.05.006. PMID: 29935653; PMCID: PMC6366451.
69. Davis PB, Yasothan U, Kirkpatrick P. Ivacaftor. *Nat Rev Drug Discov.* 2012;11(5):349–50. doi: 10.1038/nrd3723.
70. Farkona S, Diamandis EP, Blasutig IM. Cancer immunotherapy: the beginning of the end of cancer? *BMC Med.* 2016;14:73. doi: 10.1186/s12916-016-0623-5.
71. Liao X, Lochhead P, Nishihara R, Morikawa T, Kuchiba A, Yamauchi M, et al. Aspirin use, tumor PIK3CA mutation, and colorectal-cancer survival. *N Engl J Med.* 2012;367(17):1596–606. doi: 10.1056/NEJMoa1207756.
72. Nan H, Hutter CM, Lin Y, Jacobs EJ, Ulrich CM, White E, et al. Association of aspirin and NSAID use with risk of colorectal cancer according to genetic variants. *JAMA.* 2015;313(11):1133–42. doi: 10.1001/jama.2015.1815.
73. Jeon J, Du M, Schoen RE, Hoffmeister M, Newcomb PA, Berndt SI, et al. Colorectal Transdisciplinary S, Genetics, Epidemiology of Colorectal Cancer C. Determining risk of colorectal cancer and starting age of screening based on lifestyle, environmental, and genetic factors. *Gastroenterology.* 2018. doi: 10.1053/j.gastro.2018.02.021.
74. Jain D. Regulation of digital healthcare in India: ethical and legal challenges. *Healthcare.* 2023 Mar;11(6):911. MDPI.
75. Maaß L, Freye M, Pan CC, Dassow HH, Niess J, Jahnel T. The definitions of health apps and medical apps from the perspective of public health and law: qualitative analysis of an interdisciplinary literature overview. *JMIR mHealth and uHealth.* 2022;10(10):e37980.
76. Al Meslamani AZ. Technical and regulatory challenges of digital health implementation in developing countries. *Journal of Medical Economics.* 2023;26(1):1057–60.
77. Babalola O. Nigeria's data protection legal and institutional model: an overview. *International Data Privacy Law.* 2022;12(1):44–52.
78. Chaipipat S. ASEAN governance on data privacy: challenges to regional protection of data privacy and personal data in cyberspace.
79. Anjana RM, Pradeepa R, Deepa M, Jebarani S, Venkatesan U, Parvathi SJ, et al. Acceptability and utilization of newer technologies and effects on glycemic control in type 2 diabetes: lessons learned from lockdown. *Diabetes Technol Ther.* 2020;22(7):527–34.
80. Caetano R, Silva AB, Guedes ACCM, Paiva CCND, Ribeiro GDR, Santos DL, Silva RMD. Challenges and opportunities for telehealth during the COVID-19 pandemic: ideas on spaces and initiatives in the Brazilian context. *Cadernos de Saúde Pública.* 2020;36:e00088920.
81. Yehualashet DE, Seboka BT, Tesfa GA, Demeke AD, Amede ES. Barriers to the adoption of electronic medical record system in Ethiopia: a systematic review. *J Multidiscip Healthc.* 2021;2597–603.
82. Jain S, Agarwal A, Bhardwaj A, Lakshmi PVM, Singh M, Chauhan A, Singh M. Remote monitoring and holistic care of home-isolated COVID-19 positive healthcare workers through digital technology during the omicron (B1.1.529) wave: a prospective cohort study from India. *Front Public Health.* 2022;10:936000.
83. Adeloye D, David RA, Olaogun AA, Auta A, Adesokan A, Gadanya M, et al. Health workforce and governance: the crisis in Nigeria. *Hum Resour Health.* 2017;15:1–8.
84. Bressan T, Valdivia-Gago A, Silvera-Ccallo RM, Llanos-Cuentas A, Condor DF, Padilla-Huamantinco PG, et al. Challenges of design, implementation, acceptability, and potential for biomedical technologies in the Peruvian Amazon. *Int J Equity Health.* 2022;21(1):183.
85. Malkin R, Keane A. Evidence-based approach to the maintenance of laboratory and medical equipment in resource-poor settings. *Med Biol Eng Comput.* 2010;48:721–6.
86. Labrique AB, Vasudevan L, Kochi E, Fabricant R, Mehl G. mHealth innovations as health system strengthening tools: 12 common applications and a visual framework. *Global Health Sci Pract.* 2013;1(2):160–71.
87. World Health Organization (WHO). WHO developing guidelines for recommendations on digital health interventions for RMNCAH and health systems strengthening; 2019. Accessed Jan. 19, 2019. Available from: https://who.int/reproductivehealth/topics/mhealth/digital-health-interventions/en/

88. Rambaud-Althaus C, Shao A, Samaka J, Swai N, Perri S, Kahama-Maro J, et al. Performance of health workers using an electronic algorithm for the management of childhood illness in Tanzania: a pilot implementation study. *Am J Trop Med Hyg.* 2017;96(1):249.
89. Mitchell M, Hedt-Gauthier BL, Msellemu D, Nkaka M, Lesh N. Using electronic technology to improve clinical care–results from a before-after cluster trial to evaluate assessment and classification of sick children according to Integrated Management of Childhood Illness (IMCI) protocol in Tanzania. *BMC Med Inform Decis Mak.* 2013;13:1–8.
90. Perri-Moore S, Routen T, Shao AF, Rambaud-Althaus C, Swai N, Kahama-Maro J, et al. Using an eIMCI-derived decision support protocol to improve provider–caretaker communication for treatment of children under 5 in Tanzania. *Global Health Commun.* 2015;1(1):41–7.
91. Mitchell M, Lesh N, Cranmer H, Fraser H, Haivas I, Wolf K. Improving care–improving access: the use of electronic decision support with AIDS patients in South Africa. *Int J Healthc Technol Manag.* 2009;10(3):156–68.
92. Wyber R, Vaillancourt S, Perry W, Mannava P, Folaranmi T, Celi LA. Big data in global health: improving health in low-and middle-income countries. *Bull World Health Organ.* 2015;93:203–8.
93. Bram JT, Warwick-Clark B, Obeysekare E, Mehta K. Utilization and monetization of healthcare data in developing countries. *Big Data.* 2015;3(2):59–66.
94. Board on Population Health, Public Health Practice, Committee on a National Surveillance System for Cardiovascular, & Select Chronic Diseases. *A nationwide framework for surveillance of cardiovascular and chronic lung diseases.* National Academies Press; 2011.
95. Were MC. Challenges in digital medicine applications in under-resourced settings. *Nat Commun.* 2022;13:3020.

9

Polymerase Chain Reaction: A New Paradigm in Diagnosis

Blay Kwofie, Deborah Clotworthy, Emmanuel Kwaku Ofori, Benedicta Quaye, Benedicta Obenewaa Dankyi, and Seth Kwabena Amponsah

9.1 Introduction

Before the advent of molecular techniques, diagnostic tools relied heavily on culture-based methods, biochemical assays, and immunoassays, each with limitations in sensitivity, specificity, and precision [1]. Developed by the 1993 Nobel Prize winner Mullis, the polymerase chain reaction (PCR) has since become an indispensable tool in biomolecular sciences and is renowned for its applications in genetics [2]. PCR involves the denaturation and renaturation of short segments of deoxyribonucleic acid (DNA) or ribonucleic acid (RNA) sequences using DNA polymerase I enzyme. PCR has become the cornerstone of modern healthcare and provides important information for disease detection, monitoring, and treatment. The ability of PCR to amplify specific segments of DNA or RNA has transformed diagnostics, allowing for unprecedented precision in identifying pathogens, detecting genetic mutations, and quantifying disease progression [3]. This chapter will explore the principles, technical aspects, applications, and future of PCR as a diagnostic tool, highlighting its pivotal role in reshaping molecular diagnostics.

9.2 Principles of PCR

PCR involves the amplification of nucleic acids. The process entails denaturation and renaturation of short DNA or RNA sequences. There may be several cycles amplifying a specific DNA sequence using two complementary oligonucleotide primers flanking the target region. PCR allows for the in vitro detection and amplification of DNA sequences through enzymatic reactions [4, 5]. Each cycle consists of three main steps as depicted in Figure 9.1:

A. **Denaturation**: The double-stranded DNA template is separated into two single strands by heating to approximately 93–94°C. This high temperature breaks the hydrogen bonds between the strands.
B. **Annealing**: The temperature is then lowered to around 50–65°C, enabling the primers (short, synthetic DNA sequences) to bind (or anneal) to their complementary sequences on the single-stranded DNA.
C. **Extension**: DNA polymerase, typically Taq polymerase (derived from the thermophilic bacterium *Thermus aquaticus*), extends the primers by adding nucleotides to synthesize new strands of DNA. This step occurs at a temperature of 72°C, which is optimal for the activity of Taq polymerase.

DOI: 10.1201/9781003486909-9

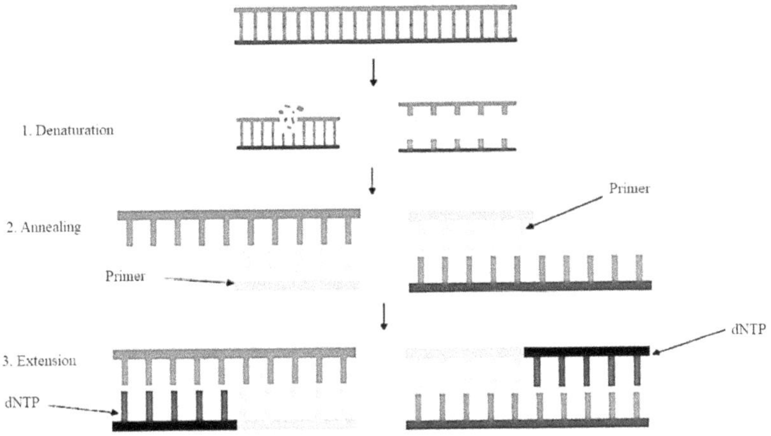

FIGURE 9.1 Steps in conventional polymerase chain reaction.

PCR amplification occurs when the nucleic acid template is combined with a mixture which includes thermostable DNA polymerase, two specific primers, magnesium chloride (which serves as a cofactor for the enzyme), deoxynucleotide triphosphates (dNTPs), and buffering agents. The primers are synthetic single-stranded oligonucleotides and are complementary to the forward and reverse strands of the target DNA, referred to as forward and reverse primers. The reaction is subjected to a series of temperature changes, starting with the denaturation step, where the double-stranded DNA template is heated to over 90°C to separate the strands. Next, the temperature is lowered to allow the primers to anneal (bind) to complementary sequences on the single-stranded DNA, which depends on the melting temperature of the primers. This is followed by the extension step, where the DNA polymerase extends the primers from their 3′ ends, synthesizing new DNA strands in the 5′ to 3′ direction [6]. In the early days of PCR technology, polymerases which were not thermostable were used, meaning more enzymes had to be added during each amplification cycle. This necessitated the introduction of thermostable DNA polymerase thus making PCR more reliable and forming the basis for how it is used today in research and diagnostics [7].

Primers are present in excess in the reaction mix to ensure they bind to the target sequences rather than to each other or the template strands. During the first PCR cycle, the original DNA template serves as the only template for amplification. In the second cycle, target fragments flanked by the primers begin to form, and by the third cycle, these fragments are available as templates for further amplification. Throughout the cycles, the amount of the target DNA sequence can become 25–30 times more abundant in the products compared to the initial amount, and the DNA can multiply exponentially, potentially resulting in millions of copies [8].

9.3 Variations of PCR

Since its invention, PCR has evolved significantly, leading to several variations that cater for different diagnostic needs. Aside conventional PCR used in diagnostics, real-time PCR, digital PCR, reverse transcription PCR, nested PCR, and multiplex PCR are other variations of PCR (Figure 9.2). Each of these PCR types has its own strengths and is chosen based on the specific diagnostic requirements, such as sensitivity needs, quantification requirements, or the complexity of the target being analyzed. Results from conventional PCR are visualized after the reaction is complete, typically using gel electrophoresis. As a primarily qualitative procedure, conventional PCR is used for detecting the presence or absence of a specific DNA sequence [9, 10].

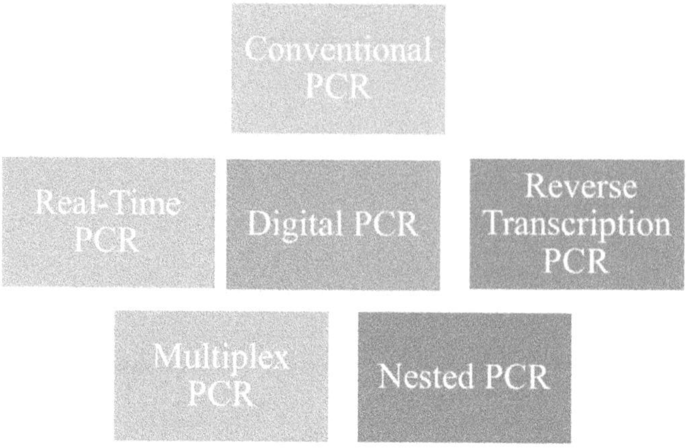

FIGURE 9.2 Variations of polymerase chain reaction.

9.3.1 Real-Time or Quantitative PCR

Unlike conventional PCR, real-time or quantitative PCR (qPCR) measures fluorescence after each PCR cycle to monitor the amplification of DNA. At the initial stages, the fluorescence may be too weak to distinguish from background noise. As amplification progresses, the intensity of fluorescence increases and becomes detectable, indicating the presence of DNA amplicons. The technique offers superior sensitivity, detecting even trace amounts of nucleic acids, and provides accurate quantification of initial template amounts. These features make qPCR an indispensable tool across diverse fields, from basic research to clinical diagnostics [11].

Despite its widespread use, qPCR has several limitations. The use of standard curves for quantification may introduce errors and potentially lead to false positives. Additionally, variations in experimental conditions, reagents, instruments, and data analysis can result in inconsistent results between laboratories. These challenges have led to the development of more advanced PCR techniques [12]

9.3.2 Digital PCR

Digital PCR (dPCR) addresses many of the limitations of qPCR by offering absolute quantification without the need for standard curves. This innovative approach represents a significant advancement in PCR technology, providing enhanced sensitivity and precision. In dPCR, the sample is partitioned into numerous nanoscale droplets, with each randomly containing zero or one copy of the target DNA. After amplification, fluorescence intensity is measured in each compartment, with positive reactions scored as 1 and negatives scored as 0 (Figure 9.3). This binary scoring system, combined with Poisson statistics, enables precise calculation of initial copy numbers. This approach grants dPCR unprecedented sensitivity, allowing absolute quantification from minute amounts of target DNA without the need for standard curves. As a result, dPCR has emerged as a powerful molecular tool, offering unparalleled precision in quantifying low-abundance targets or rare genetic variants [13].

9.3.3 Reverse transcription PCR

Reverse transcription PCR (RT-PCR) is a variation of the conventional PCR. It enables the amplification and analysis of RNA. This method has become indispensable in molecular biology and diagnostics, particularly for studying gene expression and detecting RNA viruses. The RT-PCR process occurs in two main steps. First, the target RNA is converted into complementary DNA (cDNA) using an enzyme called reverse transcriptase. This step effectively transforms the unstable RNA into more stable DNA, which can then undergo standard PCR amplification. Once the cDNA is created, traditional PCR techniques are applied to amplify the target sequence, allowing for its detection and analysis. RT-PCR has proven

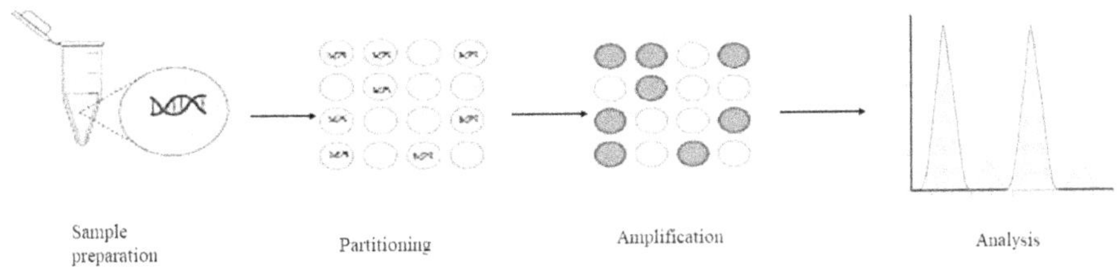

FIGURE 9.3 Steps in digital PCR.

invaluable in detecting RNA viruses. Notable examples include its use in testing human immunodeficiency virus (HIV) and, more recently, its critical role in diagnosing severe acute respiratory syndrome coronavirus 2 (SARS-CoV-2) infections during the coronavirus disease 2019 (COVID-19) pandemic.

Furthermore, RT-PCR can be combined with qPCR technology, resulting in a technique known as reverse transcription quantitative PCR (RT-qPCR). This powerful variant allows for the real-time quantitative analysis of RNA, offering a more precise measurement of gene expression or viral load. The versatility and sensitivity of RT-PCR and its variants have made it an essential tool in molecular biology, diagnostics, and biomedical research [14].

9.3.4 Multiplex PCR

Multiplex PCR allows the simultaneous amplification of multiple target sequences in a single reaction. The process uses multiple primer pairs to amplify different targets concurrently allowing the detection of multiple pathogens or genetic markers in a single test. As an advantage, this variation of PCR saves time and resources, and is especially useful in complex diagnostic scenarios [15].

9.3.5 Nested PCR

This is a two-step process designed to increase sensitivity and specificity. Nested PCR involves two sets of PCR reactions, with the second reaction using primers that bind within the first PCR product. It is particularly useful for detecting very low copy number targets or for improving specificity in complex samples; however, there is a higher risk of contamination due to the two-step process [16].

9.4 Application of PCR in Diagnostics

PCR has revolutionized diagnostic practices across various fields, from infectious diseases to genetic disorders. Its ability to amplify specific DNA or RNA sequences makes it invaluable for detecting and quantifying genetic material with high sensitivity and specificity.

9.4.1 Detection of Infectious Disease Pathogens

PCR is widely used for detecting and identifying pathogens which cause infectious diseases. The technique offers rapid and accurate diagnosis, even in cases where pathogens are present in low quantities. PCR is used to identify bacteria such as *Mycobacterium tuberculosis*, the causative agent of tuberculosis (TB). It can detect specific genetic markers of the bacteria, which is crucial for early diagnosis and treatment [17]. For example, the GeneXpert MTB/RIF assay is a PCR-based test that does not only detect TB but also identifies rifampicin resistance [18]. PCR is also essential in detecting viral infections, including HIV, hepatitis B and C, and SARS-CoV-2 [19–21]. In the case of HIV, PCR detects viral RNA in blood samples, which is critical for diagnosing infection, monitoring viral load, and assessing treatment efficacy [22]. The real-time PCR assay used during the COVID-19 pandemic enabled rapid identification of infected individuals, significantly impacting public health responses [23].

9.4.2 Genetic Disorder Screening

PCR plays an important role in diagnosing genetic disorders by amplifying and analyzing specific genes or mutations associated with certain disease conditions. For conditions such as cystic fibrosis, Duchenne muscular dystrophy, and sickle cell anemia, PCR can detect mutations in the relevant genes [24–26]. In cystic fibrosis, PCR can identify deletions in the cystic fibrosis transmembrane conductance (CFTR) gene, allowing for early diagnosis and management [27]. Non-invasive prenatal testing using PCR techniques can detect fetal DNA in maternal blood, and this can aid in the screening of conditions such as Down syndrome and other chromosomal abnormalities. This method provides a safer alternative to invasive procedures like amniocentesis [28].

9.4.3 Cancer Diagnostics and Monitoring

PCR is extensively used in oncology for the detection, diagnosis, and monitoring of cancer. PCR can detect specific genetic mutations and gene expressions associated with different types of cancer. For instance, PCR assays can identify the BCR-ABL fusion gene in chronic myeloid leukemia, guiding diagnosis and treatment decisions. PCR is employed to monitor minimal residual disease in cancer patients [29]. This involves detecting low levels of cancer cells that remain after treatment, which can indicate relapse. PCR-based measurable residual disease assays are used for various hematologic malignancies, including leukemia and lymphoma [30].

9.4.4 Forensic Science Application

In forensic science, PCR is used for DNA profiling and identification. PCR enables the amplification and analysis of DNA from crime scene samples, which can be compared to DNA profiles of suspects or databases. This has been instrumental in solving crimes and exonerating the innocent. In mass disasters, PCR can help identify victims from degraded or fragmented DNA samples. The technique aids in matching DNA profiles from victims to their relatives or existing records [31, 32].

9.5 Future Directions

So far, PCR technology has been marked by continuous innovations aimed at enhancing its efficiency, accessibility, and scope. Thus, it is expected that newer innovations would be added in the near future. One significant trend is the development of point-of-care (POC) PCR systems that allow for rapid and on-site testing. These systems are designed to be compact, user-friendly, and capable of delivering results within minutes. Portable PCR devices could revolutionize diagnostics in remote or underserved areas, providing real-time results for infectious disease detection and other applications [33].

Digital PCR is poised to become a standard tool in precision medicine due to its ability to provide absolute quantification of nucleic acids with high sensitivity. Future developments may focus on expanding its use in high-throughput settings, allowing for simultaneous analysis of large numbers of samples or targets. This could be particularly valuable in genomic research, cancer monitoring, and epidemiological studies [34].

The integration of artificial intelligence (AI) and machine learning (ML) with PCR data analysis holds promise for improving diagnostic accuracy and predictive capabilities. AI algorithms can analyze complex PCR data to identify patterns and make predictions about disease progression or treatment outcomes. This fusion of technologies could lead to more personalized and effective healthcare solutions [35].

9.6 Conclusion

PCR has undeniably transformed diagnostic sciences, offering rapid, sensitive, and accurate detection of nucleic acids. From its application in detecting infectious diseases to its role in personalized cancer treatment and forensics, PCR has made a profound impact on modern medicine. As advancements in PCR technology continue to unfold, its applications will expand, ushering new possibilities for diagnosis and treatment in healthcare. The future of diagnostics lies in the continuous evolution of techniques like PCR, ensuring better healthcare outcomes for patients worldwide.

REFERENCES

1. Buchan BW, Ledeboer NA. Emerging technologies for the clinical microbiology laboratory. *Clin Microbiol Rev.* 2014;27:783–822. https://doi.org/10.1128/CMR.00003-14.
2. Julin D. Polymerase chain reaction. *Molecular life sciences.* Springer; 2014. p. 1–3. https://doi.org/10.1007/978-1-4614-6436-5_95-4.
3. Yang S, Rothman RE. PCR-based diagnostics for infectious diseases: uses, limitations, and future applications in acute-care settings. *Lancet Infect Dis.* 2004;4:337–48. https://doi.org/10.1016/S1473-3099(04)01044-8.
4. Kadri K. Polymerase chain reaction (PCR): principle and applications. In: *Synthetic biology - new interdisciplinary science.* IntechOpen; 2020. https://doi.org/10.5772/intechopen.86491.
5. Valones MAA, Guimarães RL, Brandão LAC, Souza PRE de, Carvalho A de AT, Crovela S. Principles and applications of polymerase chain reaction in medical diagnostic fields: a review. *Braz J Microbiol.* 2009;40:1–11. https://doi.org/10.1590/S1517-83822009000100001.
6. Lorenz TC. Polymerase chain reaction: basic protocol plus troubleshooting and optimization strategies. *J Vis Exp.* 2012. https://doi.org/10.3791/3998.
7. Pestana EA, Belak S, Diallo A, Crowther JR, Viljoen GJ. Traditional PCR. *Early, rapid and sensitive veterinary molecular diagnostics - real time PCR applications.* Springer Netherlands; 2009. p. 9–25. https://doi.org/10.1007/978-90-481-3132-7_2.
8. Garibyan L, Avashia N. Polymerase chain reaction. *J Investig Dermatol.* 2013;133:1–4. https://doi.org/10.1038/jid.2013.1.
9. Adams G. A beginner's guide to RT-PCR, qPCR and RT-qPCR. *Biochem (Lond).* 2020;42:48–53. https://doi.org/10.1042/BIO20200034.
10. Shah NJ. Polymerase chain reaction. In: *Introduction to basics of pharmacology and toxicology.* Springer Singapore; 2019. p. 395–7. https://doi.org/10.1007/978-981-32-9779-1_31.
11. Kralik P, Ricchi M. A basic guide to real-time PCR in microbial diagnostics: definitions, parameters, and everything. *Front Microbiol.* 2017;8. https://doi.org/10.3389/fmicb.2017.00108.
12. Smith CJ, Osborn AM. Advantages and limitations of quantitative PCR (Q-PCR)-based approaches in microbial ecology. *FEMS Microbiol Ecol.* 2009;67:6–20. https://doi.org/10.1111/j.1574-6941.2008.00629.x.
13. Nazir S. Medical diagnostic value of digital PCR (dPCR): a systematic review. *Biomed Eng Adv.* 2023;6:100092. https://doi.org/10.1016/j.bea.2023.100092.
14. Ohan NW, Heikkila JJ. Reverse transcription-polymerase chain reaction: an overview of the technique and its applications. *Biotechnol Adv.* 1993;11:13–29. https://doi.org/10.1016/0734-9750(93)90408-F.
15. Elnifro EM, Ashshi AM, Cooper RJ, Klapper PE. Multiplex PCR: optimization and application in diagnostic virology. *Clin Microbiol Rev.* 2000;13:559–70. https://doi.org/10.1128/CMR.13.4.559-570.2000.
16. Green MR, Sambrook J. Nested polymerase chain reaction (PCR). *Cold Spring Harb Protoc.* 2019;2019:pdb.prot095182. https://doi.org/10.1101/pdb.prot095182.
17. Ahmed N, Mohanty AK, Mukhopadhyay U, Batish VK, Grover S. PCR-based rapid detection of Mycobacterium tuberculosis in blood from immunocompetent patients with pulmonary tuberculosis. *J Clin Microbiol.* 1998;36:3094–5. https://doi.org/10.1128/JCM.36.10.3094-3095.1998.
18. Zeka AN, Tasbakan S, Cavusoglu C. Evaluation of the GeneXpert MTB/RIF assay for rapid diagnosis of tuberculosis and detection of rifampin resistance in pulmonary and extrapulmonary specimens. *J Clin Microbiol.* 2011;49:4138–41. https://doi.org/10.1128/JCM.05434-11.

19. Lakshmi V, Sudha T, Rakhi D, Anilkumar G, Dandona L. Application of polymerase chain reaction to detect HIV-1 DNA in pools of dried blood spots. *Indian J Microbiol.* 2011;51:147–52. https://doi.org/10.1007/s12088-011-0135-0.
20. Filchakova O, Dossym D, Ilyas A, Kuanysheva T, Abdizhamil A, Bukasov R. Review of COVID-19 testing and diagnostic methods. *Talanta.* 2022;244:123409. https://doi.org/10.1016/j.talanta.2022.123409.
21. Brechot C. Polymerase chain reaction for the diagnosis of viral hepatitis B and C. *Gut.* 1993;34:S39–44. https://doi.org/10.1136/gut.34.2_Suppl.S39.
22. Bosevska G, Panovski N, Dokić E, Grunevska V. RT-PCR detection of HIV in Republic of Macedonia. *Bosn J Basic Med Sci.* 2008;8:350–5. https://doi.org/10.17305/bjbms.2008.2896.
23. Artika IM, Dewi YP, Nainggolan IM, Siregar JE, Antonjaya U. Real-time polymerase chain reaction: current techniques, applications, and role in COVID-19 diagnosis. *Genes (Basel).* 2022;13:2387. https://doi.org/10.3390/genes13122387.
24. Iskandar K, Dwianingsih EK, Pratiwi L, Kalim AS, Mardhiah H, Putranti AH, et al. The analysis of DMD gene deletions by multiplex PCR in Indonesian DMD/BMD patients: the era of personalized medicine. *BMC Res Notes.* 2019;12:704. https://doi.org/10.1186/s13104-019-4730-1.
25. Schwartz KM, Pike-Buchanan LL, Muralidharan K, Redman JB, Wilson JA, Jarvis M, et al. Identification of cystic fibrosis variants by polymerase chain reaction/oligonucleotide ligation assay. *J Mol Diagn.* 2009;11:211–5. https://doi.org/10.2353/jmoldx.2009.080106.
26. Singh PJ, Shrivastava AC, Shrikhande AV. Prenatal diagnosis of sickle cell disease by the technique of PCR. *Indian J Hematol Blood Transfus.* 2015;31:233–41. https://doi.org/10.1007/s12288-014-0427-8.
27. Hantash FM, Milunsky A, Wang Z, Anderson B, Sun W, Anguiano A, et al. A large deletion in the CFTR gene in CBAVD. *Genet Med.* 2006;8:93–5. https://doi.org/10.1097/01.gim.0000200945.54234.d7.
28. D'Aversa E, Breveglieri G, Boutou E, Balassopoulou A, Voskaridou E, Pellegatti P, et al. Droplet digital PCR for non-invasive prenatal detection of fetal single-gene point mutations in maternal plasma. *Int J Mol Sci.* 2022;23:2819. https://doi.org/10.3390/ijms23052819.
29. Jennings LJ, George D, Czech J, Yu M, Joseph L. Detection and quantification of BCR-ABL1 fusion transcripts by droplet digital PCR. *J Mol Diagn.* 2014;16:174–9. https://doi.org/10.1016/j.jmoldx.2013.10.007.
30. Chen J, Gale RP, Hu Y, Yan W, Wang T, Zhang W. Measurable residual disease (MRD)-testing in hematological and solid cancers. *Leukemia.* 2024;38:1202–12. https://doi.org/10.1038/s41375-024-02252-4.
31. McDonald C, Taylor D, Linacre A. PCR in forensic science: a critical review. *Genes (Basel).* 2024;15:438. https://doi.org/10.3390/genes15040438.
32. Budowle B, Sajantila A, Hochmeister MN, Comey CT. The application of PCR to forensic science. In: *The polymerase chain reaction.* Birkhäuser Boston; 1994. p. 244–56. https://doi.org/10.1007/978-1-4612-0257-8_21.
33. Zhu H, Zhang H, Xu Y, Laššáková S, Korabečná M, Neužil P. PCR past, present and future. *Biotechniques.* 2020;69:317–25. https://doi.org/10.2144/btn-2020-0057.
34. Sancha Dominguez L, Cotos Suárez A, Sánchez Ledesma M, Muñoz Bellido JL. Present and future applications of digital PCR in infectious diseases diagnosis. *Diagnostics.* 2024;14:931. https://doi.org/10.3390/diagnostics14090931.
35. Langer T, Favarato M, Giudici R, Bassi G, Garberi R, Villa F, et al. Development of machine learning models to predict RT-PCR results for severe acute respiratory syndrome coronavirus 2 (SARS-CoV-2) in patients with influenza-like symptoms using only basic clinical data. *Scand J Trauma Resusc Emerg Med.* 2020;28:113. https://doi.org/10.1186/s13049-020-00808-8.

10

Diagnostic Utility of Magnetic Resonance Imaging

Derick Seyram Sule and Godwill Acquah

10.1 Introduction

The primary benefits of magnetic resonance imaging (MRI) over other imaging modalities are its capacity to identify soft tissue lesions, whether they are located inside or outside of bone, and its three-dimensional lesion visualization capability. MRI creates high-resolution images using radio waves and strong magnetic fields instead of other imaging methods that employ ionizing radiation. This capability makes MRI particularly useful in diagnosing various conditions, from neurological disorders to musculoskeletal injuries. The functional capabilities of MRI include but are not limited to functional MRI (fMRI), real-time MRI, interventional MRI, molecular imaging, parallel MRI, quantitative MRI, magnetic resonance spectroscopy (MRS), and hyperpolarized gas MRI.

10.1.1 Functional MRI

By identifying variations in blood flow, a specialized method called functional magnetic resonance imaging (fMRI) maps and quantifies brain activity [1]. It is frequently utilized to study neurological disorders and brain function in research and therapeutic settings. Regarding pre-surgical planning for patients with brain tumors or epilepsy, fMRI is very helpful since it may identify and retain important functional domains including language, motor abilities, and sensory processing [2]. Mapping these areas enables surgeons to minimize the risk of postoperative deficits. Additionally, fMRI is used to study cognitive processes, including memory, attention, and emotion, providing insights into normal brain function and the effects of various neurological and psychiatric conditions [3]. Research applications of fMRI include understanding brain plasticity, studying the effects of neuropsychiatric disorders, and evaluating the impact of therapies [4]. The non-invasive nature of fMRI, combined with its ability to generate real-time functional information, makes it a powerful tool for advancing our understanding of the human brain and improving patient care.

10.1.2 Real-time MRI

Continuous real-time imaging of anatomical structures in motion, like the heart, is referred to as real-time magnetic resonance imaging. Based on radial Fast Low-Angle Shot Magnetic Resonance Imaging (FLASH MRI) and iterative algorithms, this approach is one of many that have been developed since the early 2000s. This results in images with an in-plane resolution between 1.5 mm and 2.0 mm with a temporal resolution between 20 ms and 30 ms [5]. Although FLASH MRI produces worse contrast of images between the myocardial and blood pool, balanced Steady-State Free Precession (bSSFP) imaging causes extreme banding artifacts when the magnetic field heterogeneity is strong. In the past, real-time MRI was feasible only with low image quality or low temporal resolution since MRI is based on the laborious scanning of k-space. These restrictions have lately been removed owing to an iterative reconstruction

DOI: 10.1201/9781003486909-10

approach now being used. Real-time MRI holds great potential to provide valuable insights into musculoskeletal and cardiac disorders. In numerous instances, patients may now find MRI exams becoming simpler and more comfortable. Real-time MRI may offer valuable information on heart and joint problems and, in many situations, make MRI exams more comfortable and easy for patients, particularly those with arrhythmias or difficulty holding their breath [6].

10.1.3 Interventional MRI

MRI is a good option for interventional radiology because it doesn't negatively affect the patient or the operator. During interventional MRI, the images generated by the MRI scanner are used to guide less invasive procedures. These less invasive procedures don't require any ferromagnetic equipment [7]. Intraoperative MRI, in which an MRI is used during surgery, is a specialized and expanding subset of interventional MRI. Concurrent imaging with the surgical operation is possible with certain sophisticated MRI equipment. Usually, an MRI is used to evaluate the procedure's success or direct further surgical work, therefore the surgical process is briefly stopped [8]. Interventional magnetic resonance imaging is frequently used to guide heat ablation of tissue, remove tumors, take lesion samples, and perform other treatments. It is frequently employed in neurosurgery, where a patient's prognosis might vary depending on every millimeter of tissue preserved after operation [7].

10.1.4 Molecular Imaging By MRI

MRI is highly recommended for morphological and functional imaging and has very high spatial resolution. However, MRI does have a number of drawbacks. Initially, MRI's sensitivity can be highly restrictive compared to other imaging modalities, which ranges between 10^{-3} mol/L and 10^{-5} mol/L [9]. The extremely tiny population difference between the nuclear spin states at ambient temperature accounts for this. For instance, the difference between the high- and low-energy states is around 9 mol/2 million at 1.5 Tesla, which in clinical MRI is the normal magnetic field (BO) strength [9]. Enhancements to augment BO intensity and induce hyperpolarization through optical pumping or dynamic nuclear polarization are two ways to enhance magnetic resonance sensitivity. Numerous chemical exchange-based signal amplification techniques are available to further boost sensitivity [9]. A high degree of specificity and relaxivity (sensitivity) in targeted MRI contrast agents is necessary to obtain molecular imaging of disease biomarkers by MRI. A great deal of research has been done to enable molecular imaging by MRI and create targeted MRI contrast agents. Typically, targeting is accomplished by using small protein domains, antibodies, peptides, and tiny ligands. These targeting moieties are typically coupled to high payload or high relaxivity MRI contrast agents to increase the contrast agents' sensitivity [10]. A novel group of gene-targeting magnetic resonance contrast media has been developed to highlight the distinct mRNA and gene transcription factor protein gene actions [11, 12]. Viral, mRNA, and microRNA-specific cells may all be traced using these novel contrast agents, which can also detect a living brain's tissue reaction to inflammation [13]. According to TaqMan analysis, optical, and electron microscopy, the MR indicates a change in gene expression that is positively correlated [14].

10.1.5 Parallel MRI

Using successive applications of magnetic field gradients to collect MRI data is time-consuming. The gradient switching rate has physiological and physical limits, even for the most efficient MRI sequences [15, 16]. Parallel MRI gets around these restrictions by collecting part of the data concurrently rather than sequentially as is customary. Broadband radiofrequency (RF) detector coil arrays, each featuring a different depiction of the body, are used to achieve this. By using a smaller number of gradient steps, the residual spatial data is completed by merging signals from different coils according to their established patterns of spatial sensitivity [15]. Parallel MRI can be used to achieve 2–4 times the initial acceleration with suitable coil array configurations, and significantly higher accelerations have been demonstrated with specialized coil arrays [15]. The main limitations are the total number of coils and the signal-to-noise ratio, which decreases with increasing acceleration [15, 16].

Following the introduction of the Simultaneous Acquisition of Spatial Harmonics (SMASH) technology in 1997, parallel imaging was the subject of much research and application. Prior to this, the MRI field largely ignored numerous early recommendations for using detector arrays to accelerate imaging [15]. The parallel imaging techniques that are now most often used in medical practice are Generalized Autocalibrating Partially Parallel Acquisitions (GRAPPA) and SENSitivity Encoding (SENSE) [16, 17]. Since the introduction of parallel MRI, a significant amount of research and development has been conducted on RF coil design and image reconstruction. Additionally, the number of receiver channels accessible on commercial MR systems has rapidly increased. Nowadays, a variety of anatomical structure investigations and research procedures use parallel MRI on a regular basis [16].

10.1.6 Quantitative MRI

The primary goal of most MRIs is to obtain spatial maps of relative differences in signal strength that are "weighted" by specific parameters [18]. This allows for the qualitative interpretation of MR data. Rather than using qualitative approaches, quantitative methods aim to quantify specific geographical features or create spatial maps with accurate tissue relaxometry parameter values and magnetic fields [18].

T1-mapping, which is mostly utilized in cardiac magnetic resonance imaging, is one example of a quantitative MRI technique [19]; T2-mapping [20]; the process of mapping quantitative susceptibility (QSM); certain forms of cerebrospinal fluid flow MRI are quantitative fluid flow MRI [21]; and MR elastography (MRE) [22].

Prior to recently, lengthier scan periods were necessary for quantitative MRI, which strives to improve the reliability of MR images and interpretations [18]. Sometimes, multiparametric quantitative MRI – which maps several tissue relaxometry parameters in a single imaging session – is more precisely referred to as quantitative MRI (or qMRI) [23]. Sequences that map many parameters simultaneously have been generated in an attempt to expedite multiparametric quantitative MRI. This has been achieved by fitting the MR signal's evolution to a multiparameter model or using distinct encoding techniques for each parameter in the sequence [24–26].

10.1.7 Magnetic Resonance Spectroscopy

By using a range of single-voxel or imaging-based methods, magnetic resonance spectroscopy (MRS) is utilized to quantify the concentrations of several metabolites in bodily tissues [2]. An isotope being "excited" can have various chemical configurations represented in the resonance spectrum produced by the MR signal. In addition to providing information about tumor metabolism [4], this signature is utilized in the diagnosis of certain metabolic diseases, particularly those that impact the brain.

MRSI, or magnetic resonance spectroscopic imaging, creates spatially localized spectra from within the patient or material by combining both spectroscopic and imaging techniques. Each voxel's spectra include information on several metabolites, despite the significantly reduced spatial resolution (which is restricted by the available SNR) [27]. Higher field strengths are necessary for MRSI to achieve high SNR since the available signal is utilized in encoding spectral and spatial data [27]. Their expensive acquisition and maintenance is a major barrier to the acceptance of MRIs with very high field strengths. Suggested software techniques (like SAMV) that utilize compressed sensing can attain super-resolution even at high field strengths [28].

10.1.8 Hyperpolarized Gas MRI

Hyperpolarized gases are used to increase the sensitivity and spatial resolution of MRI, which is often referred to as hyperpolarized helium-3 MRI or HPHe-3 MRI. Imaging the lungs and other body parts with low tissue density is just one of the possible medical uses of this imaging technique. Nowadays, spirometric pulmonary function testing (PFT) is the gold standard for identifying lung illnesses and tracking their trajectory. However, these tests are typically not sensitive enough to identify functional alterations in the gas exchange areas and small airways; instead, they only evaluate the lung as a whole. This insensitivity has earned these areas the moniker "silent zone"[1].

Due to the reduced number of water molecules containing protons that the magnetic field can activate, traditional magnetic resonance imaging produces subpar images of lung tissue. Lung ventilation abnormalities can be detected using an MRI scan using hyperpolarized gas. Prior to the scan, the patient is instructed to breathe in a mixture of hyperpolarized xenon and either nitrogen or helium buffer gas. Compared to a typical MRI, the resultant lung images are of far greater quality.

10.2 Applications of MRI in Medical Specialties

10.2.1 Neuroimaging

MRI is a cornerstone of neuroimaging, providing unparalleled detail and clarity in the visualization of the brain and spinal cord. It is especially effective in diagnosing a variety of neurological disorders, including brain tumors, multiple sclerosis, stroke, and neurodegenerative diseases such as Alzheimer's. The ability to produce detailed images of both the brain's structure and function sets MRI apart. Techniques like diffusion-tensor imaging (DTI) and functional MRI (fMRI) offer insights into brain connectivity and activity, respectively [29]. For example, fMRI measures changes in blood flow to different brain areas, indicating neuronal activity and thus enabling the mapping of brain functional areas [30]. This is crucial in pre-surgical planning for brain tumor resections, where it is important to avoid critical areas involved in speech or motor function [31]. Moreover, advanced MRI techniques like perfusion and spectroscopy provide additional layers of information about brain metabolism and physiology, further aiding in the diagnosis and management of complex neurological conditions [32]. The application of MRI images in neuroimaging is shown in Figure 10.1 and Figure 10.2.

10.2.2 Musculoskeletal MRI

MRI excels in musculoskeletal imaging due to its superior contrast resolution and ability to visualize soft tissue structures [33]. It is particularly valuable in diagnosing sports injuries, arthritis, infections, and tumors. For instance, MRI can detect tears in ligaments and tendons, cartilage defects, bone marrow edema, and other soft tissue abnormalities that are not visible on X-rays or CT scans. This detailed imaging is critical for planning surgeries and other interventions. For example, in the diagnosis of Osteochondritis Dissecans (OCD), MRI can determine the stability of the lesion and the condition of the cartilage, guiding treatment decisions between conservative management and surgical intervention [34]. Additionally, MRI is invaluable in assessing chronic conditions like rheumatoid arthritis and osteoarthritis, providing detailed images of joint anatomy, including the synovium, cartilage, and bone [35, 36]. This helps in monitoring disease progression and evaluating the effectiveness of treatments [37].

10.2.3 Cardiovascular Imaging

Cardiovascular MRI (CMR) is a powerful tool for assessing cardiac anatomy and function. It provides high-resolution images of the heart and great vessels, enabling the detailed evaluation of myocardial structure, function, and viability. CMR is particularly useful in diagnosing cardiomyopathies, congenital heart disease, valvular heart disease, and coronary artery disease [38, 39]. For instance, in patients with myocardial infarction, CMR can differentiate between viable and non-viable myocardium, which is crucial for determining the best treatment approach [40]. Techniques such as late gadolinium enhancement (LGE) highlight areas of myocardial scarring, providing essential information for risk stratification and management [41]. Additionally, CMR can assess myocardial perfusion and blood flow, offering insights into ischemic heart disease and guiding revascularization strategies [19]. The ability to visualize blood-flow dynamics without the need for ionizing radiation makes CMR a preferred modality for repeated evaluations and long-term follow-up of cardiac patients.

10.2.4 Abdominal and Pelvic MRI

MRI is highly effective in diagnosing a range of abdominal and pelvic conditions, providing excellent soft tissue contrast and the ability to image in multiple planes. It is particularly useful for evaluating liver lesions, pancreatic disorders, renal masses, and gastrointestinal conditions like Crohn's disease [42]. In liver imaging, MRI with contrast agents like gadolinium can characterize lesions, distinguishing between benign and malignant tumors with high accuracy [43]. For example, hepatocellular carcinoma (HCC) and haemangiomas have distinct enhancement patterns on MRI, aiding in their differentiation [43]. Additionally, MRI is the modality of choice for evaluating pelvic conditions such as uterine fibroids, endometriosis, and ovarian masses [44, 45]. It provides detailed images that guide surgical planning and treatment strategies. For patients with renal impairment, MRI offers a safer alternative to CT, as it does not require nephrotoxic contrast agents [46]. Visualizing structures in multiple planes and providing functional information, such as bowel motility in Crohn's disease, enhances its diagnostic utility [47].

10.2.5 Breast Imaging

MRI has become an indispensable tool in breast imaging, especially for high-risk patients and those with dense breast tissue. It is highly sensitive in detecting breast cancer, often identifying lesions that are not visible on mammography or ultrasound. Breast MRI is used to screen high-risk patients, evaluate the extent of cancer, assess treatment response, and monitor recurrence. The use of contrast-enhanced MRI helps differentiate benign and malignant lesions by analyzing the pattern of contrast uptake and washout. For example, malignant tumors typically show rapid uptake and washout of contrast, whereas benign lesions exhibit different enhancement characteristics [48, 49]. MRI is also valuable in evaluating breast implants for rupture and in planning surgeries, particularly in patients undergoing breast-conserving surgery or mastectomy [50]. Its ability to image the entire breast and adjacent structures in three dimensions provides a comprehensive assessment that enhances surgical planning and treatment outcomes.

10.3 Accuracy and Sensitivity of MRI in Disease Detection

MRI is known for its high accuracy and sensitivity in detecting a wide range of diseases, making it a reliable diagnostic tool in healthcare.

10.3.1 Cerebrovascular Accident (Stroke)

Cerebrovascular accidents (CVAs), commonly known as strokes, are major contributors to global illness and death [51, 52]. The role of MRI in diagnosing CVAs is vital for early detection and treatment. MRI is essential in managing stroke patients by offering detailed brain images that help doctors identify the

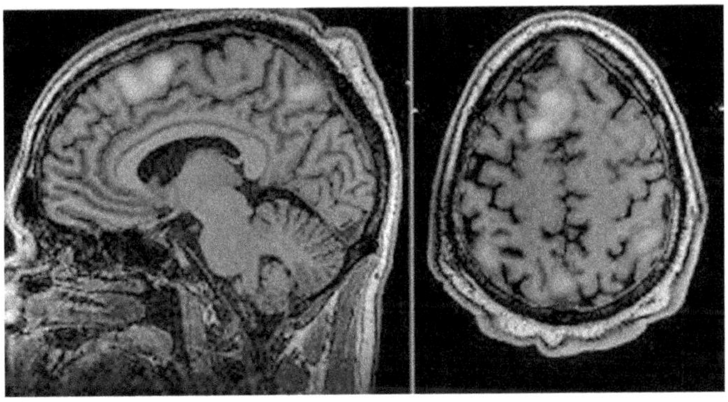

FIGURE 10.1 Diffusion-weighted imagery.

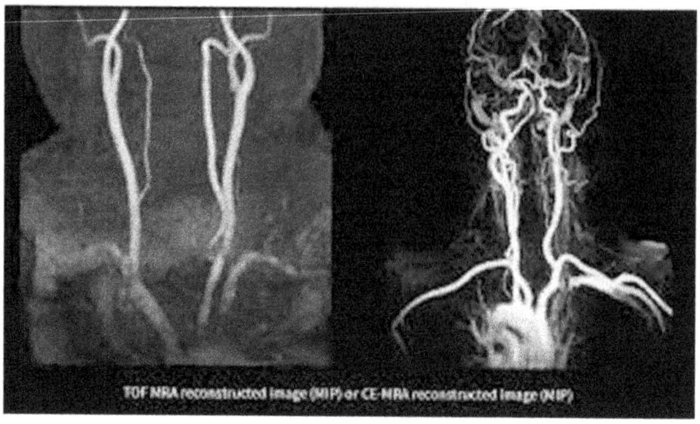

FIGURE 10.2 Images from the time-of-flight (TOF) effect during MRA.

type of stroke and determine the appropriate treatment [51, 52]. MRI is non-invasive, painless, and free from ionizing radiation [53]. It can detect ischemic strokes, which are caused by a sudden drop in blood flow to the brain, and can also visualize the penumbra, the at-risk but not yet damaged brain tissue [51]. MRI provides more accurate diagnoses than other imaging methods. For example, Vessel Wall MRI (VW-MRI) surpasses lumen-based imaging techniques and enhances the etiological assessment of ischemic stroke [51].

MRI's sensitivity, specificity, and accuracy in diagnosing strokes are remarkable [51, 52]. MRI is approximately five times more sensitive and twice as accurate as immediate non-contrast CT for identifying ischemic stroke [53], with a sensitivity of 99% and a specificity of 92% [52]. These statistics highlight MRI's reliability in diagnosing ischemic strokes, which comprise most CVAs [51, 52]. Thus, MRI's high sensitivity and specificity establish it as an essential tool in stroke diagnosis and management [51, 52]. Nonetheless, MRI use must be balanced with factors such as patient safety, resource availability, and time constraints. It is also known to be more complex and time-consuming than CT scans. MRI's diagnostic utility in strokes is substantial, providing detailed and precise information crucial for patient management. Despite its limitations, its advantages in diagnosing and managing strokes are clear.

10.3.2 Lung Nodule

Lung nodules, also called pulmonary nodules, are abnormal lung growths often found during imaging tests. The use of MRI to diagnose lung nodules is an area of ongoing research [54]. MRI is increasingly used to evaluate pulmonary nodules. MRI provides detailed soft tissue images, making it effective for detecting and characterizing lung nodules [55]. MRI can help distinguish between malignant and benign tumors using techniques like diffusion-weighted imaging [54]. However, its use is limited by technical challenges such as low signal-to-noise ratios and motion artifacts [54].

MRI's sensitivity, specificity, and accuracy in diagnosing lung nodules are critical considerations [56]. A meta-analysis indicated that both CT and MRI have high diagnostic accuracy for pulmonary nodules, but CT outperforms MRI in accuracy. Specifically, the detection accuracy in MRI, compared to the reference CT, was 100% for lesions measuring 6 mm or larger, 80% for those between 4 and 6 mm, and 23% for those smaller than 4 mm [56]. These results suggest that while MRI can be helpful in some cases, it may not be as reliable as CT for diagnosing lung nodules. Therefore, the choice of imaging method should depend on the individual patient's situation and available resources. Recent advancements in MRI technology have enhanced its effectiveness in evaluating pulmonary nodules, making it a valuable diagnostic tool despite its limitations. However, MRI cannot currently replace CT in diagnosing these nodules. In conclusion, while MRI shows promise in evaluating lung nodules, further research is needed to fully understand its diagnostic utility compared to other methods like CT.

10.3.3 Spondyloarthritis

Spondyloarthritis (SpA) is a group of complex disorders characterized by inflammatory back pain, primarily affecting younger male patients [57]. The diagnostic utility of MRI in SpA is increasingly recognized [58, 59]. MRI is essential for diagnosing and managing SpA [58, 59]. MRI offers detailed images of the sacroiliac joints (SIJ) and spine, detecting active inflammation, new bone formation, erosive bone damage, and fusion of facet joints. These detailed images allow for more accurate diagnoses than other imaging methods [59]. MRI can identify SIJ changes that appear years before they are visible on radiographs [58].

MRI's sensitivity, specificity, and accuracy in diagnosing SpA are significant [60, 61]. Diagnoses of axial spondyloarthritis with sacroiliitis by MRI have a 97.2% sensitivity and 94.2% specificity when paired with at least one particular clinical characteristic in a young adult with chronic back pain [36]. These high figures indicate that MRI is highly reliable for diagnosing SpA, representing a major field advancement [62]. Therefore, MRI's high sensitivity and specificity make it indispensable for diagnosing and managing SpA. It aids in early detection and guides treatment plans, potentially mitigating the debilitating effects of SpA.

A standardized examination of MR imaging of the SIJ can allow patients with non-specific back pain (NSBP) and those with spondyloarthritis (SpA) to be differentiated from one another [63]. Ordinarily, when young patients present with plain radiographs of the sacroiliac joints and exhibit normal results, it is still challenging to diagnose early spondyloarthritis (SpA). It may take several years for conventional radiography to reveal post-inflammatory structural changes in the SIJ's subchondral bone, despite these changes being there. [64, 65].

Widely acknowledged as the most sensitive imaging technique for sacroiliitis detection – the hallmark of SpA – MRI can identify inflammatory alterations in bone marrow and soft tissues [65]. As a result, before radiography, anomalies in SIJ may be identified. MRI's overall sensitivity and specificity for diagnosing SpA were 0.90 with a positive likelihood ratio (LR+) of 9.0, according to a 2004 systematic literature review [66] that reviewed studies that examined the diagnostic utility of MRI in patients with either established AS or IBP. Since then, this estimation of diagnostic usefulness has been included in clinical practice diagnostic algorithms for SpA diagnosis, which depend on estimations of the extent to which a positive MRI raises the pre-test chance of SpA [66].

However, there are a few reasons why this diagnostic utility estimate needs to be reevaluated. Because dynamic (as opposed to standard) contrast-enhanced magnetic resonance imaging is expensive, unreliable, and not commonly used in clinical practice, most of the studies included in the systematic review did not have age- or sex-matched controls [77–71]. Furthermore, the need to incorporate specific methodological elements into study designs is becoming more widely acknowledged. Examples of these elements include agreement on definitions of abnormalities visible on MRIs, standardization of MR image acquisition and reading techniques, and uniform training and calibration of readers from various sites. These requirements aim to ensure the external validity of study conclusions [69].

First of all, a positive MRI showing sacroiliitis is now considered an acceptable imaging criterion indicative of axial spondyloarthritis [72]. However, this criterion requires the presence of at least one clinical feature of spondyloarthritis. This information was recently published in the Assessment of SpondyloArthritis (ASAS) International Society classification criteria. A working group within ASAS has also put forth a consensus definition of a positive MRI for sacroiliitis, which is based solely on the existence of osteitis on the T1-weighted gadolinium-enhanced sequence (T1 post-Gd) or bone marrow edema on the short tau inversion recovery (STIR) sequence [73].

Many discoveries have consequential clinical impacts on the utilization of MRI in SpA [63]. MRI has substantially more diagnostic usefulness than previously described, as demonstrated by implementing a systematic and consistent method for examining SIJ [63]. Second, individuals with SIJ who have had symptoms for less than a year can still clearly see the early disease course structural alterations. Third, comparatively non-specific BME and fat infiltration that extends into successive slices or is present in more than one SIJ quadrant can happen to healthy, asymptomatic people [63]. Fourth, SpA is somewhat unique when it comes to erosion. The fifth drawback of restricting evaluation to BME is that it can miss important diagnostic data from MR sequences acquired during standard screening [63].

Clinical practice frequently employs MRI protocols that use T1-weighted and STIR sequences to evaluate SIJ in patients with clinically suspected SpA; however, two recent studies found that the evaluation of SIJ in this clinical setting does not benefit from the additional, costly, and prolonged contrast-enhanced MRI sequences over STIR and T1-weighted sequences alone [74]. The primary diagnostic tool for patients exhibiting clinical symptoms of SpA with equivocal radiographs should be T1W and STIR MRI of the SIJ imaged in the tilted coronal orientation [75].

10.3.4 Multiple Sclerosis Lesions

A considerable fraction of lesions in multiple sclerosis (MS) are found in the cerebral cortex, and this location is correlated with the severity of disability felt by the patient, according to a number of magnetic resonance imaging studies [76]. In a recent study, Abdelrahman et al. [77] showed that double inversion recovery (DIR) is more sensitive in identifying the various forms of cortical lesions. In addition to being found to be more effective than Fluid-Attenuated Inversion Recovery (FLAIR) in detecting the MS plaque numbers of cortical plaque types, DIR was also found to be significantly more effective than FLAIR in detecting the MS plaque numbers of overall cortical types (juxtacortical and juxtacortical extended MS plaques) and in detecting the MS plaque numbers in the infratentorial region, subcortical white matter, periventricular white matter, and overall multiple sclerosis plaques burden [77].

According to the findings of their study, there is a substantial link between the total cortical MS plaque types and the overall MS plaque burden, as well as the duration of the MS disease, the frequency of episodes, and EDSS. This means that 3D DIR MRI imaging is a superior delineator and a dependable tool for identifying cortical subtypes [77].

10.3.5 Demyelinating and Infectious Brain Lesions

While the T1-weighted sequence is generally considered the gold standard for post-contrast MRI exams, CE-FLAIR is becoming more and more popular these days [78]. The synergistic effects of gadolinium's T1 shortening and the lesions' combined T2 lengthening can account for the contrast enhancement seen on FLAIR [79]. Contrast enhancement is possible because FLAIR images come with an innate T1-weighting component. As a result of the slow-flowing superficial blood arteries, the T1-shortening effect of gadolinium, and perhaps magnetization transfer effects, CE-FLAIR is especially sensitive when depicting leptomeningeal enhancement [80]. In an attempt to increase diagnostic sensitivity, a variety of intracranial diseases have been investigated with post-contrast FLAIR [81]. CE-FLAIR has been a valuable sequence for assessing a variety of diseases over the past ten years. Meningeal enhancement in CE-FLAIR images is easily identifiable due to the abrogation of cerebrospinal fluid signal, subtle vascular augmentation compared to T1WI, and a degree of T1 relaxation effect [82]. Additionally, compared to CET1WI, CE-FLAIR is more sensitive in detecting low gadolinium concentrations [83]. This suggests that lesions that show faint enhancement on CE-T1WI may be easier to distinguish on CE-FLAIR [84]. Therefore, when compared to the routine CE-T1W sequence, CE-FLAIR offers greater lesion identification capabilities, enhanced contrast-to-background resolution, and higher image enhancement. As a result, it provides improved diagnostic information directly supporting prompt diagnoses and improved patient management [84].

10.4 Conclusion

The book chapter has explored the diverse forms of MRI imaging (functional MRI – fMRI, real-time MRI, interventional MRI, molecular imaging, parallel MRI, quantitative MRI, magnetic resonance spectroscopy – MRS, hyperpolarized gas MRI) and has presented the applications and diagnostic capabilities of MRI technology, highlighting its significant role in facilitating accurate disease detection, treatment planning, and monitoring of therapeutic interventions. An extensive overview of MRI in Neuroimaging, Musculoskeletal MRI, Cardiovascular Imaging, Abdominal and Pelvic MRI, and Breast Imaging has been presented. The discussion showed the accuracy and sensitivity of MRI in the detection of disease conditions such as cerebrovascular accidents, lung nodules, spondyloarthritis, multiple sclerosis lesions, and demyelinating and infectious brain lesions.

REFERENCES

1. Hogg JC, Chu F, Utokaparch S, et al. The nature of small-airway obstruction in chronic obstructive pulmonary disease. *N Engl J Med.* 2004;350(26):2645–53.
2. Landheer K, Schulte RF, Treacy MS, Swanberg KM, Juchem C. Theoretical description of modern 1H in vivo magnetic resonance spectroscopic pulse sequences. *J Magn Reson Imaging.* 2020;51(4):1008–29.
3. Rosen Y, Lenkinski RE. Recent advances in magnetic resonance neurospectroscopy. *Neurotherapeutics.* 2007;4(3):330–45.
4. Golder W. Magnetic resonance spectroscopy in clinical oncology. *Onkologie.* 2004;27(3):304–9.
5. Uecker M, Zhang S, Voit D, Karaus A, Merboldt KD, Frahm J. Real-time MRI at a resolution of 20 ms. *NMR Biomed.* 2010;23(8):986–94.
6. Uyanik I, Lindner P, Tsiamyrtzis P, Shah D, Tsekos NV, Pavlidis IT. Applying a level set method for resolving physiologic motions in free-breathing and non-gated cardiac MRI. *Funct Imaging Model Heart.* 2013;7945:466–73.
7. Lewin JS. Interventional MR imaging: concepts, systems, and applications in neuroradiology. *AJNR Am J Neuroradiol.* 1999;20(5):735–48.
8. Sisk JE. *The gale encyclopedia of nursing and allied health.* 3rd ed. Gale; 2013.
9. Gallagher FA. An introduction to functional and molecular imaging with MRI. *Clin Radiol.* 2010;65(7):557–66.
10. Xue S, Qiao J, Pu F, Cameron M, Yang JJ. Design of a novel class of protein-based magnetic resonance imaging contrast agents for the molecular imaging of cancer biomarkers. *Wiley Interdiscip Rev Nanomed Nanobiotechnol.* 2013;5(2):163–79.
11. Liu CH, Kim YR, Ren JQ, Eichler F, Rosen BR, Liu PK. Imaging cerebral gene transcripts in live animals. *J Neurosci.* 2007;27(3):713–22.
12. Liu CH, Ren J, Liu CM, Liu PK. Intracellular gene transcription factor protein-guided MRI by DNA aptamers in vivo. *FASEB J.* 2014;28(1):464–73.
13. Liu CH, You Z, Liu CM, et al. Diffusion-weighted magnetic resonance imaging reversal by gene knockdown of matrix metalloproteinase-9 activities in live animal brains. *J Neurosci.* 2009;29(11):3508–17.
14. Liu CH, Yang J, Ren JQ, Liu CM, You Z, Liu PK. MRI reveals differential effects of amphetamine exposure on neuroglia in vivo. *FASEB J.* 2013;27(2):712–24.
15. Sodickson DK, Manning WJ. Simultaneous acquisition of spatial harmonics (SMASH): fast imaging with radiofrequency coil arrays. *Magn Reson Med.* 1997;38(4):591–603.
16. Griswold MA, Jakob PM, Heidemann RM, et al. Generalized autocalibrating partially parallel acquisitions (GRAPPA). *Magn Reson Med.* 2002;47(6):1202–10.
17. Pruessmann KP, Weiger M, Scheidegger MB, Boesiger P. SENSE: sensitivity encoding for fast MRI. *Magn Reson Med.* 1999;42(5):952–62.
18. Gulani V, Nicole S. Quantitative MRI: rationale and challenges. In: Seiberlich N, Gulani V, Campbell-Washburn A, Sourbron S, Doneva MI, Calamante F, Hu HH. *Quantitative magnetic resonance imaging.* Academic Press; 2020. p. xxxvii-li.
19. von Knobelsdorff-Brenkenhoff F, Schulz-Menger J. Cardiovascular magnetic resonance imaging in ischemic heart disease. *J Magn Reson Imaging.* 2012;36(1):20–38.
20. Cobianchi BF, De Marino L, Arrigoni F, et al. T2-mapping MRI evaluation of patellofemoral cartilage in patients submitted to intra-articular platelet-rich plasma (PRP) injections. *Radiol Med.* 2021;126(8):1085–94.
21. Battal B, Kocaoglu M, Bulakbasi N, Husmen G, Tuba Sanal H, Tayfun C. Cerebrospinal fluid flow imaging by using phase-contrast MR technique. *Br J Radiol.* 2011;84(1004):758–65.
22. Hirsch S, Braun J, Sack I. Magnetic Resonance Elastography. Wiley Online Books; 2016.
23. Seiler A, Nöth U, Hok P, et al. Multiparametric Quantitative MRI in Neurological Diseases. *Front Neurol.* 2021;12:640239.

24. Warntjes JB, Leinhard OD, West J, Lundberg P. Rapid magnetic resonance quantification on the brain: optimization for clinical usage. *Magn Reson Med.* 2008;60(2):320–9.
25. Ehses P, Seiberlich N, Ma D, et al. IR TrueFISP with a golden-ratio-based radial readout: fast quantification of T1, T2, and proton density. *Magn Reson Med.* 2013;69(1):71–81.
26. Ma D, Gulani V, Seiberlich N, et al. Magnetic resonance fingerprinting. *Nature.* 2013;495(7440):187–92.
27. Chakeres DW, Abduljalil AM, Novak P, Novak V. Comparison of 1.5 and 8 tesla high-resolution magnetic resonance imaging of lacunar infarcts. *J Comput Assist Tomogr.* 2002;26(4):628–32.
28. Abeida H, Zhang Q, Li J, Merabtine N. Iterative sparse asymptotic minimum variance-based approaches for array processing. *IEEE Trans Signal Process.* 2013;61(4):933–44.
29. Scaccianoce E, Laganà MM, Baglio F, et al. Combined DTI–fMRI analysis for a quantitative assessment of connections between WM bundles and their peripheral cortical fields in verbal fluency. *Brain Topogr.* 2016;29:814–23.
30. Chen S, Li X. Functional magnetic resonance imaging for imaging neural activity in the human brain: the annual progress. *Comput Math Methods Med.* 2012;2012:613465.
31. Lakhani DA, Sabsevitz DS, Chaichana KL, Quiñones-Hinojosa A, Middlebrooks EH. Current State of Functional MRI in the Presurgical Planning of Brain Tumors. *Radiology Imaging Cancer.* 2023;5(6):e230078.
32. Abdelgawad MS, Kayed MH, Reda MI, Abdelzaher E, Farhoud AH, Elsebaie N. Contribution of advanced neuro-imaging (MR diffusion, perfusion and proton spectroscopy) in differentiation between low grade gliomas GII and MR morphologically similar non neoplastic lesions. *Egypt J Radiol Nucl Med.* 2022;53(1):20.
33. Shapiro L, Harish M, Hargreaves B, Staroswiecki E, Gold G. Advances in musculoskeletal MRI: technical considerations. *J Magn Reson Imaging.* 2012;36(4):775–87.
34. Brittberg M. Knee osteochondritis dissecans-treatment technical aspects. *J Orthop.* 2022;34:104–10.
35. Hayashi D, Roemer FW, Jarraya M, Guermazi A. Imaging of osteoarthritis. In: Guglielmi G, Peh WCG, Guermazi A. *Geriatric imaging.* 2013:93–121.
36. Sudoł-Szopińska I, Jans L, Teh J. Rheumatoid arthritis: what do MRI and ultrasound show? *J Ultrasonogr.* 2017;17(68):5–16.
37. Drake-Pérez M, Boto J, Fitsiori A, et al. Clinical applications of diffusion-weighted imaging in neuroradiology. *Insights Imaging.* 2018; 9:535–547.
38. Stacey RB, Hundley WG. The role of cardiovascular magnetic resonance (CMR) and computed tomography (CCT) in facilitating heart failure management. *Curr Treat Options Cardiovasc Med.* 2013;15:373–86.
39. von Knobelsdorff-Brenkenhoff F, Schulz-Menger J. Cardiovascular magnetic resonance in the guidelines of the European Society of Cardiology: a comprehensive summary and update. *J Cardiovasc Magn Reson.* 2023;25(1):42.
40. Shabana A, El-Menyar A. Myocardial viability: what we knew and what is new. *Cardiol Res Pract.* 2012;2012:607486.
41. Meier C, Eisenblätter M, Gielen S. Myocardial late gadolinium enhancement (LGE) in cardiac magnetic resonance imaging (CMR)—An important risk marker for cardiac disease. *J Cardiovasc Dev Dis.* 2024;11(2):40.
42. Sun B, Liu J, Li S, Lovell JF, Zhang Y. Imaging of gastrointestinal tract ailments. *J Imaging.* 2023;9(6):115.
43. Heiken JP. Distinguishing benign from malignant liver tumours. *Cancer Imaging.* 2007;7(Special Issue A):S1.
44. Nikolic O, Basta Nikolic M, Spasic A, Otero-Garcia MM, Stojanovic S. Systematic radiological approach to utero-ovarian pathologies. *Br J Radiol.* 2019;92(1099):20180439.
45. Wilde S, Scott-Barrett S. Radiological appearances of uterine fibroids. *Indian J Radiol Imaging.* 2009;19(3):222–31.
46. Andersen PE. Patient selection and preparation strategies for the use of contrast material in patients with chronic kidney disease. *World J Radiol.* 2012;4(6):253.
47. Maccioni F, Busato L, Valenti A, Cardaccio S, Longhi A, Catalano C. Magnetic resonance imaging of the gastrointestinal tract: current role, recent advancements, and future perspectives. *Diagnostics.* 2023;13(14):2410.

48. O'Flynn EA, DeSouza NM. Functional magnetic resonance: biomarkers of response in breast cancer. *Breast Cancer Res.* 2011;13:1–10.
49. El Khouli RH, Macura KJ, Jacobs MA, et al. Dynamic contrast-enhanced MRI of the breast: quantitative method for kinetic curve type assessment. *Am J Roentgenol.* 2009;193(4):295–300.
50. Zingaretti N, Cordaro ER, Parodi PC, et al. Determinants of surgeon choice in cases of suspected implant rupture following mastectomy or aesthetic breast surgery: clinical implications. *Medicine.* 2020;99(27):e21134.
51. Vymazal J, Rulseh AM, Keller J, Janouskova L. Comparison of CT and MR imaging in ischemic stroke. *Insights Imaging.* 2012;3:619–27.
52. Wintermark M, Sanelli PC, Albers GW, et al. Imaging recommendations for acute stroke and transient ischemic attack patients: a joint statement by the American society of neuroradiology, the American college of radiology, and the society of neurointerventional surgery. *AJNR Am J Neuroradiol.* 2013;34(11):E117–27.
53. Chalela JA, Kidwell CS, Nentwich LM, et al. Magnetic resonance imaging and computed tomography in emergency assessment of patients with suspected acute stroke: a prospective comparison. *Lancet.* 2007;369(9558):293–8.
54. Tietz E, Müller-Franzes G, Zimmermann M, Kuhl CK, Keil S, Nebelung S, Truhn D. Evaluation of pulmonary nodules by radiologists vs. radiomics in stand-alone and complementary CT and MRI. *Diagnostics.* 2024;14(5):483.
55. Liu H, Chen R, Tong C, Liang XW. MRI versus CT for the detection of pulmonary nodules: a meta-analysis. *Medicine.* 2021; 100(42):e27270.
56. Hinsen M, Nagel AM, May MS, Wiesmueller M, Uder M, Heiss R. Lung nodule detection with modern low-field MRI (0.55 T) in comparison to CT. *Invest Radiol.* 2024; 59(3):215–22.
57. Diekhoff T, Lambert R, Hermann KG. MRI in axial spondyloarthritis: understanding an 'ASAS-positive MRI' and the ASAS classification criteria. *Skeletal Radiology.* 2022 Sep;51(9):1721–30.
58. Maksymowych WP, Weber U. Diagnostic utility of MRI in early spondyloarthritis. *Curr Rheumatol Rep.* 2011; 13:402–8.
59. Mandl P, Navarro-Compán V, Terslev L, et al. EULAR recommendations for the use of imaging in the diagnosis and management of spondyloarthritis in clinical practice. *Ann Rheum Dis.* 2015 Jul 1;74(7):1327–39.
60. Canella C, Schau B, Ribeiro E, Sbaffi B, Marchiori E. MRI in seronegative spondyloarthritis: imaging features and differential diagnosis in the spine and sacroiliac joints. *Am J Roentgenol.* 2013; 200(1):149–57.
61. Pohlner T, Deppe D, Ziegeler K, et al. Diagnostic accuracy in axial spondyloarthritis: a systematic evaluation of the role of clinical information in the interpretation of sacroiliac joint imaging. *RMD Open.* 2024; 10(2):e004044.
62. Lukas C, Cyteval C, Dougados M, Weber U. MRI for diagnosis of axial spondyloarthritis: major advance with critical limitations 'Not everything that glisters is gold (standard)'. *RMD Open.* 2018; 4(1):e000586.
63. Weber U, Lambert RG, Ostergaard M, Hodler J, Pedersen SJ, Maksymowych WP. The diagnostic utility of MRI in spondyloarthritis: an international multicentre evaluation of 187 subjects (The MORPHO study). *Arthritis Rheumatol.* 2010;62(10):3048–58.
64. Mau W, Zeidler H, Mau R, et al. Clinical features and prognosis of patients with possible ankylosing spondylitis. Results of a 10-year follow-up. *J Rheumatol.* 1988; 15:1109–14.
65. Bennett AN, McGonagle D, O'Connor P, et al. Severity of baseline magnetic resonance imaging-evident sacroiliitis and HLA-B27 status in early inflammatory back pain predict radiographically evident ankylosing spondylitis at eight years. *Arthritis Rheum.* 2008; 58:3413–8.
66. Rudwaleit M, van der Heijde D, Khan MA, Braun J, Sieper J. How to diagnose axial spondyloarthritis early. *Ann Rheum Dis.* 2004; 63:535–43.
67. Braun J, Bollow M, Eggens U, Koenig H, Distler A, Sieper J. Use of dynamic magnetic resonance imaging with fast imaging in the detection of early and advanced sacroiliitis in spondyloarthropathy patients. *Arthritis Rheum.* 1994; 37:1039–45.
68. Hanly JG, Mitchell MJ, Barnes DC, MacMillan L. Early recognition of sacroiliitis by magnetic resonance imaging and single photon emission computed tomography. *J Rheumatol.* 1994; 21:2088–95.
69. Bollow M, Braun J, Hamm B, et al. Early sacroiliitis in patients with spondyloarthropathy: evaluation with dynamic gadolinium-enhanced MR imaging. *Radiology.* 1995; 194:529–36.

70. Blum U, Buitrago-Tellez C, Mundinger A, et al. Magnetic resonance imaging (MRI) for detection of active sacroiliitis: a prospective study comparing conventional radiography, scintigraphy, and contrast-enhanced MRI. *J Rheumatol.* 1996; 23:2107–15.
71. Puhakka KB, Jurik AG, Egund N, et al. Imaging of sacroiliitis in early seronegative spondylarthropathy. Assessment of abnormalities by MRI in comparison with radiography and CT. *Acta Radiol.* 2003; 44:218–29.
72. Rudwaleit M, van der Heijde D, Landewé R, et al. The development of Assessment of SpondyloArthritis international Society classification criteria for axial spondyloarthritis (part II): validation and final selection. *Ann Rheum Dis.* 2009; 68:777–83.
73. Rudwaleit M, Jurik AG, Hermann KGA, et al. Defining active sacroiliitis on magnetic resonance imaging (MRI) for classification of axial spondyloarthritis: a consensual approach by the ASAS/OMERACT MRI group. *Ann Rheum Dis.* 2009; 68:1520–7.
74. Madsen KB, Egund N, Jurik AG. Grading of inflammatory disease activity in the sacroiliac joints with magnetic resonance imaging: comparison between short tau inversion recovery and gadolinium contrast-enhanced sequences. *J Rheumatol.* 2010; 37:393–400.
75. Maksymowych WP, Weber U. Diagnostic Utility of MRI in Early Spondyloarthritis. *Curr Rheumatol Rep.* 2011; 13:402–8.
76. Herranz E, Giannì C, Louapre C, et al. Neuroinflammatory component of gray matter pathology in multiple sclerosis. *Ann Neurol.* 2016; 80(5):776–90.
77. Abdelrahman AS, Khater NH, Barakat MMK. Diagnostic utility of 3D DIR MRI in the estimation of MS lesions overall load with special emphasis on cortical subtypes. *Egypt J Radiol Nucl Med.* 2022;53(47):1–9.
78. Fukuoka H, Hirai T, Okuda T, et al. Comparison of the added value of contrast-enhanced 3D fluid-attenuated inversion recovery and magnetization-prepared rapid acquisition of gradient echo sequences in relation to conventional postcontrast T1-weighted images for the evaluation of leptomeninges. *Am J Neuroradiol.* 2010; 31(5):868–73.
79. Kim SC, Park SW, Ryoo I, Jung SC, Yun TJ. Contrast-enhanced FLAIR (Fluid-Attenuated Inversion Recovery) for evaluating mild traumatic brain injury. *PLoS One.* 2014; 9(7):102229.
80. McKinney A, Palmer C, Short J, Lucato L, Truwit C. Utility of fat-suppressed FLAIR and subtraction imaging in detecting meningeal abnormalities. *Neuroradiology.* 2006; 48(12):881–5.
81. Dickinson PJ, Jones-Woods S, Cissell DD. Abrogation of fluid suppression in intracranial postcontrast fluid-attenuated inversion recovery magnetic resonance imaging: a clinical and phantom study. *Vet Radiol Ultrasound.* 2008; 59(4):432–43.
82. Ahmad A, Azad S, Azad R. Differentiation of leptomeningeal and vascular enhancement on post-contrast FLAIR MRI sequence: role in early detection of infectious meningitis. *J Clin Diagn Res.* 2015; 9(1):TC08–12.
83. Park YW, Ahn SJ. Comparison of contrast-enhanced T2 FLAIR and 3D T1 black-blood fast spin-echo for detection of leptomeningeal metastases. *Invest Magn Resonance Imaging.* 2018; 22(2):86.
84. Lee EK, Lee EJ, Kim S, Lee YS. Importance of contrast-enhanced fluid-attenuated inversion recovery magnetic resonance imaging in various intracranial pathologic conditions. *Korean J Radiol.* 2016; 17(1):127–41.

11

Utility of High-Performance Liquid Chromatography in Complementary Medicine

Parixit Prajapati, Megha Chavda, Chandni Chandarana, and Bhupendra Prajapati

11.1 Complementary Medicine

Complementary medicine encompasses a range of therapeutic and diagnostic practices that predominantly operate beyond the confines of conventional healthcare. Initially emerging in the 1970s and 1980s, these disciplines primarily served as alternatives to conventional healthcare, earning them the collective label of "alternative medicine". Over time, the term "complementary medicine" gained prominence as both systems began to be utilized in tandem, complementing each other's approaches [1].

Complementary medicine and therapies represent healthcare approaches that have originated outside the mainstream Western medical paradigm. Three terms, often used interchangeably but with distinct meanings, warrant clarification: complementary, alternative, and integrative. "Alternative" refers to non-mainstream practices utilized instead of conventional medicine. "Complementary" denotes non-mainstream practices employed alongside conventional medicine. "Integrative" signifies the integration of conventional and complementary approaches in a coordinated manner.

Presently, the use of alternative medicine is rare, with most individuals opting for complementary approaches in conjunction with conventional treatments [2]. Commonly employed complementary and alternative medicine therapies encompass non-vitamin, mineralogy products, practice deep breathing, meditation, chiropractic care, yoga, massage, and diet-based therapies [3].

The National Institutes of Health have categorized complementary and alternative medicine into five domains, which, to some extent, overlap, as outlined below:

1. Biologically based practices encompass a broad spectrum of approaches. These may involve the utilization of various vitamins and mineral supplements, as well as natural products like chondroitin polysulfate sodium sourced from shark cartilage. Additionally, herbals such as ginkgo biloba, are commonly included in this category. Unconventional dietary strategies, such as the low-carbohydrate approach popularized by Robert Atkins, also fall under this umbrella.
2. Manipulative and body-based therapies encompass a range of practices, including massage, with roots tracing back throughout history. In the 19th century, the United States witnessed the emergence of formal manipulative disciplines: chiropractic medicine and osteopathic medicine. These disciplines arose from efforts to alleviate structural pressures on vertebrae and spinal nerve roots.
3. Mind-body medicine draws upon the age-old belief across various cultures that the mind profoundly impacts bodily functions, and vice versa.
4. Alternative medical systems offer diverse perspectives on health and healing. While the ancient Greeks emphasized the equilibrium of vital humors, Asian customs placed a strong emphasis

DOI: 10.1201/9781003486909-11

on the body's vital energy circulation and equilibrium. For instance, acupuncture, a practice rooted in this philosophy, aims to restore the flow of vital energy by strategically placing needles at key points on the body.

There is also energy medicine that employs therapies utilizing energy, whether through biofield or bioelectromagnetic-based interventions. An instance of the former is Reiki therapy, where the goal is to rebalance and enhance the flow of beneficial energies by harnessing the energy emitted from the hands of a skilled practitioner [4].

11.1.1 History of Complementary and Alternative Medicine

11.1.1.1 Traditional Chinese Medicine

Emerging from ancient China, traditional Chinese medicine (TCM) has undergone millennia of evolution. TCM encompasses the utilization of herbs, dietary therapy, and mind-body practices such as acupuncture and tai chi. While the precise count of TCM users in the United States remains elusive, the National Center for Complementary and Integrative Health (NCCIH) estimated in 1997 that over 10,000 practitioners attended to more than 1 million patients annually. Among the various TCM modalities, acupuncture and tai chi emerged as the most prevalent choices.

11.1.1.2 Homeopathy

Homeopathy, the most ancient form of complementary and alternative medicine in Europe, traces its roots back to Samuel Hahnemann and emerged in Germany in the late 18th century. Two fundamental principles guide homeopathic medicine: "like cures like" and the "law of minimum dose". Homeopathic preparations are made up from herbs, minerals, or animals, often administered in the form of sugar pellets. It's important to note that treatments can differ among individuals with the same ailment, as homeopathic remedies are typically customized to meet each person's specific requirements.

11.1.1.3 Ayurvedic Medicine

Ayurveda, with its roots tracing back over 3,000 years to India, stands as one of the most ancient medical systems globally. Numerous practices within Ayurveda have been transmitted orally, predating written documentation. This holistic approach to health comprises three main categories of action: elimination therapies, pacification therapies, and nourishing therapies. Practitioners tailor customized treatments, incorporating a blend of herbal compounds, dietary adjustments, exercise regimes, yoga practices, physical manipulations, and lifestyle advice.

11.1.1.4 Native American Traditional Healing

In contrast to conventional Western methods, Native American wellness and traditional healing prioritize the harmony of mental, physical, and spiritual well-being. The fundamental connection that exists between Native American communities, the natural world, customs, and the Great Spirit is the basis of this approach and ensures the continued life of these traditions. While specific practices may vary among tribes, fundamental aspects of Native American healing encompass the use of plants, storytelling, tobacco, music, smudging, and ceremonies. Although healers or medicine men play a role in guiding these treatments within communities, there's a deep-rooted belief that maintaining health and well-being ultimately rests on individual responsibility [5]. The terms "complementary" and "alternative" refer to practices and products individuals adopt either in conjunction with or in lieu of Western medical methods. Many of these practices lack scientific evidence and are met with skepticism by medical authorities. To streamline research efforts into these approaches, the United States requires a structured agenda.

11.1.2 Safety of Complementary and Alternative Medicine

After thorough analysis, several complementary and alternative medicine treatments were shown to be usually safe and beneficial. These consist of, among other things, yoga, meditation, and acupuncture. Others, on the other hand, could cause adverse effects or adversely interact with conventional drugs.

Complementary and alternative medicine encompasses a diverse range of botanicals and nutritional products, including herbal supplements, dietary supplements, and vitamins. Unlike conventional medications, these products do not require approval from the Food and Drug Administration (FDA) before use in the population, and a prescription is not necessary for their purchase. Consequently, the responsibility falls on individuals to determine what is most suitable for them. Despite advertisements or historical usage claims, these factors alone do not guarantee safety or effectiveness, especially when used in conjunction with medications [6].

11.2 High-Performance Liquid Chromatography

High-performance liquid chromatography (HPLC) is an analytical technique to separate, identify, and quantify components in a mixture. HPLC works by forcing a liquid mobile phase through a column that is filled with a stationary phase under high pressure. Chromatography has developed over time using a variety of stationary phase materials. It is a technique for separating mixtures according to how their constituents interact with stationary and mobile phases. The need for quicker, more effective methods for the analysis of particular classes of analytes is increasing due to developments in adsorbent materials. One of the most popular, up-to-date, reliable, and flexible chromatographic techniques for separating ingredients in herbal extracts or products is HPLC. It makes it possible to identify and measure individual components and to create chemical fingerprints, or profiles, for crude mixtures.

The herbal product industry and its regulatory agencies use HPLC extensively for the identification and measurement of both known and unknown chemicals in herbal product quality assurance. Its flexibility includes the ability to accurately identify and measure secondary metabolites found in both source materials and derived products while analyzing a wide range of consumables, including food, drinks, and fragrances. Additionally, HPLC is an essential instrument for detecting and quantifying pollutants arising from adulteration.

11.2.1 Normal Phase HPLC

This method mirrors that of thin-layer chromatography or column chromatography. Despite its label as "normal", it isn't the most prevalent type of HPLC. Utilizing tiny silica particles packed within the column and a non-polar solvent such as hexane, this technique employs columns typically with an internal diameter of about 4.6 mm or smaller and lengths ranging from 150 to 250 mm. Polar compounds within the sample adhere more strongly to the polar silica, causing them to elute from the column at a slower rate compared to non-polar compounds, which pass through more rapidly [7].

11.2.2 Reversed Phase HPLC

In this case, the column dimensions stay the same, but the silica is modified to become non-polar by long hydrocarbon chains connected, typically with 8 to 18 carbon atoms, to its surface. Using a polar solvent, a mixture of water and methyl alcohol, for example, creates a sturdy bond between the solvent and the polar molecules in the sample. On the other hand, there is very little interaction between the polar molecules and the hydrocarbon chains that are attached to the silica (the stationary phase). Polar molecules therefore tend to travel with the solvent, whereas non-polar chemicals interact with the hydrocarbon through van der Waals dispersion forces. Moreover, non-polar chemicals must break hydrogen bonds in order to move between molecules of water or methyl alcohol since they are less soluble in the solvent, which results in a shorter period in solution and a slower flow along the column. Additionally, polar molecules traverse the column at a swifter pace. Reversed-phase HPLC has emerged as the predominant HPLC due to these operational principles [8].

11.2.3 Principles of HPLC

The separation principle of HPLC is based on the distribution of the analyte (sample) between a mobile phase (eluent) and a stationary phase (packing material of the column). Depending on the chemical structure of the analyte, the molecules are retarded while passing the stationary phase. The specific intermolecular interactions between the molecules of a sample and the packing material define their time "on-column". Hence, different constituents of a sample are eluted at different times. Thereby, the separation of the sample ingredients is achieved. A detection unit, for example, ultraviolet (UV) detector recognizes the analytes after leaving the column. The signals are converted and recorded by a data management system (computer software) and then shown in a chromatogram. After passing the detector unit, the mobile phase can be subjected to additional detector units, a fraction collection unit, or waste. In general, an HPLC system contains the following modules: a solvent reservoir, a pump, an injection valve, a column, a detector unit, and a data processing unit. The solvent (eluent) is delivered by the pump at high pressure and constant speed through the system. To keep the drift and noise of the detector signal as low as possible, a constant and pulseless flow from the pump is crucial. The analyte (sample) is provided to the eluent by the injection valve [9].

The processing of a crude source material to provide a sample suitable for HPLC analysis as well as the choice of solvent for sample reconstitution can have a significant bearing on the overall success of natural product isolation [10]. The source material, for example, dried powdered plant, will initially need to be treated in such a way as to ensure that the compound of interest is efficiently liberated into solution. In the case of dried plant material, an organic solvent (methanol or chloroform) may be used for the initial extraction following a period of maceration. Afterward, the solid material is then removed by decanting off the extract by filtration [11, 12]. The filtrate is then concentrated and injected into HPLC for separation.

The usage of guard columns is necessary in the analysis of crude extract. Many natural product materials contain a significant level of strongly binding components, such as chlorophyll and other endogenous materials that may in the long term compromise the performance of analytical columns. Therefore, the guard columns will significantly protect the lifespan of the analytical columns. To begin compound identification with HPLC, the initial step entails choosing a suitable detector. Once the detector is chosen and optimized for detection, the next phase involves crafting a separation assay. This assay's parameters should be carefully adjusted to ensure the chromatograph exhibits a distinct, unadulterated peak corresponding to the known sample [13].

11.2.4 Instrumentation of HPLC System

A reservoir for the mobile phase or solvent, a system for delivering the solvent, a device for introducing samples, a column, post-column apparatus, a detector, a system for data collection and output, post-detector eluent processing, and tubing with fittings for connectivity are the nine basic components of an HPLC system. All of these elements are necessary for the performance of an HPLC system, with the exception of the post-column equipment [14].

11.2.4.1 Solvent Reservoir

The mobile phase storage can be any clean, inert container. It can carry anywhere from 0.5 and 2 L of solvent. It includes a cap that fits over a tubing input line so that the mobile phase may be delivered to the solvent delivery system more easily. This cap does several tasks: it prevents dust from entering the container, reduces solvent evaporation, allows pressurization of the container, provides ports for extra intake lines, and facilitates sparging, which is the process of distributing argon or helium into the mobile phase to decrease dissolved air. Depending on the application, the material selection for the mobile phase reservoir is frequently critical. When doing tiny molecule analysis, glass is typically chosen over plastics to avoid any potential material leaching [14].

11.2.4.2 Pump

The operating pressure range for the high-pressure pump is 500 to 20,000 psi. Its main purpose is to provide the column with a mobile phase that is pulsation-free, precise, accurate, consistent, and repeatable. At the moment, syringe-based or displacement pumps, constant flow pumps, and constant pressure pumps are the three main types of HPLC pumps used. Constant flow pumps are the most popular option because of their adaptability and versatility, whereas constant pressure and syringe-based pumps provide difficulties when adjusting to gradient solvent delivery [14].

11.2.4.3 Sample Injector

The injector can function as either a standalone unit or as part of an automated system. Specifically tailored for HPLC applications, it ensures precise liquid sample injections ranging from 0.1 to 100 mL, maintaining high reproducibility even under pressures reaching 4000 psi. It is also designed to endure the severe pressures of the liquid system. As an alternative, an autosampler offers automatic functionality. This is especially helpful when managing a large number of samples or when manual injection is not feasible. In order to maintain precision at a high degree, injectors must be inert and repeatable in order to deliver samples into the mobile phase stream consistently [15].

11.2.4.4 Columns

Columns typically have internal diameters of 2 to 5 mm and lengths ranging from 50 to 300 mm. They are typically composed of polished stainless steel. They are often filled with a stationary phase made up of particles that range in size from 3 to 10 µm. Additionally, microbore columns, characterized by internal diameters smaller than 2 mm, are widely used in the field. Maintaining consistent temperatures for both the mobile phase and the column is optimal during analysis. Frequently referred to as the "core element" of the chromatograph, the column employs a stationary phase with varied physical and chemical properties to effectively separate target sample constituents. Under normal flow circumstances, the presence of tiny particles in the column causes a rise in back pressure; this suggests that a considerable amount of pumping effort is required to drive the mobile phase across the column [16]. This component is crucial and requires proper maintenance according to the supplier's instructions to achieve consistent separation efficiency from one run to the next. The main column types are:

1. Guard column: To prolong the lifespan of the analytical column, a guard column is installed upstream. Particulate particles, pollutants from solvents, and sample elements that create permanent bindings with the stationary phase are its main functions likewise it eliminates solvent losses from the analytical column by saturating the mobile phase alongside the stationary phase. Similar to the analytical column, the packing material in the guard column frequently has greater particle sizes. The guard column can be completely replaced with a new one or repacked in the event of contamination.
2. Analytical columns: The central component of HPLC is the liquid-chromatographic column, usually ranging from 100 to 300 mm in length. These columns are frequently straight but, when necessary, they can be connected to form longer columns. Liquid columns typically have inside diameters between 4 and 10 mm, and the most typical packing particle sizes are 5 or 10 µm. A typical column configuration is 250 mm long, 4.6 mm in diameter inside, and filled with 5 µm-sized particles. Columns that satisfy these requirements usually show between 40,000 and 60,000 plates per meter of plates [17].

11.2.4.5 Detectors

HPLC analysis requires a detector to track the substances that are separated in the column in order to quantify and identify them. The particular substance being detected determines which detector is best. Solute and bulk property detectors are the two types of detectors.

1. Solute Property HPLC Detectors
    a. Mass Spectroscopic Detectors

       Mass spectroscopy detectors are extremely accurate and precise. Its identification is contingent upon the splitting of molecules by an electric field, and its separation depends on the mass-to-charge ratio of these broken molecules. Interestingly, this detector is thought to be harmful [18].

    b. UV/VIS HPLC Detectors

       The ultraviolet (UV) or visible (VIS) detector stands as the prevalent choice in HPLC due to its excellent stability, user-friendly operation, and high sensitivity. Within this category, one finds fixed wavelength detectors, variable wavelength detectors, and diode array detectors [19].

    c. Photodiode Array (PDA) Detectors

       With many individual diodes, resolution components, or pixels, the PDA can detect multiple wavelengths at once when used as a UV detector. It functions as the perfect detector in a UV/VIS dispersive spectrophotometer to capture the whole spectrum [20].

    d. Fluorescence Detectors

       Excellent sensitivity is provided by fluorescence detectors for certain component groups. They use a specific wavelength to activate the component atoms, causing them to release a light signal. The component's concentration can be measured by assessing the intensity of the light that is released. Clinical samples, pharmaceuticals, natural materials, and petroleum products are all known to exhibit fluorescent absorbance [21].

2. Bulk Property HPLC Detectors
    a. Electrical Conductivity Detectors

       Since conductivity detectors are used to measure conductivity, they are categorized as bulk property detectors. The ability to detect charged species and surfactants with great sensitivity is one of their main characteristics. They work by measuring electrical resistance, and the amount of ions in the solution is proportionate to the result that is seen [22].

    b. Refractive Index Detectors (RID)

       A refractive index detector assesses the analyte's refractive index concerning the solvent. It operates based on the principles of light deflection and reflection within the solution. Various types of RID detectors include the thermal lens detector, the Christiansen effect detector, the dielectric constant detector, and the interferometer [23].

    c. Electrochemical Detectors

       The purpose of the electrochemical detector is to detect and quantify the electric currents generated by oxidation-reduction reactions in substances. The oxidation-reduction reaction of each molecule requires a different voltage, which is why the electrochemical detector has such excellent selectivity and sensitivity. Interestingly, the way this detector works is harmful [24].

    d. Light Scattering Detectors

       The scattered light that the eluent emits is picked up by a light scattering detector. It works especially well with compounds that have a large molecular weight, such as carbohydrates, lipids, and surfactants. The low-angle laser light scattering detector and the multiple-angle laser light scattering detector are the two types of light scattering detectors that are accessible [25].

11.2.4.6 Detectors Hyphenated with HPLC

Hyphenated procedures are those that combine an HPLC system with an independent analytical approach. Although other techniques like infrared spectroscopy (LC-IR) and nuclear magnetic resonance (LC-NMR) are also often used, mass spectrometry (LC-MS) stands out as the principal approach. Although mass spectrometry is increasingly adopted as a routine HPLC detector, comprehensive reviews detailing its utility and other hyphenated techniques are accessible for further insights [26].

11.2.4.7 System for Data Collection and Output

A computer, integrator, recorder, or other data gathering and output device is connected to the detector's electronic output. This device receives the detector's electronic signal and generates a graphical representation of the response over time, known as a chromatogram. This chromatogram provides both qualitative and quantitative information upon evaluation. Although standalone recorders are rarely utilized nowadays, integrators and computers provide the capability to integrate chromatogram peaks and store data for subsequent processing. Computer-based collection systems enable data export to diverse programs and applications. Furthermore, computers commonly oversee and regulate the entire HPLC system, making computer-controlled data collection and output systems prevalent in modern HPLC setups.

11.2.4.8 Post-detection Eluent Processing

The eluent is normally sent to a designated trash container after exiting the detector; this container has to be appropriately labeled for disposal in an ecologically responsible manner. A mobile phase recycling device may be put after the detector in isocratic chromatography cases. The clean mobile phase is returned to the reservoir by this device, which runs during instrument runtime, when no injections are being produced, or at times when no peaks are eluted. After the detector, a fraction collecting device is installed if it is necessary to collect the eluted peaks. Fixed time intervals, movable phase volume, or detector signal output can all be used as the basis for this collection. Furthermore, for enhanced usability, fraction collectors may be managed by the HPLC's computer.

11.2.4.9 Connective Tubing

When it comes to materials inert to solvents and components of the mobile phase, tubing used in HPLC systems must be composed of stainless steel or polymer-based materials such as Teflon or PEEK. Tubing is connected to HPLC components using fittings and unions in an effort to reduce dead volume and surplus volume. Fittings with low dead volume (LDV) and zero dead volume (ZDV) are essential to minimizing band-broadening effects. Since more column volume reduces the effectiveness of separation, assembly of the columns and fittings must be done carefully to guarantee correct matching and flat fitting. A nut and ferrule are commonly seen on fittings, and they function in tandem to provide leak-proof connections with tubing openings. Due to its impermeability, buffer and solvent tolerance, adaptability, and simplicity of handling, polymer-based (PEEK) tubing and fittings are commonly used [27].

11.3 Applications of HPLC in Complementary Medicine

Medicinal plants serve as vital reservoirs of new natural compounds, offering a rich chemical diversity crucial for pharmaceutical development. They form the foundation for numerous complementary and alternative medicines, dietary supplements, cosmetics, and even medical devices. However, the intricate nature of herbs and extracts, catering to diverse markets and regulatory frameworks, presents significant challenges in classification and quality assurance. This underscores the necessity for robust analytical methods for their identification, standardization, and detection of adulterants and contaminants. Customs laboratories frequently encounter herbal samples, spanning herbal medicines, dietary supplements, tobacco, cannabis, and more, prompting inquiries ranging from identity verification to contamination assessment, risk mitigation, and legal compliance. Recent years have witnessed notable progress in the processing and investigation of medicinal plants, facilitated by modern extraction techniques and the identification of key components. Analytical methods such as HPLC and hyphenated HPLC have emerged as indispensable tools for assessing the identification and quality of herbal products [28].

11.3.1 Quality Control of Herbal Medicine

In the discovery domain, the identification (quantitative and qualitative) of active compounds from the herbal extract is the most difficult and challenging task. In modern discovery, processes like isolation with preparative bio-activity do not match the pace as they are slow and tedious, whereas modern systems prefer easy, accurate, and fast processes to be utilized. Traditional techniques, which use multiple isolations, can lead to a decrease or complete vanishing of the activity of the active compound. So to overcome the drawbacks, profiling of compounds with HPLC analytical technique is done in modern discovery to identify the multiple compounds accurately due to the versatility of the analytical technique [29].

For quality assurance, herbs and traditional medicinal products obtained from the extract of plants can be estimated for the chemical components with the HPLC technique. In the identification of phytoconstituents in herbal medicine products, the standardization technique with the marker profile is of greater benefit as the quantifications of the multiple constituents from the herbal medicinal formulations have issues related to safety and efficacy [30].

Separation of components using traditional polyherbal medicinal formulation is a convincing analytical technique and it has been gaining importance in the quality control of herbs for qualification, quantification, and authentication. Further, harvesting season, drying techniques, plant origin, presence of heavy metals, and microbial contents are the major reasons which vary the quality of the herbs [31].

11.3.2 Detection and Quantification of Active Constituents

When it comes to HPLC detectors, the UV detector is the most often used and simple choice. It is not without limits, especially when it comes to herbal constituents that do not include UV chromophores, all things considered, it offers the finest combination of sensitivity, linearity, flexibility, and reliability of any LC detector that has been made to date. The majority of natural goods absorb UV light between 200 and 550 nm, which includes compounds that have unshared electrons or double bonds. Therefore, compounds with moderate chromophores, such as triterpene glycosides, can be effectively detected by UV at short wavelengths (203 nm). However, as they may make it more difficult to identify natural compounds with weak chromophores, care must be taken to avoid mobile phase components with high UV cut-offs [32].

The crude extracts that have been distinguished frequently necessitate gradient elution, which modifies baseline at low wavelengths. Modifiers such as trifluoroacetic acid (TFA) or phosphate buffers with low UV cut-offs can be used to get around this problem. Such modifiers are not the best choice for multi-hyphenated systems that need HPLC-MS, though, and they should be avoided in such situations due to their non-volatility and tendency for ion suppression [33].

Due to its simplicity and cost-effectiveness, HPLC-UV finds widespread use in numerous pharmacopoeias for quantifying individual natural products in quality control processes for herbal drugs, as well as for detecting and quantifying active constituents. In both the European and United States pharmacopoeias [34], HPLC-UV (at 203 nm) systems are employed to ascertain the total ginsenoside content of ginseng roots and measure the ratio of ginsenosides [35]. Some clinical applications of these are shown in Figure 11.1.

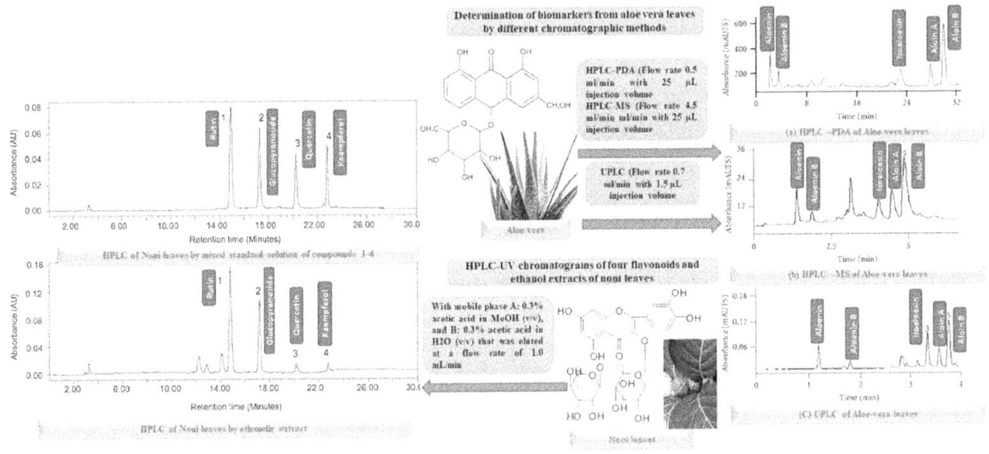

FIGURE 11.1 Application of HPLC in the detection of compounds in plants.

11.3.3 Identification of Adulterants and Contamination

The integrity of both raw herbal materials and their derived formulations is compromised by substitutions and adulterations. Adulterants, originating from various sources, encompass heavy metals, microbial agents, radioactive materials, synthetic compounds, and undisclosed substances. Additionally, chemical ingredients and prescription drugs, posing health risks, may be present as adulterants. Herbal products span diverse categories such as weight loss aids, blood pressure regulators, cholesterol-lowering agents, skin lighteners, and sexual performance enhancers. Unfortunately, these formulations often harbor undeclared synthetic drugs, steroids, and hazardous substances. Instances of contamination include arsenic in cancer treatment formulations, mercury in skin whitening creams, and carcinogenic and mutagenic compounds like β Asarone, Xanthotoxin, Berberine, Benzyl cyanide, and Digitalis glycosides in herbal medicine. Synthetic adulterants, spanning analgesics, antibiotics, antidiabetic drugs, aphrodisiacs, hormones, and anabolic substances, are sometimes added to enhance the efficacy of herbal medicine. Various studies have detected benzodiazepines, tricyclic antidepressants, cyproheptadine, ibuprofen, and dipyrone in different herbal formulations, underscoring the pervasiveness of adulteration across categories [36]. A comprehensive list of common adulterants in each category is provided in Table 11.1 [37–39].

HPLC is a frequently used chromatographic technique aimed at identifying medicine adulteration. MS and UV are two examples of the detectors that may be connected to HPLC. The sensitive and repeatable analytical findings provided by HPLC-UV analysis techniques are enhanced by their quick analysis

TABLE 11.1

Categories of adulterants

Adulterant	Examples
Heavy metal	Lead, Arsenic, Mercury, Cadmium, Aluminum, Nitrate and nitrite, Calcium, Copper, Iron, Potassium, Sodium
Microbial/biological	*Aspergillus flavus*, *Aspergillus funigatus*, *Astralagus sarcocolla*, Coliform and fecal coliform, *Bacillus cereus*, *Aeromonas hydrophilia*, *Shigella* spp., *Enterobacter* sp., *Escherichia coli*, *Vibrio fluvialis*
	Earthworms, Amoeba, Moulds, Protozoa, Yeasts, Nematode.
	Viruses
	Insects
Synthetic drugs	Tramadol, Caffeine, Fluoxetine, Rizatriptan, Venlafaxine, Methadone, Glibenclamide, Sibutramine hydrochloride, Sildenafil, Fenproporex

times, low sample needs, and excellent accuracy and precision when identifying several chemicals in a sample at once. For example, HPLC-UV can be used to analyze undeclared synthetic pharmaceuticals in herbal items such as phenolphthalein, sildenafil, and butramine. HPLC may be coupled not only with a UV detector but also with tandem mass spectrometry (MS/MS) [40, 41]

11.3.4 Standardization of Complementary Medicine

It is necessary to define qualitative and quantitative values, set consistent standards, and guarantee quality, safety, efficacy, and repeatability in order to standardize herbal medications. This entails identifying the distinctive qualities of the medications through testing and observation in order to establish and align technical standards. Thus, standardization is an essential tool for quality control [42].

The World Health Organization (WHO) states that a thorough procedure of physicochemical examination of raw materials is required for the standardization and quality control of herbal products. In this process, raw materials are chosen and handled, the finished product's stability, safety, and effectiveness are assessed, safety and risk information is documented based on experience, consumer product information is given, and the product is promoted. These evaluations use a range of analytical techniques and instruments to conduct physical, chemical, and biological analyses [43].

Pharmaceutical companies commonly utilize preparative and analytical HPLC for the extraction and purification of herbal constituents. Preparative HPLC can be categorized into low pressure usually less than 5 bar and high pressure greater than 20 bar systems. High-pressure preparative HPLC involves larger stainless steel columns and packing materials with particle sizes ranging from 10 to 30 micrometers. Analytical HPLC prioritizes resolution, sensitivity, and rapid analysis. While preparative HPLC is geared toward isolating or purifying compounds, analytical HPLC focuses on obtaining information about the sample, which is essential for the swift release of new natural and synthetic products into the pharmaceutical market. This efficient purification method enables reduced synthesis time for optimal synthesis conditions [44].

11.3.5 Determination of Marker Compound

A marker compound is a chemical component found in a medicinal substance that helps determine its strength or authenticity. These flag chemicals are sometimes referred to as active components or substances that verify the original material's proper botanical identification. Finding appropriate marker compounds for traditional medicinal substances is challenging, as some medicines contain unidentified active constituents, while others consist of several active components.

Analytical methods are pivotal for ensuring the quality, safety, and effectiveness of plant materials. These approaches often involve the use of spectroscopic techniques like fluorescence, MS, and differential absorption spectrum (DAD) in conjunction with chromatographic methods like HPLC and gas chromatography (GC). Additionally, they may involve the use of generic detectors like charged aerosol, or specific detectors like electrochemical and ion capture. Although these approaches have inherent limits, the correct identification of elements depends on reference standards and composite database sources. It is well known that, although important, main chemical markers cannot include all of the active metabolites in an extract. One notable example of an easy-to-use and reasonably priced analytical method for identifying low-molecular-weight chemicals in a variety of pharmaceutical, environmental, and dietary samples is thin-layer chromatography (TLC). Its popularity surpasses that of other chromatographic methods like GC and HPLC owing to its versatility, cost-effectiveness, accessibility, simplicity, minimal solvent and reagent usage, and ability to analyze multiple samples concurrently [45].

Identifying marker compounds using HPLC involves several steps:

1. Sample Preparation: Prepare your sample for analysis. This might involve extraction, filtration, dilution, or other sample pretreatment steps to ensure compatibility with the HPLC system.

2. Instrument Configuration: Configure the HPLC system in accordance with the specific demands of your analysis. This entails selecting the suitable column, mobile phase, detector, and operational parameters such as flow rate, temperature, and injection volume.
3. Method Optimization: Develop an HPLC protocol tailored to effectively separate and detect the target marker compound(s). This process entails fine-tuning parameters such as column selection, mobile phase composition, elution method, and detector wavelength.
4. Sample Evaluation: Introduce your prepared sample into the HPLC system and execute the analysis following the established method. Gather data from the detector, typically acquiring chromatograms displaying compound retention times and peak areas.
5. Compound Verification: Contrast the retention time and spectral attributes (if accessible) of peaks in your sample chromatogram with those of established standards or references in the literature. Validation may additionally encompass fortifying your sample with recognized standards to authenticate the existence of the marker compounds [46, 47].

11.3.6 Ensuring Batch-to-Batch Consistency

In pharmaceutical manufacturing, products are made using standard operating procedures which are specific for each product. As a result, it is expected that any number of batches of the same product selected at random for evaluation should either have the same results for all tested criteria or the difference between them should be within the acceptable limits. Batch-to-batch consistency study of herbal products is an important quality control parameter for assessing their reproducibility, efficacy, and safety profile. To assess the batch-to-batch consistency of a herbal product, parameters such as color, odor, taste, pH, and total solid residue can be utilized.

11.3.7 HPLC Fingerprints for Herbal Medicine

As the herbal medicine market continues to grow, the use of HPLC chromatogram fingerprinting has become essential for analyzing plant-based remedies both qualitatively and quantitatively. Methods like principal component analysis and hierarchical clustering analysis, which typically rely on particular biomarkers or reference standards, are commonly used in the qualitative identification and validation of unknown plant extracts. However, in the absence of a suitable reference standard, a simple and standard chromatographic fingerprint of the herbal product will suffice to pass regulatory requirements [48].

11.3.8 Pharmacokinetic Studies

Pharmacokinetic investigation offers a pragmatic method for pinpointing potentially significant compounds, those bioavailable at target sites with substantial exposure levels following herbal medicine administration. Enhancing comprehension of the pharmacokinetic characteristics of these absorbable substances is crucial for assessing the medicinal advantages and possible drawbacks of herbal remedies, in addition to their interplay with pharmacokinetics. This becomes more important when conventional therapy is combined with herbal medication [49].

11.3.9 Bioavailability and Metabolism of Herbal Compounds

Bioavailability pertains to how quickly and to what extent the phytochemical or active component is absorbed from the ingested matrix, enabling it to arrive to the intended action point. This definition stems from two primary factors governing the efficacy of any compound in vivo: first, the active compound must reach the site of action to exert its biological effect, and second, the concentration and duration of exposure of the active compound at the site of action influence the level of activity [50].

It is generally recognized that bioactive substances have the ability to elicit biological reactions that result in changes in metabolism that are beneficial to human health. These reactions might entail enhancing particular physiological processes or reducing the likelihood of certain diseases. Bioactive chemicals, which vary greatly in their chemical makeup and biological function, are abundant in plants. Minerals, vitamins, and other non-nutrient elements known as phytochemicals are a few examples of these health-promoting substances that may be found in plants. Among other things, phytochemicals include glucosinolates, phytosterols, phenolic compounds, carotenoids, and terpenoids [51].

The bioavailability, pharmacokinetics, and metabolism of bioactive chemicals have been investigated using a variety of experimental models, with in vitro models being widely used for this purpose. When hyphenated techniques are used, they play a crucial role in metabolomics. This combination reduces complexity and matrix effects, improves selectivity, and makes it easier to separate chemicals beforehand. Although analytical techniques are versatile, most studies on bioavailability and metabolism primarily employ high- or ultrahigh-performance liquid chromatography coupled with mass spectrometry. Given the significant advantages of LC-MS detection, the utilization of the DAD in such studies is declining. Nonetheless, some studies still integrate DAD, often in conjunction with an MS detector (LC–DAD–MS) [52].

Standard parameters including maximum plasma concentration (C_{max}), the area under the plasma concentration-time curve (AUC), time to achieve C_{max} (t_{max}), and elimination half-life ($t_{1/2}$) are routinely calculated in studies concentrating on bioavailability and pharmacokinetics [53].

11.3.10 Studying Interaction between Different Components

Herb-drug interactions can have significant clinical consequences and increase the risk of microbial resistance when using herbal products contaminated with conventional medications. The complex content of herbal remedies renders it challenging to positively identify adulterants. An analytical technique is recommended for identifying adulteration in herbal products [54]. Combined methods, such as HPLC-MS/MS, offer enhanced selectivity and sensitivity, making it possible to definitively screen herbal products for adulterants [55]. Instances of herb-drug interactions are provided in Table 11.2 [56–60].

11.3.11 HPLC Analysis of Common Plant Products

Complementary and alternative therapies that fall within the category of herbal medicine can be analyzed using HPLC. Several studies have been conducted in this regard [61–71]. A summary of these studies is shown in Table 11.3.

11.3.12 Comparisons of Traditional and Modern Analytical Techniques

There are several important phases involved in the standardization and quality assurance processes for herbal medicine. These include analyzing the finished product's stability, efficacy, and safety; evaluating the physical and chemical properties of the raw materials; and offering comprehensive information

TABLE 11.2

Some common herb-drug interactions

Herb	Drug	Interaction
Garlic	Antihypertensive drugs	Herb may decrease blood pressure
Ginkgo bibola	Acetaminophen, anticonvulsants/tricyclic antidepressants, thiazides	Subarachnoid hemorrhage Increase seizures May lead to hypertension
Grape fruit	Calcium channel blockers and many drugs	Increase oral bioavailability
St. John's Wort	Zolpidem	Likely increases CYP3A4 activity, leading to a reduction in the plasma concentration of zolpidem
Andrographis paniculata	Glipizide	Alter the pharmacokinetic of glipizide

TABLE 11.3

A summary of plant products analyzed using HPLC

No.	Plant name/ biological source	Parts used	Column used	Mobile phase/ stationary phase	Detector	Phytochemicals	Retention time
1	Turmeric (*Curcuma longa*)	Rhizomes	C18 column (250 × 4.6 mm, Eurospher 100 with 5 µm)	Ethyl Nitrile -methanol-water-at a volume ratio of 65:5:30	UV-VIS detectors	Bis-demethoxycurcumin (BDMC),	RT:4.82 Rs:4.74 T:0.95
						Demethoxycurcumin (DMC),	RT:5.18 Rs:1.48 T:1.12
						Curcumin (C)	RT:5.58 Rs:1.68 T:1.16
2	Black pepper (*Piper nigrum*)	Dried unripe fruit	C18 column (250 × 4.6 mm, with 5 µm) with a pre-column	Ethyl Nitrile -methanol-water-at a volume ratio of 65:5:30	UV-VIS detectors	Piperin	RT:7.91 Rs:3.57 T:1.06
3	Garlic (*Allium sativum* L.)	Bulb	C18 column (250 × 4.6 mm i.d., 5 µm particle size) (A kromasil)	Isocratic mode Methanol: water (50:50)	UV detector	Allicin	RT:5.07 Rs:1.3
4	Liqorice (*Glycyrrhiza lensis* Fisch., *Glycyrrhiza inflata* Bat., and *Glycyrrhiza glabra* L.)	Dried root and rhizome	Column: C8 reversed-phase (150 × 4.6 mm i.d.; 5 µm) and a Phenomenex (Torrance, CA, USA) Guard C8 pre-column (4.0 × 3.0 mm i.d.; 5 µm)	Methanol: Acetonitrile :water: glacial acetic acid (35:35:29:1, by volume)	PAD detector	Glycyrrhizin	RT:2.9
						Glycyrrhetic acid	RT:16
5	Ginger (*Zingiber officinale* Roscoe)	Rhizomes	(4.6 mm × 250 mm; particle size 5 µm) C-18 column, temperature of 30°C	Acetonitrile: 0.1% Phosphoric acid: Methanol (55:44:1)	UV-VIS detectors	6-Gingerol	RT:4.11 Rs:17.6 T:1.1
						6-Shogaol	RT:10.51 T:1.07

(Continued)

TABLE 11.3 (CONTINUED)

A summary of plant products analyzed using HPLC

No.	Plant name/ biological source	Parts used	Column used	Mobile phase/ stationary phase	Detector	Phytochemicals	Retention time
6	Green Tea (*Camellia sinensis*)	Leaves	C18 column (4.6 mm × 250 mm)	Mobile phases included an aqueous solution of methanol (A) and 1.0% phosphoric acid solution (B). Gradients of 20–42% of methanol for 0–5 min, 42–43% of methanol for 15–5 min, 43–90% of methanol for 25–45 min, keeping 90% of methanol for 45–55 min, decreasing to 20% of methanol for 55–60 min, and keeping 20% of methanol for 60–70 min	UV detector	Epigallocatechin Catechin Epicatechin EpigallocatecHin gallate Epicatechin gallate	RT: 13.013 RT: 13.780 RT: 16.494 RT: 17.696 RT: 20.754
7	Cinnamon	Bark	C18 Column (4.6 × 250 mm, 5 µm)	Isocratic elution, Ethanol: Ethyl Nitrile (0.5% v/v) flow rate: 1 mL/min	UV-VIS detector	Cinnamaldehyde	RT: 6.989
8	Fenugreek (*Trigonella foenum-graecum*)	Seeds	C18 column (4.6 mm × 250 mm, 5 µm particle size)	Acetonitrile: water (90:10 v/v)	UV detector	Diosgenin (aq.) Diosgenin (methanol)	RT: 24.927 RT: 25.033

(Continued)

TABLE 11.3 (CONTINUED)

A summary of plant products analyzed using HPLC

No.	Plant name/ biological source	Parts used	Column used	Mobile phase/ stationary phase	Detector	Phytochemicals	Retention time
9	Aloe vera (*Aloe-barbadensis*)	Leaves	C-18 column	Methanol: acetic acid (98 : 2)	PDA detector	Aloenin Aloenin Isoaloesin Aloin A Aloin B	RT: 7.9 RT: 9.0 RT: 25.1 RT: 29.0 RT: 30.7
10	Ashwagandha	Roots	C18Eclipse, XDB, 4.6mm × 150mm, 5 µm particle size Agilent Column	Acetonitrile: Buffer (35:65)	Diode Array Detector (DAD)	Withaferin A	RT: 5.090
11	Noni	Fruit	C-18-E (150 mm × 4.6 mm) particle size: 3.5 µm	15% ACN in water	DAD detector	Scopoletin	RT: 19.69 T: 1.002
12	Ephedra (*Ephedra sinica*)	Arial Part	HS F5 column (15 cm × 4.6 mm ID, 5 µm particles)	Acetic acid, ammonium salt: Acetonitrile–water (90:10, v/v),	Photodiode Array Detector (PAD)	Norephedrine Norpseudoephedrine Synephrine Methyl ephedrine Ephedrine Pseudoephedrine	RT:8.82 RT:9.60 Rs:2.38 RT:10.51 Rs:2.49 RT:12.65 Rs:4.85 RT:13.43 Rs:1.56 RT:14.48 Rs:1.92

RS = Resolution; RT = Retention Time; T = Tailing factor.

to help customers. The evaluation process typically includes visual examinations, chemical analyses, and biological tests of samples. There are three main approaches to analytical evaluation: analyzing marker compounds or individual components, creating fingerprints or profiles of the herbal material, and conducting metabolomic studies. Marker compounds act as references for potency and are frequently selected from the variety of chemicals found in the plant. However, depending just on marker chemicals to standardize data might occasionally produce inaccurate findings, particularly if the marker of choice is not a good representation of the active components of the plant.

Furthermore, the therapeutic benefits of herbal medicine may arise from complex interactions among various constituents, making one or a few markers insufficient predictors of overall effectiveness. In contrast, fingerprinting methods analyze the complete chemical makeup of the botanical sample. When combined with statistical analysis of multivariate data or chemometrics, this intricate profile may be compressed to a unique pattern that correlates with particular biological or pharmacological action. This offers a starting point for evaluating certain materials or formulas. The origins of plant species may be determined and genuine herbal treatments can be distinguished from fakes using fingerprinting techniques. The creation of phytochemical patterns frequently involves the use of chromatographic methods like TLC and HPLC. Other technologies such as capillary electrophoresis, molecular spectroscopy, and DNA-based methods can also generate molecular or chemical fingerprints for comparable objectives [72].

11.3.13 Improving the Quality and Safety of Complementary Medicine Products

One of the biggest challenges facing researchers is creating dependable analytical techniques for complex herbal medicines that can precisely profile their phytochemical content. These techniques include quantitative studies of marker/bioactive molecules and other important elements. Standardization is essential for the production of herb medicines to ensure consistent biological activity, a consistent chemical profile, and the execution of quality assurance processes. Due to the fact that HPLC can assess active indicators that are chemical or biological in origin both subjectively and quantitatively, it has become a regularly used method in the standardization of complicated herbal remedies. Through the efficient removal of instrumental interference, correction of retention time shifts, enhancement of selectivity, increase of chromatographic separation capabilities, and assurance of measurement precision, hyphenated chromatographic and spectrometric procedures provide significant gains in performance [73].

11.4 Challenges and Future Perspectives

The pursuit of sensitive, all-encompassing HPLC detection with consistent response factors for every analyte remains unfulfilled. Currently, there is no perfect answer, and the kind of natural products being examined must be considered while selecting certain detectors. One reason why it is still difficult to create universally applicable HPLC techniques is the lack of a sensitive and universal detection approach suited for qualitative and quantitative analysis under various circumstances. Approximately, 20% of HPLC applications are HPLC-MS (with roughly one-third pertaining to MS-MS), whereas over 70% of HPLC applications are carried out utilizing HPLC-UV and HPLC-DAD [74]. Evaporative light scattering detector (ELSD) accounted for 1.5%, HPLC-electrochemical detection (ECD) for 3%, and HPLC-NMR for 2%. Other detection methods are mentioned in fewer than 1 percent of all HPLC applications. Most analyses are still carried out with HPLC-UV, which is a popular choice in many labs.

HPLC-MS is a powerful and adaptable instrument renowned for its sensitivity and ability to function as both a particular and an all-purpose detection technique. Its popularity across several fields of herbal product research is expected to expand with the introduction of more user-friendly benchtop equipment, even if they are currently rather expensive. However, because HPLC-MS is susceptible to the ionization process, it is still not as robust as other techniques for quantitative analysis. This might cause problems with ionization suppression when working with complicated matrices. The increased separation speed

TABLE 11.4

Overview of the benefits and constraints of each liquid-chromatographic detection methods

No.	Hyphenated technique	Benefits	Constraints	Utilization
1	UV	Widespread, affordable, simple to use, and suited to a sizable variety of natural compounds, with low-wavelength detection	Not suitable for substances lacking chromophores, not particularly selective, and incompatible with components of the mobile phase that have strong UV cut-offs	All natural products with chromophores (even weak chromophores: 203 nm)
2	DAD	Recording of all wavelengths, the ability to modify provided spectra for dereplication, and simultaneous monitoring of several wavelengths	UV spectra only provide little structural information for dereplication	Every natural substance that has a distinctive chromophore, particularly polyketides, alkaloids, quinones, and polyphenols
3	FD	Excellent selectivity and sensitivity	Restricted to natural products that naturally glow or need a laborious derivatization process	Mostly aflatoxins, with fluorescent tags used to selectively detect other NPs following derivation
4	EC	Low cost, perceptive, and somewhat discerning	Redox response understanding and possible optimization are required, involvement, the sample is changed by detecting	Any and all natural products with electroactive groups, including ethers, quinones, phenols, aromatics, amines, thiols, olefins, and ester
5	RID	Universal, affordable	Sensitive to temperature, pressure, and flow rate variations; poor sensitivity; not suitable to gradients	Polymers, certain terpenes, and carbohydrates
6	ELSD	Adaptable, widely used, simple to operate, and consistent with gradient elution	Non-linear response, requiring drift tube temperature and gas flow optimization	Every natural product, mostly employed for identifying natural products with weak chromophores, such as terpenes and carbs
7	CAD	Wide dynamic range, higher sensitivity than ELSD, and universality (4 orders of magnitude)	Non-linear reaction	Used for lipids, polysaccharides, and medicines; not yet used for natural products
8	MS	Broadly applicable, precise, sensitive, and able to deliver molecular formula (HR mode) or structural MW information (LR mode)	Response depending on the compound, incompatible with buffers which are not volatile, susceptible to ion suppression effects in intricate matrix systems, and costly	All natural products; limited sensitivity for non-polar Natural products
9	MS-MS	Universal, pervasive, sensitive, offering very precise detection (MRM mode) and fragmented information	Similar to MS, the MS-MS spectra's reliance on the instrument and the absence of an MS-MS database for Natural products	Similar to MS, fragment information provides valuable details mostly on glycosides and/or polyphenols

(*Continued*)

TABLE 11.4 (CONTINUED)

Overview of the benefits and constraints of each liquid-chromatographic detection methods

No.	Hyphenated technique	Benefits	Constraints	Utilization
10	NMR	All-encompassing and crucial structural data for real-time de novo structure determination	Inexpensive, poor sensitivity, response dependent on the mode of operation (on-flow, stop-flow, at-line)	All natural products, on-flow for identifying those with a distinctive 1H pattern, and on-line for determining the detailed structure (1D and 2D)

CAD = Charged aerosol detector; DAD = Differential absorption spectrum; EC = electrochemical; ELSD = Evaporative light scattering detector; FD = Fluorescence detection; UV = Ultraviolet; MS = Mass spectrometry; MS/MS = Tandem mass spectrometry; NMR = Nuclear magnetic resonance; RID = Refractive index detection.

provided by these new separation techniques presents a problem for LC detectors hoping to provide quicker answers.

HPLC-DAD-MS is an essential strategic tool for online structure determination; it is mostly utilized for dereplication in drug development laboratories. Nevertheless, the possibilities for automation and prediction in the dereplication process are constrained by the absence of extensive HPLC-MS datasets. Recent years have seen significant progress in this field, especially in the areas of HPLC-based on-flow bioassays and activity profiling. These strategies offer completely integrated lead-finding platforms by progressively integrating with multi-hyphenated methodologies. Detection in HPLC is still a difficult problem because of the increasing need for metabolomics, dereplication, quality assurance, profiling, and fingerprinting. Table 11.4 presents a summary outlining the benefits and constraints of each LC detection method [74, 75].

Conventional analytical methods struggle to meet the demands of modern natural product research due to increasing complexities. Hyphenated techniques offer an advanced solution, merging separation and spectroscopic methods to leverage their respective strengths. Notable progress in hyphenated systems has greatly expanded their utility in analyzing natural products. Combining separation and spectroscopic systems has proven effective in both quantifying and identifying unknown phytoconstituents in extracts or fractions. These techniques facilitate the thorough characterization of chemical profiles in herbal extracts, medicines, and formulations.

Currently, infrared or Fourier-transform (IR or FTIR) spectroscopy serves as a valuable technique for identifying organic compounds, utilizing the mid-IR region where organic compound structures exhibit characteristic absorption bands corresponding to specific functionalities such as –OH, –COOH, and more. Although less sensitive than techniques like UV and MS, IR spectroscopy remains effective in compound identification. Recent advancements in HPLC-IR techniques, achieved through the integration of two fundamental approaches, form the basis of HPLC-IR or HPLC-FTIR techniques [75].

LC-MS denotes the pairing of a mass spectrometer with liquid chromatography. The utilization of LC-MS-MS is experiencing rapid growth due to its effectiveness in combining biological screening with natural products. This encompasses techniques like HPLC coupled with UV and mass spectrometry, which are considered the most compatible interfaces in phytochemical analysis [76].

Among spectrometric techniques, NMR stands out as the least sensitive but highly advantageous for elucidating the structure of natural products. These studies may be carried out with systems operating at 0.5, 0.6, and 0.8 GHz and equipped with ^{1}H, ^{13}C, ^{2}H, ^{19}F, and ^{31}P probes. They can be carried out in together continuous-flow and stop-flow modes. New developments in hardware and software have improved this hyphenated technology by creating new avenues for the direct connection of LC and NMR [77].

11.5 Conclusion

This chapter highlights key considerations when using HPLC in the analysis of complementary medicines. The complex nature associated with the separation of compounds in plant products remains a significant challenge with the use of HPLC. Nevertheless, this approach is recognized as an adaptable and reliable method for examining secondary metabolites in plants, providing a range of uses in the isolation, as well as the quantitative and qualitative evaluation of active molecules. Furthermore, HPLC offers insights into advanced extraction methods aimed at isolating and purifying compounds from plant sources.

REFERENCES

1. Zollman C, Vickers A. ABC of complementary medicine. *BMJ.* 1999 Sep 11;319(7211):693. https://doi.org/10.1136/bmj.319.7211.693
2. https://guides.library.duq.edu/complementary_medicine/research_methods
3. Barnes PM, Bloom B, Nahin RL. Complementary and alternative medicine use among adults: United States, 2002. *Natl Health Stat Report.* 2008 Jun;(12):1–23.
4. Alleyne G, Breman J, Claeson M, Evans D, Jamison D, Jha P, Measham A, Mills A, Musgrove P. *Disease control priorities in developing countries.* 2nd ed. World Bank, Washington DC; 2006.
5. Kalariya Y, Kumar A, Ullah A, Umair A, Neha FN, Madhurita FN, Varagantiwar V, Jaffari SM, Ahmad A, Aman M, Sapna FN. Integrative medicine approaches: bridging the gap between conventional and renal complementary therapies. *Cureus.* 2023 Sep 26;15(9):e48523.
6. National Cancer Institute. Complementary and integrative medicine. Available from: https://www.cancer.gov/about-cancer/treatment/cam#top
7. Malviya R, Bansal V, Pal O, Sharma P. High performance liquid chromatography: a short review. *J Global Pharma Technol.* 2010;2(3):22–6.
8. Abidi SL. High-performance liquid chromatography of phosphatidic acids and related polar lipids. *J Chromatogr A.* 1991;587(2):193–203. https://doi.org/10.1016/0021-9673(91)85156-A.
9. Gupta MK, Biswas PK. Chapter 10 - Chromatography: basic principle, types, and applications. In: Bhatt AK, Bhatia RK, Bhalla TC, editors. *Basic biotechniques for bioprocess and bio-entrepreneurship.* Academic Press; 2023. p. 173–82. ISBN 9780128161098. https://doi.org/10.1016/B978-0-12-816109-8.00010-6.
10. Barbosa Filho VM, Waczuk EP, Kamdem JP, Abolaji AO, Lacerda SR, Costa JGM, et al. Phytochemical constituents, antioxidant activity, cytotoxicity and osmotic fragility effects of Caju (Anacardium microcarpum). *Ind Crops Prod.* 2014;55:280–8.
11. Janovik V, Boligon AA, Athayde ML. Antioxidant activities and HPLC/DAD analysis of phenolics and carotenoids from the barks of *Cariniana domestica* (Mart.) Miers. *Res J Phytochem.* 2012;6:105–12.
12. Sasidharan S, Chen Y, Saravanan D, Sundram KM, Yoga Latha L. Extraction, isolation and characterization of bioactive compounds from plants' extracts. *Afr J Tradit Complement Altern Med.* 2011;8:1–10.
13. Boligon AA, Athayde ML. Importance of HPLC in analysis of plant extracts. *Austin Chromatogr.* 2014;1(3):2.
14. LaCourse WR. *HPLC instrumentation.* Elsevier Inc., Amsterdam; 2017.
15. Fredj G, Paillet M, Aussel F, Brouard A, Barreteau H, Divine C, Micaud M. Determination of sulbactam in biological fluids by high-performance liquid chromatography. *J Chromatogr.* 1986 Nov 28;383(1):218–22. https://doi.org/10.1016/s0378-4347(00)83464-7. PMID: 3029153.
16. Polite L. Liquid chromatography: basic overview. In: Miller J, Crowther JB, editors. *Analytical chemistry in a GMP environment: a practical guide.* John Wiley & Sons, Hoboken, New Jersey; 2000.
17. The United States Pharmacopoeia, USP 27, NF 22, United States Pharmacopeial Convention, Rockville, Md, USA, 2004.
18. Watson DG. *Pharmaceutical analysis.* 2nd ed. Elsevier, Amsterdam; 2007. p. 281–6.
19. Beckett AH, Stenlake JB. *Practical pharmaceutical chemistry, part 2.* 1st ed. CBS Publishers and Distributors, New Delhi; 2007. p. 157–66.

20. Fourkaridis GN, Muntingh GL, Osuch E. Application of diode array detection for the identification of poisoning by traditional medicines. *J Ethnopharmacol.* 1994;41(3):135–46.
21. Chatwal GR, Anand SK. *Instrumental methods of chemical analysis.* 5th ed. Himalaya Publishing House, Shaniwar Peth; 2007. p. 2624–39.
22. Ashrani S, Goyal A, Vaishnav R. HPLC detectors, their types and use: a review. *Org Med Chem IJ.* 2018;6(5):555700. https://doi.org/10.19080/OMCIJ.2018.06.555700.
23. Kenmore CK, Ersline SR. Refractive index detection by interferometric backscatter in packed-capillary high performance liquid chromatography. *J Chromatogr.* 1997;762(1–2):219–25.
24. Ismail H, Kassandra K, Dernik G. Electrochemical imaging of fusion pore openings by electrochemical detectors arrays. *Cent Sci Stud.* 2005;102:13879–84.
25. Wang D, Abate D. HPLC: past and present. *Angew Chem Int Ed.* 2010;49:1300–2312.
26. Swartz M. HPLC detectors: a brief review. *J Liq Chromatogr Relat Technol.* 2010;33:9–12:1130–50.
27. LaCourse ME, LaCourse WR. General instrumentation in HPLC. In: *Liquid chromatography: fundamentals and instrumentation*, 2nd ed. Elsevier; 2017. Vol. 1, pp. 417–29. https://doi.org/10.1016/B978-0-12-805393-5.00017-8.
28. Nonga W, Mutombo Shakalenga C, Sheridan H, Nachtergael A, Duez P. Quality control of herbal drugs and preparations: the methods of analysis, their relevance and applications. *Sci Rep.* 2021;4:100070.
29. Hamburger M. HPLC-based activity profiling for pharmacologically and toxicologically relevant natural products–principles and recent examples. *Pharm Biol.* 2019;57(1):328–34.
30. Nag M, Kar A, Chanda J, Mukherjee PK. RP-HPLC analysis of methanol extract of *Viscum articulatum*–a plant from Ayurveda. *J Ayurveda Integr Med.* 2019. https://doi.org/10.1016/j.jaim.2018.02.135.
31. Raclariu AC, Paltinean R, Vlase L, Labarre A, Manzanilla V, Ichim MC, de Boer H. Comparative authentication of *Hypericum perforatum* herbal products using DNA metabarcoding, TLC and HPLC-MS. *Sci Rep.* 2017;7(1):1–12.
32. Gao XF, Dan M, Zhao AH, Xie GX, Jia W. Simultaneous determination of saponins in flower buds of *Panax notoginseng* using high-performance liquid chromatography. *Biomed Chromatogr.* 2008;22:244–9.
33. Leitner A, Emmert J, Boerner K, Lindner W. Influence of solvent additive composition on chromatographic separation and sodium adduct formation of peptides in HPLC-ESI MS. *Chromatographia.* 2007;65:649–53.
34. European Pharmacopoeia 5.1, 5th ed. Strasbourg: Council of Europe; 2002.
35. Fuzzati N. Analysis methods of ginsenosides. *J Chromatogr B.* 2004;812:119–33.
36. Dharan Arya, Solanki Kalpesh, Gaur J. Detection of adulterants in herbal formulations: a review. *Int J Forensic Sci Leg Med.* 2021;1(1):33–9.
37. Alwakeel SS. Microbial and heavy metals contamination of herbal medicines. *Res J Microbiol.* 2008;3:683–91. https://doi.org/10.3923/jm.2008.683.691.
38. Kosalec I, Cvek J, Tomić S. Contaminants of medicinal herbs and herbal products. *Arh Hig Rada Toksikol.* 2009 Dec;60(4):485–501. https://doi.org/10.2478/10004-1254-60-2009-2005. PMID: 20061249.
39. Dastjerdi AG, Akhgari M, Kamali A, Mousavi Z. Principal component analysis of synthetic adulterants in herbal supplements advertised as weight loss drugs. *Complement Ther Clin Pract.* 2018 May;31:236–41. https://doi.org/10.1016/j.ctcp.2018.03.007. Epub 2018 Mar 15. PMID: 29705461.
40. Hemdan A, Tawakol SM. HPLC–UV chromatographic methods for detection and quantification of undeclared withdrawn synthetic medications in counterfeit herbal medicines with confirmation by HPLC–PDA and mass spectrometry. *Chromatographia.* 2018;81:777–83.
41. Al Lawati HA, Al Busaidi I, Kadavilpparampu AM, Suliman FO. Determination of common adulterants in herbal medicine and food samples using core-shell column coupled to tandem mass spectrometry. *J Chromatogr Sci.* 2017;55:232–42.
42. Kunle FO, Egharevba OH, Ahmadu PO. Standardization of herbal medicines: a review. *Int J Biodivers Conserv.* 2012;4:101–12.
43. World Health Organization (WHO). *Quality assurance of pharmaceuticals: a compendium of guidelines and related materials, good manufacturing practices and inspection.* World Health Organization; 1996. p. 1–413.
44. Lamichhane S, Sahariah BJ, Das B, Khatiwara D, Sola P, Adhikari RP, Gogoi B, Alam T. Herbal drug standardization: a systemic review. *J Drug Deliv Ther.* 2023;13(4):149–53.

45. Ma T, Huang C, Meng X, et al. Fingerprint analysis of Hawk-tea by high-performance liquid chromatography. *Food Chem.* 2011;129(2):551–6.
46. Maimaiti Z, Turak A, Ma Q, Liu G, Aisa H. Quantitative determination of marker compounds and fingerprint analysis of the seeds of *Vernonia anthelmintica. Int J Anal Chem.* 2020:1–12. https://doi.org/10.1155/2020/8859425.
47. Kim JH, Doh EJ, Lee G. Quantitative comparison of the marker compounds in different medicinal parts of *Morus alba L.* using high-performance liquid chromatography-diode array detector with chemometric analysis. *Molecules.* 2020;25:5592. https://doi.org/10.3390/molecules25235592.
48. Archer M, Kumadoh D, N'guessan B, Adase E, Sarkodie J. Batch-to-batch consistency in the quality attributes of a phyto-pharmaceutical MA001 used to treat typhoid in Ghana. *J Med Biomed Sci.* 2023;9:1–17. https://doi.org/10.54106/249509.jmbs7z.
49. Jia WW, Lu C, Lin G, Ge GB. Editorial: pharmacokinetics of herbal medicines and herb-drug interactions. *Front Pharmacol.* 2022;13:1107777. https://doi.org/10.3389/fphar.2022.1107777.
50. Neilson A, Goodrich K, Ferruzzi M. Bioavailability and metabolism of bioactive compounds from foods. In: Coulston AM, Boushey CJ, Ferruzzi MG, Delahanty LM. *Bioavailability and metabolism of bioactive compounds from foods.* Academic Press, Cambridge; 2017. p. 301–19.
51. Hosseinzadeh S, Jafarikukhdan A, Hosseini A, Armand R. The application of medicinal plants in traditional and modern medicine: a review of *Thymus vulgaris. Int J Clin Med.* 2015;6:635–42.
52. Fernández-Ochoa Á, Cádiz-Gurrea MDL, Fernández-Moreno P, Rojas-García A, Arráez-Román D, Segura-Carretero A. Recent analytical approaches for the study of bioavailability and metabolism of bioactive phenolic compounds. *Molecules.* 2022;27:777. https://doi.org/10.3390/molecules27030777.
53. Kumar BR. Application of HPLC and ESI-MS techniques in the analysis of phenolic acids and flavonoids from green leafy vegetables (GLVs). *J Pharm Anal.* 2017;7:349–64.
54. Haider AJ, Al Lawati HJ, Al Busaidi I, Kadavilpparampu AM, Suliman FO. Determination of common adulterants in herbal medicine and food samples using core-shell column coupled to tandem mass spectrometry. *J Chromatogr Sci.* 2017;55:232–42. https://doi.org/10.1093/chromsci/bmw175.
55. Mwankuna CJ, Uwamaliya GA, Mariki EE, Mabiki F, Malebo HM, Mdegela R, Styrishave B. A HPLC-MS/MS method for screening of selected antibiotic adulterants in herbal drugs. *Anal Methods.* 2022 Mar 10;14(10):1060–8. https://doi.org/10.1039/d1ay01966j. PMID: 35195137.
56. Asdaq SM, Inamdar MN. Pharmacodynamic and pharmacokinetic interactions of propranolol with garlic (*Allium sativum*) in rats. *Evid Based Complement Alternat Med.* 2011.
57. Tang J, Sun J, Zhang Y, Li L, Cui F, He Z. Herb–drug interactions: effect of *Ginkgo biloba* extract on the pharmacokinetics of theophylline in rats. *Food Chem Toxicol.* 2007;45(12):2441–5. https://doi.org/10.1016/j.fct.2007.05.023.
58. Glesby MJ, Aberg JA, Kendall MA, Fichtenbaum CJ, Hafner R, Hall S, Grosskopf N, Zolopa AR, Gerber JG. Pharmacokinetic interactions between indinavir plus ritonavir and calcium channel blockers. *Clin Pharmacol Ther.* 2005 Aug;78(2):143–53.
59. Hojo Y, Echizenya M, Ohkubo T, Shimizu T. Drug interaction between *St John's wort* and zolpidem in healthy subjects. *J Clin Pharm Ther.* 2011 Dec;36(6):711–15.
60. Sundhani E, Nugroho AE, Nurrochmad A, Puspitasari I, Amalia Prihati D, Lukitaningsih E. Pharmacokinetic herb-drug interactions of glipizide with *Andrographis paniculata* (Burm. f.) and andrographolide in normal and diabetic rats by validated HPLC method. *Molecules.* 2022;27:6901. https://doi.org/10.3390/molecules27206901.
61. Pellati F, Benvenuti S. Determination of ephedrine alkaloids in *Ephedra* natural products using HPLC on a pentafluorophenylpropyl stationary phase. *J Pharm Biomed Anal.* 2008;48(2):254–63. https://doi.org/10.1016/j.jpba.2007.10.034.
62. Bose S, Laha B, Banerjee S. Quantification of allicin by high performance liquid chromatography-ultraviolet analysis with effect of post-ultrasonic sound and microwave radiation on fresh garlic cloves. *Phcog Mag.* 2014;10:288–93.
63. Sabbioni C, Ferranti A, Bugamelli F, Forti GC, Raggi MA. Simultaneous HPLC analysis, with isocratic elution, of glycyrrhizin and glycyrrhetic acid in liquorice roots and confectionery products. *Phytochem Anal.* 2006 Jan-Feb;17(1):25–31. https://doi.org/10.1002/pca.877. PMID: 16454473; PMCID: PMC7167644.

64. Sahul Hamid LS, Jalil J, Abdul Wahab SM, Azmi N, Yaakob NS. Comparative HPLC analysis of 6-Gingerol and 6-Shogaol in soil-based and soilless-grown ginger. *J Med Plants By-prod.* 2023;12(4):319–28. https://doi.org/10.22034/jmpb.2023.362686.1577.
65. Maslov OY, Komisarenko MA, Kolisnyk YS, Kostina TA. Determination of catechins in green tea leaves by HPLC compared to spectrophotometry. *J Org Pharm Chem.* 2021 Oct 20;19(3(75)):28–33. Available from: https://ophcj.nuph.edu.ua/article/view/238177.
66. Dhillon A, Sardana S, Thakkar AR. Development and validation of HPLC and UV spectrophotometric method for the quantification of cinnamaldehyde in cinnamon bark extract. *J Nat Remedies.* 2023.
67. Priyadarshini CH, Eswara Prasad P, Aswani Kumar K, Nagalakshmi D, Madhuri D. Quantitative determination of diosgenin in *Trigonella foenum graceum* seeds by HPLC method. *The Pharma Innovation J.* 2022;11(9S):932–6.
68. Azaroual L, Liazid A, Barbero G, Brigui J, Palma M, Barroso C. Improved chromatographic methods for determination of bioactive compounds from *Aloe vera* leaves. *ISRN Chromatogr.* 2012. https://doi.org/10.5402/2012/609095.
69. Meena A, Prabhu R, Esakki A, Marimuthu G, Narasimha Bhat S, Raju I. Estimation of Withaferin-A by HPLC and standardization of the Ashwagandhadi lehyam formulation. *Heliyon.* 2021;7:e06116. https://doi.org/10.1016/j.heliyon.2021.e06116.
70. Nur Tasfiyati A, Dwi Antika L, Wira Septama A, Hikmat H, Hendris Hendarsyah Kurniawan, Ariani N. A validated HPLC-DAD method and comparison of different extraction techniques for analysis of scopoletin in noni-based products. *Kuwait J Sci.* 2023;50(3):276–81. https://doi.org/10.1016/j.kjs.2023.02.023.
71. Pellati F, Benvenuti S. Determination of ephedrine alkaloids in *Ephedra* natural products using HPLC on a pentafluorophenylpropyl stationary phase. *J Pharm Biomed Anal.* 2008 Sep 29;48(2):254–63. https://doi.org/10.1016/j.jpba.2007.10.034. Epub 2007 Nov 6. PMID: 18077120.
72. Noviana E, Indrayanto G, Rohman A. Advances in fingerprint analysis for standardization and quality control of herbal medicines. *Front Pharmacol.* 2022;13:853023. https://doi.org/10.3389/fphar.2022.853023.
73. Govindarajan R, Tejas V, Pushpangadan P. High-performance liquid chromatography (HPLC) as a tool for standardization of complex herbal drugs. *J AOAC Int.* 2019;102(4):986–92. https://doi.org/10.5740/jaoacint.18-0378.
74. Wolfender JL. HPLC in natural product analysis: the detection issue. *Planta Med.* 2009 Jun;75(7):719–34. https://doi.org/10.1055/s-0028-1088393. Epub 2009 Jan 14. PMID: 19145552.
75. Potterat O, Hamburger M. Natural products in drug discovery – concepts and approaches for tracking bioactivity. *Curr Org Chem.* 2006;10:899–920.
76. Patel KN, Patel JK, Patel MP, Rajput GC, Patel HA. Introduction to hyphenated techniques and their applications in pharmacy. *Pharm Methods.* 2010 Oct;1(1):2–13. https://doi.org/10.4103/2229-4708.72222. PMID: 23781411; PMCID: PMC3658024.
77. Cramer B, Humpf HU. Applications of HPLC-MS techniques for the analysis of chemical contaminants and residues in food. In: Schrenk D. *Chemical contaminants and residues in food.* Woodhead Publishing, Sawton; 2012. p. 62–78.

12

Advanced Diagnostics for Personalized Medicine: A New Paradigm

Benjamin Tagoe, Louisa Quainoo, Deborah Clotworthy, Emmanuel Kwaku Ofori, and Seth Kwabena Amponsah

12.1 Introduction

Personalized medicine is an evolving field that takes into account the clinical, genetic, and environmental factors of a patient. It involves a strategic and evidence-based approach to customizing patient care, spanning from maintaining health to managing disease. By leveraging on molecular insights, personalized medicine enhances preventative health and enables the early initiation of drug therapy. The ultimate goal is to tailor medical care and improve outcomes for each patient [1]. The concept of personalized medicine is not entirely new; it has deep historical roots. Over two and a half millennia ago, Hippocrates, often referred to as the "Father of Medicine", acknowledged the uniqueness of each individual by stating, "Every human is unique, and this affects both disease prediction and treatment". This early concept laid the foundation for the principle that treatments should be tailored to each patient; an idea that remains central to personalized medicine today [2].

The evolution of personalized medicine continued through the 20th century, marked by significant scientific breakthroughs. One such milestone occurred in 1956 when researchers discovered the genetic basis of "favism", a condition in which certain individuals experience severe reactions to fava beans. This adverse reaction was found to be caused by a deficiency in the enzyme glucose-6-phosphate dehydrogenase (G6PD), a crucial metabolic enzyme. The identification of G6PD deficiency as a genetic factor as the basis for this condition highlighted the importance of genetics in determining health outcomes and reinforced the idea of customizing treatments [2].

Another pivotal moment in the development of personalized medicine occurred in 1985 when Nobel laureate Renato Dulbecco proposed that sequencing the human genome could significantly advance cancer research. Dulbecco highlighted the genetic basis of diseases, and the need to develop more targeted and effective therapies. The Human Genome Project, a scientific breakthrough that mapped the entire human genome, was inspired by Dulbecco. This project has since provided invaluable insights into genetic variations that contribute to diseases, paving the way for more precise and personalized treatment [2].

Overall, the journey of personalized medicine from Hippocrates' early insights to the modern era of genomic research reflects a long-standing commitment to understanding health and disease. As this field continues to develop, it holds the promise of revolutionizing healthcare by providing customized treatments that consider each patient's unique genetic makeup, environment, and lifestyle, ultimately improving the quality of care and patient outcomes [2]. The human genome is the foundation of personalized medicine and is viewed as the future of diagnosis and therapy.

The treatment of malaria, which is regarded as the first personalized therapeutic strategy, emphasizes the necessity of novel diagnostic technologies and treatment approaches. Advanced biochemical

DOI: 10.1201/9781003486909-12

advancements, including biochips, genotyping, and single-nucleotide polymorphisms (SNPs), have brought personalized medicine into practice [2]. Furthermore, extensive molecular and clinical data over the past few decades has transformed personalized medicine, raising expectations for its ability to propel biomedical research and healthcare [3, 4]. Indeed, personalized medicine involves utilizing an individual's genetic profile to guide decisions related to disease prevention, diagnosis, and treatment [5]. Personalized medicine, a related data-driven approach, integrates an individual's medical, genetic, behavioral, and environmental information to deliver tailored therapies [6]. This overview charts the evolution of customized medicine and highlights key milestones [2].

12.2 Relevance of Personalized Medicine

While there are considerable challenges to overcome before personalized medicine can be widely adopted in everyday clinical practice, its principles are increasingly being applied across various fields of medicine, with oncology at the forefront [4]. Significant advancements have been made in eye care by identifying genetic variants associated with both simple and complex ocular diseases, such as glaucoma and macular degeneration. While differences in therapeutic responses to eye treatments have been noted for many years, practical application of personalized ocular therapy in clinical settings is not widespread. The primary advantage of personalized medicine lies in its ability to transform clinical management and drug delivery approaches. When properly implemented, personalized medicine can be preventive, precise, and cost-effective [7].

With personalized medicine, emphasis is often given to preventive care. For instance, genetic screening for BRCA1 and BRCA2 mutations is commonly used to identify women at high risk of developing breast cancer [8]. Women with these mutations are informed about their risk and possible preventive measures, such as more frequent mammograms, prophylactic surgery, and chemoprevention, following the guidelines of the National Cancer Institute [8]. Currently, there are more than 2,000 genetic tests available in clinical settings to identify risks for a wide range of diseases, from mild to severe. Although not every test is linked to a specific treatment, knowing hereditary risks can enable proactive and targeted prevention strategies [7].

Personalized medicine can offer more effective treatments, as seen in the management of specific subtypes of breast cancers. A notable example is the treatment of breast cancer characterized by high levels of human epidermal growth factor receptor 2 (HER2), which represents up to 30% of all breast cancer cases [9]. Standard treatments are not effective for these patients; however, the antibody Herceptin (trastuzumab), when used alongside chemotherapy, can significantly lower tumor recurrence by 52%. Indeed, a molecular diagnostic test for HER2 expression is routinely performed as part of the standard care to identify these patients before starting treatment [9].

As a matter of fact, personalized medicine will be fully realized when doctors can accurately provide the right treatment to the right patient at the right time. This has always been a priority for physicians, but the necessary scientific knowledge and technological advancements were not available until the recent discovery of the human genome [7]. It took 50 years to progress from identifying deoxyribonucleic acid (DNA)'s four repeating nucleotides to fully sequencing the human genome. Personalized medicine involves working with a much more complex subject: an individual whose genetic variations and phenotypic expressions change in response to environmental factors. Indeed, achieving personalized medicine as a component of clinical practice will require significant collaborative efforts [7].

12.3 Advanced Diagnostic Techniques in Personalized Medicine

At the heart of personalized medicine are advanced diagnostic techniques that offer detailed insights into the genetic and molecular foundations of diseases. These diagnostic tools play an important role in customizing healthcare to meet the needs of each patient. There are a number of diagnostic approaches that aid personalized medicine, some of these include: computational tools, machine learning tools, bioprinting technology, and stereolithography, among others.

12.3.1 Computational Approaches

Personalized medicine involves treating patients according to their distinct clinical characteristics [1]. This approach customizes treatment plans by considering a patient's unique traits, making it more sophisticated than standard methods [10]. Recent studies indicate that genetic differences may account for inter-individual variability in drug response [11]. Advances in high-throughput technology have generated a large amount of molecular data, uncovering new insights into cellular processes. Additionally, computational tools utilize this extensive data to understand disease mechanisms, enhance patient diagnosis, and explore treatment options. These tools can categorize patients into subgroups based on their genomic and treatment response profiles, which helps in predicting diseases, making clinical decisions, and providing personalized treatments [2].

Several research groups have applied computational methods (disease models) to various aspects of personalized medicine [12]. Additionally, these approaches not only enhance existing disease models but also assist in developing predictive models for a range of diseases [2]. Such analyses help differentiate between the molecular mechanisms in normal or control states from those in disease conditions. These technologies enable the development of predictive models for rare diseases, ensuring that patients with these diseases receive the most appropriate therapy.

Computational models play an important role in medicine and drug development, encompassing areas such as disease modeling, biomarker research, and evaluations of therapeutic efficacy and safety [13]. Both the scientific community and regulatory agencies like the Food and Drugs Authority (FDA) and European Medicines Agency (EMA) acknowledge the importance of these models, often referred to as digital evidence, in medical research [14, 15] There are two main types of models: data-driven and mechanistic. Mechanistic models use equations to represent physiological processes, offering insights into their underlying mechanisms. In contrast, data-driven approaches depend on artificial intelligence (AI) techniques and algorithms [16, 17].

12.3.1.1 Molecular Interaction Maps

Molecular interaction maps (MIMs) are networks that illustrate the physical and causal relationships between biological entities using knowledge-based information [18]. They explore the molecular pathways and regulatory modules involved in diseases such as Parkinson's [19] and cancer [20]. MIMs apply graph theory to uncover static features of networks, such as identifying crucial nodes, detecting communities, and predicting unseen connections. These maps enable visualization of interactions between regulators and their targets [13].

12.3.1.2 Genome-Scale Metabolic Models

Genome-scale metabolic models (GEMs) offer a mathematical framework to understand a cell's metabolic capabilities, facilitating comprehensive analysis of genetic changes, exploring diseases, and identifying enzymatic reactions and potential drug targets [21]. This modeling approach is commonly used across medical conditions such as cancer, obesity, and Alzheimer's disease [2].

12.3.1.3 Boolean Models

Basic logic-based models, or Boolean models (BMs), assign nodes to either activation or inactivation [22, 23]. Logical operators like AND, OR, and NOT are used to define the regulatory relationship between targets (downstream nodes) and regulators (upstream nodes). Big biological systems can benefit from BM's capacity to estimate parameters without requiring a great deal of kinetic data. This approach is frequently employed in medicine-based cancer research [22].

12.3.1.4 Quantitative Models

Quantitative Models (QMs) examine the quantitative dynamics of biological reactions over time. QMs involve a series of differential equations that describe how a system responds to different stimuli or disturbances [23]. This approach focuses on individual pathways and necessitates detailed kinetic data to estimate parameters accurately. In personalized medicine, such a model is employed in identifying biomarkers [24], assessing medication responses, and developing customized therapies [25].

12.3.1.5 Pharmacokinetic Models

Pharmacokinetic models describe the concentrations of medications in plasma and tissues. These models are frequently used to anticipate drug-induced reactions. Pharmacokinetics can be modeled using compartmental approaches or physiologically based approaches [26, 27].

12.3.2 Machine Learning Approaches

Machine learning excels at detecting rules, patterns, and statistical relationships within large datasets [28]. The application of machine learning in personalized medicine is expanding, with a strong emphasis on genomic and proteomic data. By analyzing genome sequencing data, machine learning helps identify the most effective treatment strategies for individuals [29]. This approach has enhanced our understanding of disease mechanisms and the development of biomarkers for various diseases.

Machine learning aids in unlocking the full potential of personalized medicine in clinical settings. It has facilitated the creation of algorithms tailored to specific diseases. For example, the FDA has approved the MammaPrint predictive test for breast cancer, which utilizes 70 gene signatures [30]. Using a microarray, MammaPrint analyzes fresh tissue samples or formalin-fixed paraffin-embedded (FFPE) samples [31]. Additionally, the BluePrint test provides expression data that could support personalized treatment strategies in the Microarray In Node negative Disease may Avoid ChemoTherapy (MINDACT) and IMPACt trials [32].

Machine learning and AI can integrate different data types including metabolomic, genetic, epigenomic, transcriptomic, genomic, medical images biobanks, and electronic health records [28, 33]. Machine learning has two main functions: regression and classification. Regression seeks to forecast continuous and real-valued outcomes, such as cholesterol levels in the blood, based on other biomarkers. Classification aims to predict the category of a large group of individuals, such as patients who have longer survival times than the average. Indeed, using machine learning can assist in identifying genetic networks responsible for diseases and speed up the drug discovery process [34].

12.3.3 Bioprinting Technology

The two primary elements of bioprinting are the materials and the printing procedures. The ideas and developments in these fields to improve performance are covered in this section. The four main technologies used in bioprinting are inkjet, extrusion, laser-assisted, and stereolithography. While each approach has pros and cons of its own, it can be customized for particular uses to promote personalized treatment [35].

12.3.3.1 Inkjet Printing

The innovative bioprinting method known as inkjet makes use of a cartridge that holds bio-ink. It is renowned for being inexpensive and simple to use since commercial printers can frequently be modified to work with this technology [35–37]. Inkjet printing also demonstrates high cell viability, with 80–90% of cells remaining functional [38]. This method uses either thermal or piezoelectric actuators to consistently eject droplets of bio-ink. In addition, the thermal actuator generates pressure through heat-induced bubble formation to expel the droplet, with temperatures typically ranging from 100 to 300°C. However, the high temperatures involved in thermal inkjet printing can induce cellular stress in the bio-ink [39].

12.3.3.2 Extrusion Printing

Extrusion-based bioprinting is a variation of inkjet printing that applies constant force to the bio-ink during deposition [40]. This technique produces a cylindrical stream of bio-ink that forms a continuous line on the surface being printed [41, 42]. Extrusion-based bioprinting has some drawbacks and these include reduced cell viability due to mechanical stress and lower resolution beyond 100 μm [40].

12.3.3.3 Laser-Assisted Printing

A high-pressure bubble is used in laser-assisted printing, a bioprinting method, to project bio-ink onto a printing surface [43, 44]. An energy-absorbing layer is included in the "donor layer", or ribbon, which is the first step in this process. This layer is evaporated at a focal point by a high-energy laser pulse [43]. The bio-ink is mixed with a thin layer of glass or metal to form the donor layer, which is vaporized into a high-pressure bubble that pushes the bio-ink onto the surface [45]. The process can have a 4000 μm^2 spot size at a laser intensity of 1.4 J/cm^2 [46]. This technique provides great cell viability and excellent resolution [42].

12.3.3.4 Stereolithography

Stereolithography utilizes ultraviolet (UV) or visible light to solidify bio-ink layer by layer [43]. This technique is notable for its ability to eliminate shear pressure during nozzle-based printing due to its fast and highly accurate resolution, ranging from 5 to 300 μm [44]. The solidification occurs through photopolymerization as the light exposure hardens each layer [45]. Gauvin and colleagues successfully created 3D structures using UV light and a gelatin-based prepolymer solution [46]. However, exposure to UV light can pose a risk of cytotoxic damage to the bio-ink cells from photo-initiators, potentially decreasing cell viability [43]. To tackle this issue, researchers experimented with adding two monomers containing thiol or alkene groups, which react spontaneously under UV light at 266 nm. After three days, they observed a significant improvement in cell viability compared to the control, achieving a level of 95% [47]. The high cost of 3D bioprinters has been a barrier to progress in personalized medicine. Enhanced technology may result in higher costs, making it difficult for medical laboratories and institutions to access equipment like laser-assisted printers, which could restrict advanced research in personalized medicine [43].

12.3.4 Clustered Regularly Interspersed Short Palindromic Repeats-Based Diagnostics

Early clustered regularly interspersed short palindromic repeats (CRISPR)-based diagnostic techniques utilize variations of Cas9 that target double-stranded DNA. Cas9-based DNA detection methods involve strategies such as the guided reassembly of split proteins by inactive fragments, cleavage of protospacer adjacent motif (PAM)-containing sequences, and the unwinding of the non-target DNA strand to enable isothermal amplification [48].

The Cas9-based technique, called nucleic acid sequence-based amplification (NASBA)-CRISPR cleavage, makes use of a toehold sensor for output, PAM-dependent detection by Cas9 cleavage, and isothermal pre-amplification of targets via NASBA [49]. Toehold triggers are connected to NASBA-amplified ribonucleic acid (RNA) fragments through reverse transcription. If the RNA fragment contains a PAM sequence, Cas9-mediated cleavage results in a shortened RNA without the trigger sequence. Conversely, if the PAM sequence is absent, the full-length RNA with the trigger activates the toehold switch, causing a color change. This technique differentiates viral lineages by detecting strain-specific PAM sites [49].

The main aim of CRISPR-based diagnostics is to identify pathogens by detecting their DNA or RNA, including viruses, bacteria, and parasites. These methods have been used to detect RNA viruses such as parvovirus B19, members of the Flaviviridae family (like dengue, Zika, and Japanese encephalitis virus), Ebola, and Coronaviridae. The SHERLOCK technique for detecting severe acute respiratory syndrome coronavirus 2 (SARS-CoV-2) involves two steps: first, recombinase polymerase amplification

(RPA)-based pre-amplification, and then T7 transcription followed by Cas13a-mediated target detection [48]. In a clinical study validated by qPCR, 154 samples were tested using both fluorescence readouts and lateral flow, while an additional 380 PCR-negative samples were tested using fluorescence only [50]. The assay demonstrated a limit of detection (LOD) of 42 RNA copies per reaction, with a sensitivity of 96% for fluorescence readouts and 88% for lateral-flow readouts. Both methods showed 100% specificity.

CRISPR-based diagnostics are capable of detecting RNA molecules associated with non-infectious diseases. For instance, CRISPR-based detection of human CXCL9 messenger RNA (mRNA) identified acute cellular rejection in kidney transplants with 93% sensitivity and 76% specificity in 31 urine cell pellet samples [48]. MicroRNAs (miRNAs) have also been detected utilizing these diagnostics; examples of this include the electrochemical detection of miR-19b in serum samples from medulloblastoma patients and the rolling-circle transcription-based detection of miR-17 and miR-21 in RNA isolated from breast cancer cell lines [48].

CRISPR-based diagnostics are particularly effective at identifying point mutations and small deletions due to the single-nucleotide specificity of Cas enzymes. This high level of specificity allows for the detection of various genetic changes, including mutations linked to Duchenne muscular dystrophy, antimicrobial resistance markers, and SNPs in the E3 ubiquitin ligase gene that influence eye color [51]. Additionally, CRISPR-based techniques can detect circulating variants of SARS-CoV-2 that have different levels of pathogenicity and transmissibility [48].

12.3.5 Genomic Sequencing

New technologies, such as genetic testing, are enhancing the ability to predict and prevent diseases. Familial hypercholesterolemia, which is characterized by heterozygous gene mutations found in approximately 1 in 500 people, is a notable example of this advancement in disease prediction and prevention. This condition significantly raises the risk of cardiovascular disease and is inherited in an autosomal dominant manner [52]. Since 2007, the National Institute for Health and Care Excellence (NICE) has recommended risk-reducing strategies for individuals with hypercholesterolemia. Molecular diagnosis and familial cascade testing through genotyping can identify those who need intensive lipid-lowering treatment, representing a promising approach for primary prevention [1]. Additionally, secondary genetic testing results for unrelated conditions could help identify more families affected by familial hypercholesterolemia. Table 12.1 highlights the clinical applications of some genomic tests carried out in clinical settings.

Personalized medicine focuses on customized treatments and targeted therapies, moving away from a one-size-fits-all approach. Advancements in technologies like genomics enhance our understanding of diseases and their underlying biological processes, enabling more individualized interventions. Additionally, other testing methods, such as transcriptomics (RNA-based analysis), metabolomics (the study of a person's metabolites), and proteomics (the analysis of all expressed proteins), are expected to play an increasingly significant role [1].

12.3.5.1 Targeted Therapy Based on Efficacy

Mutations in BRCA1 and BRCA2 have long been used in oncology to predict cancer progression and to offer personalized risk-reduction strategies. These insights are increasingly shaping therapeutic practices. Understanding the molecular effects of specific mutations in the cancer genome can aid in predicting responses to treatment. For example, the BRAF V600E mutation, commonly associated with malignant melanoma, activates downstream signaling pathways that enhance cellular proliferation [15]. NICE recommends vemurafenib, a drug that inhibits the mutant BRAF protein, as it provides better overall survival compared to standard treatments [15].

12.3.5.2 Development of New Targeted Therapies and Prediction of Adverse Drug Reactions

Many diseases have seen advancements through gene identification, understanding their causes, and developing treatments. For instance, the discovery of FGFR3 signaling pathways has shed light on impaired bone growth in achondroplasia. BMN111, a treatment now in phase III clinical trials, has shown promising results in preclinical and early-phase studies, indicating potential improvement in bone development [16, 17]. Genetic variations can predict therapeutic responses and adverse effects in various clinical contexts. For example, with the use of the drug abacavir for human immunodeficiency virus (HIV), genetic testing can forecast the likelihood of severe adverse reactions. This approach has led to the successful use of alternative antiretroviral medications.

12.4 Application of Advanced Diagnostic Tools in Personalized Medicine

Advanced diagnostic tools are pivotal in the application of personalized medicine, enabling healthcare providers to tailor treatments and interventions to individual patient profiles. These tools, including genomic sequencing, proteomics, and advanced imaging techniques, provide detailed insights into a patient's genetic predispositions, disease mechanisms, and potential responses to therapy. By leveraging these technologies, clinicians can identify the most effective treatments for each patient, minimize adverse effects, and improve overall health outcomes.

12.4.1 Biomarker-Based Personalized Medicine

Biomarker-based personalized medicine represents a significant advancement in tailoring medical treatment to the unique characteristics of each patient. This method is based on biomarkers, which are biological molecules that can be discovered in tissues, blood, or other bodily fluids and can show aberrant or normal processes or conditions. In personalized medicine, biomarkers are utilized to aid prediction of disease progression, identify patients who will benefit from specific therapies, and monitor treatment responses [24].

The identification of biomarkers has been significantly enhanced by diagnostic technologies such as next-generation sequencing (NGS) and mass spectrometry. These advanced tools provide deep insights into genetic, proteomic, and metabolomic profiles, allowing for the discovery of biomarkers linked to a

TABLE 12.1

Clinical applications of genomic tests [53]

Test	Indication	Clinical application	Ethical concerns
Cytogenomics	Utilized in the diagnosis of congenital defects, chromosomal abnormalities, and intellectual impairments	Diagnosis and counseling	May identify copy number variation (CNV) in the parents of the impacted child
Tumor genetic testing	Used to determine which cancer treatment to use depending on the existence of a certain mutation or genetic rearrangement that indicates how a particular medicine will work	Identifies the most effective medicine for treating specific tumor types	Identifies non-cancer-related germline mutations
Genome/exome sequencing	Utilized where indications and symptoms suggest a genetic illness, but there isn't a single gene that accounts for the entire phenotype	Specific therapy, diagnosis, and counseling	Potential for identifying medically relevant incidental observations

range of diseases, including cancer, cardiovascular diseases, and neurological disorders. By analyzing these profiles, researchers and clinicians can pinpoint specific biomarkers associated with various conditions, paving the way for more targeted and effective treatments [54].

Diagnostics also play a crucial role in patient stratification, which involves classifying patients based on their biomarker profiles. This process is essential for selecting individuals who are most likely to respond positively to particular therapies. By doing so, personalized medicine aims to optimize treatment efficacy while minimizing adverse effects [24]. For instance, in oncology, the presence of specific genetic mutations, such as HER2-positive status in breast cancer, allows for the use of targeted therapies designed to inhibit the pathways affected by these mutations. This approach not only improves the likelihood of a successful treatment outcome but also reduces the risk of unnecessary side effects [24].

Furthermore, monitoring treatment response through regular diagnostic testing is integral to personalized medicine. By measuring changes in biomarker levels over time, clinicians can evaluate the effectiveness of treatments and make necessary adjustments. Liquid biopsies, which analyze circulating tumor DNA in blood samples, illustrate the benefits of non-invasive monitoring methods. These biopsies enable real-time tracking of cancer progression and response to treatment, providing valuable information that helps clinicians refine and optimize therapeutic strategies [54]. This approach represents a significant leap in medical practice, one where treatments are more precisely aligned with individual patient needs, ultimately leading to better outcomes and reduced adverse effects (Figure 12.1).

12.4.2 Cell and Gene Therapies

Cell and gene therapies are at the cutting edge of medical innovation, offering the potential to cure conditions that were previously deemed untreatable. These therapies work by altering a patient's cells or genes to treat or prevent diseases, promising long-lasting effects [54]. Additionally, genetic testing helps pinpoint specific mutations or deficiencies that therapies are designed to address. For instance, gene therapy can be considered for patients with certain inherited retinal diseases by delivering a functional version of defective gene. Before administering cell and gene therapies, thorough diagnostic testing is necessary to ensure the treatments are both safe and effective. This process involves evaluating the genetic integrity of modified cells, assessing potential immune reactions, and verifying that therapeutic genes are delivered accurately to intended tissues [54].

During treatment, diagnostics are still important to detect any side effects and evaluate long-term efficacy. This involves tracking the persistence and functionality of the modified cells, identifying any adverse immune responses, and confirming that the therapeutic benefits remain effective over time. Advanced techniques such as imaging, flow cytometry, and molecular assays are commonly used to perform these evaluations [29].

12.4.3 Combining Diagnostics with AI and Machine Learning

The integration of AI and machine learning with diagnostic technologies is ushering in a transformative era for personalized medicine. These advanced computational tools enable analysis of extensive diagnostic data, uncovering patterns and insights that traditional methods might miss [54]. AI and machine learning significantly enhance data analysis by efficiently processing complex datasets from genomics, proteomics, and imaging studies. These algorithms surpass the analytical capabilities of human analysts, facilitating a deeper understanding of biomarkers and disease mechanisms. As a result, the development of targeted therapies is accelerated, leading to more precise and effective treatments [54].

Predictive analytics is another area where AI and machine learning are making substantial contributions. AI-driven predictive models leverage diagnostic data to forecast disease progression and treatment outcomes. This allows for the early identification of patients who are at risk of adverse reactions or who may not respond to certain therapies. Such foresight enables timely interventions and personalized adjustments to treatment plans, optimizing patient care and enhancing therapeutic efficacy [54].

Moreover, AI-powered image analytic tools are revolutionizing fields like radiology and pathology. These tools are capable of detecting subtle changes and anomalies with remarkable accuracy. By improving the diagnosis and monitoring of diseases, AI-driven image analysis supports more informed clinical decisions, ultimately leading to better patient outcomes [29]. In summary, the fusion of AI and machine learning with diagnostic technologies represents a major leap in personalized medicine. These advancements enhance data analysis, enable predictive analytics, and improve image analysis, collectively driving forward the development of personalized treatments.

12.5 New Diagnostic Tools for Personalized Medicine

12.5.1 Digital Tools to Access Genetic Information and Navigate Care

According to a 2020 Canadian study, access to internet health data increased by 35% in 2019, and 79% of participants said they would prefer to have electronic access to their personal health information [55]. Digital tools, such as patient portals and various applications, provide direct access to personalized health data for clinicians, patients, and their families. In the realm of personalized medicine, these technologies facilitate access to genetic test results, help users understand the findings, and offer opportunities for meaningful discussions with healthcare professionals that could enhance health outcomes [55, 56]. With the rise of comprehensive tests like whole-genome sequencing or extensive gene panels that analyze numerous genes or biomarkers, the complexity of information can be overwhelming. Also, tools that simplify this complexity and provide platforms for patients, families, and healthcare professionals to interpret genetic information could enhance patient experiences, support patient-centered care, and promote shared decision-making [57].

As these and future digital tools become more widely adopted, they may present new opportunities and challenges for health systems [58]. For example, these technologies may make patient counseling services offered by clinical geneticists, genetic counselors, or primary care physicians more accessible in light of the growing need for genetic testing. Certain digital technologies have the potential to enhance workflow efficiency by decreasing administrative duties, such as creating charts and other documents [58].

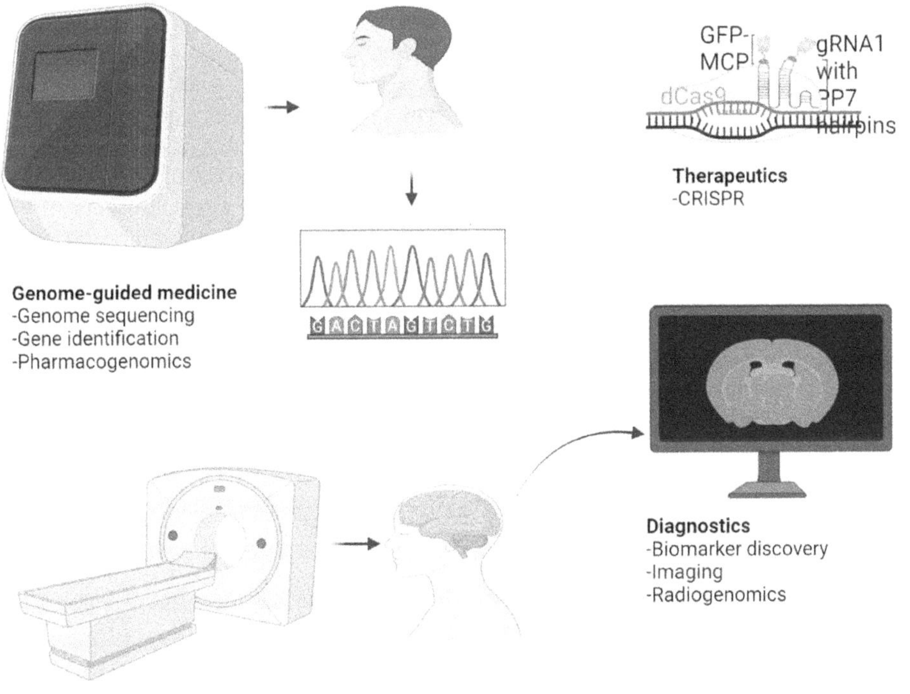

FIGURE 12.1 Engineering precision medicine technology platforms.

The proliferation of digital genomics tools underscores the need to prioritize patient data privacy and security, which are major concerns for patients, as is the case with the larger digital health space. Ensuring that genetic test results from medical records may seamlessly connect with patient-facing digital tools while protecting sensitive information, such as genetic risk factors, would need strengthening data privacy regulations in order to meet safety concerns [59]. Additionally, the broader adoption of these technologies across the globe will likely depend on considerations of digital health equity, including efforts to improve health literacy, the potential for technology to overcome geographical barriers, and the enhancement of technological infrastructure, such as internet access in rural and remote areas. ShareDNA, a new technology from Seattle, United States, is a free smartphone application that enables patients to securely upload and share their genetic test results while also learning how to interpret those results without requiring extensive personal information [60]. An initial user-testing survey indicated that users felt comfortable using the application, though there was a need for more detailed information about data security. The project is partially funded by the Kaiser Permanente Washington Health Research Institute and National Institutes of Health in the United States [61].

12.5.2 Omics-Based Sequencing Technologies

Whole-genome sequencing, exome sequencing, and transcriptome sequencing are considered "omics-based" personalized medicine technologies because they provide a comprehensive overview of the molecular information present in an individual's cells and tissues [62]. This contrasts with focused methods that solely analyze a subset of genes, genomic areas, or proteins. Due to the wide range of applications for omics-based sequencing, it is possible to perform a single test instead of several separate ones at the time of clinical presentation, which may enhance the precision of the diagnostic data and expedite the diagnostic procedure [63]. While exome, whole-genome, and transcriptome sequencing have been widely used in research settings, these technologies may become much more common in routine clinical care over the next five years due to their ability to provide more detailed and broader information compared to targeted or single-gene tests [64].

Whole genome and exome sequencing are particularly valuable for diagnosing rare diseases, pediatric conditions, and adult conditions that involve multiple organ systems. These technologies, for instance, might speed up the diagnosis of seriously unwell newborns with unidentified illnesses, potentially improving outcomes in acute care settings [65]. Furthermore, actionable mutations (genetic alterations that can be selectively targeted by medicines) in patients with uncommon or undetected cancers can be found by profiling tumors utilizing these methods. Omics-based sequencing has clinical benefits for common malignancies, but its wide use in normal treatment is hindered by issues including cost and system compatibility [66]. However, with decreasing costs of sequencing, the increasing availability of personalized-based therapies targeting specific mutations, and ongoing research into their real-world application, omics-based technologies could significantly transform diagnostic and treatment pathways [64].

Emerging technologies and initiatives in omics-based sequencing that may be useful in the future include ultrarapid nanopore genome sequencing, which aims to provide whole-genome sequencing results in under eight hours, potentially reducing the need for additional diagnostic procedures in critical care settings like neonatal intensive care units [67], and the Marathon of Hope Cancer Centres Network, which is expanding access to whole-genome and transcriptome sequencing across Canada through interprovincial networks and pilot projects, potentially benefiting thousands of cancer patients by integrating personalized medicine into routine care [68].

12.5.3 Liquid Biopsy for Informing Cancer Treatments

Liquid biopsy is an emerging technology that detects genomic information from bodily fluids and has the potential to transform traditional cancer care. Unlike traditional personalized-based testing, which often requires surgical biopsies, liquid biopsies offer a less invasive alternative by primarily targeting cell-free DNA in the blood [69]. Moreover, DNA can be found in other fluids like saliva, urine, and cerebrospinal fluid using these technologies. This method is based on mounting evidence that suggests that certain malignancies' tumor cells leak DNA into body fluids. When examined using the right equipment, these DNA fragments can have different genomic profiles from DNA from healthy cells and offer vital information about the features of the cancer [69].

While there are many different liquid biopsy technologies available, one of the most promising developments in personalized medicine is the development of technologies expressly intended to inform treatment choices following a cancer diagnosis, as opposed to screening. The majority of currently accessible methods use polymerase chain reaction (PCR)-based single-gene assays or multigene panels, although NGS technologies, which can evaluate many genomic targets, are becoming more developed and widely used [69].

Through minimally invasive techniques like blood-based assays, liquid biopsies can also provide information regarding possible therapeutic targets (as a companion diagnosis), therapeutic response (including drug resistance), cancer progression, and symptoms of recurrence [70]. Liquid biopsies may be used as a substitute or addition to tissue-based diagnostics for patients who are at high risk for surgical biopsies or for whom it is not practical to do many surgical biopsies throughout the course of their clinical journey. This could improve patient outcomes and quality of life [71]. Although liquid biopsy technology is most widely used in the management of non-small cell lung cancer (NSCLC) due to the cancer's heterogeneity and variety of treatment options, it is expected to become commonly used for other types of cancer [70].

12.6 Challenges with Implementation of Advanced Diagnosis in Personalized Medicine

The integration of advanced diagnostic tools into personalized medicine presents several challenges that need to be addressed to fully realize its potential. One major issue is the high cost of these cutting-edge technologies, which can limit their accessibility and widespread adoption in routine clinical practice. Additionally, there are significant concerns regarding the standardization and validation of diagnostic methods, as variations in techniques and interpretations can lead to inconsistent results. Ethical and legal considerations, such as data privacy and the handling of genetic information, also pose substantial barriers, requiring robust regulatory frameworks to protect patient confidentiality and ensure ethical use. Furthermore, there is a need for comprehensive education and training for healthcare professionals to effectively utilize these complex tools. Overcoming these challenges will require coordinated efforts across the healthcare ecosystem, including advancements in technology, policy development, and education.

12.6.1 Disparities in the Implementation of Personalized Medicine Technologies and Mitigation Strategies

In many health systems, there are disparities in access to and use of personalized medicine technologies. These disparities can stem from various factors such as cost, availability, geographic location, and awareness. These can be exacerbated as personalized medicine technologies become more widespread. For instance, geographic inequalities might arise if new tests are mainly reimbursed through specialized research centers with more funding, restricting access for those not treated at these centers. Implementing personalized medicine in lower-resource settings, especially in areas with geographically dispersed populations, presents unique challenges compared to higher-resource settings [71].

Health systems are developing targeted approaches to improve personalized medicine and address disparities. For instance, the Silent Genomes Project of Genome British Columbia aims to enhance the presence of First Nations, Inuit, and Métis communities in pediatric cancer genomics databases [70]. Comparably, the National Institutes of Health-funded US All of Us project seeks to create a broad and inclusive collection of social, environmental, and genetic data [72]. Both projects involve active community engagement and oversight. Additionally, efforts to enhance diversity and inclusivity in healthcare involve workforce planning, education, and co-designing personalized medicine services with underrepresented groups [73]. These initiatives also focus on collecting data to address disparities in access and outcomes of personalized medicine.

12.6.2 Increased Demands on Health System Capacity and Mitigation Strategies

Healthcare systems will face increased pressure as a result of the growth of customized treatment, including a requirement for more personnel, infrastructure, and physical resources. Physical resources include hospital space, freezers, and the equipment needed to analyze and store genetic samples. Throughout a patient's treatment, continuous testing may be required for certain malignancies and other illnesses; this emphasizes the growing significance of having a suitable infrastructure to retain samples. Enhancing the system's capability and workflow to carry out and handle testing, maintain information databases, and offer strong information technology (IT) support are additional potential infrastructure modifications. Furthermore, it will be essential to have an adequate number of experts who can conduct and interpret tests related to customized medicine, such as sequencing tests that need to adhere to tight quality control guidelines [71].

The adoption and application of personalized medicine, as well as its long-term sustainability, may be impacted by these heightened expectations. However, with the right application, customized medicine technologies can decrease needless medical intervention, enhance patient outcomes, and eventually increase the effectiveness of healthcare. Beyond merely building out infrastructure and resources, there are ways to improve customized medicine. In addition to hiring more skilled workers, improving clinical workflows, investing in technology-enabled care, and building new care models that take genetics-based patient care into account are all potential ways to increase the capacity of the health system [71].

To address health systems' capacity issues in genetic testing, several approaches are being pursued. For instance, the GenCOUNSEL project by the BC Children's Hospital Research Institute focuses on scaling up genetic counseling services by developing decision support tools and assessing the needs of genetic counseling services [71]. In England, the NHS Genomic Medicine Service is advancing genomic medicine by centralizing laboratories, integrating workforce training, and co-designing services with patients and the public [59]. Additionally, implementing alternative models of care, such as centralized testing infrastructures and technology-enabled communication tools like e-consult, can enhance coordination between healthcare professionals and streamline workflows. Supporting the adoption of digital platforms and patient portals also facilitates better information sharing across clinics and among patients and providers [59].

12.6.3 Complexity in Interpreting Test Results and Mitigation Strategies

Healthcare providers face difficulties in obtaining and interpreting the findings of the growing number of customized medicine tests available at every stage of the care; from diagnosis and screening to treatment and prognosis. Test results for customized medicine can have varying therapeutic importance, and not all of them are actionable, which means they don't always immediately guide a particular course of treatment [52]. Many medical personnel claim to be unaware of how to order and interpret test findings for customized treatment, including pharmacists, oncologists, and primary care physicians. Additionally, they find it difficult to interpret these findings in a way that makes them therapeutically relevant when placed alongside other phenotypic data, such as social and environmental determinants of health [74]. These difficulties are often intensified when caring for individuals who are underrepresented in healthcare [73]. Additionally, the potential for incidental and secondary findings (unexpected information not directly related to the reason for testing) and their implications for patients and family members add further complexity.

The difficulties in deciphering intricate genetic data may have an impact on the extent to which medical practitioners use personalized medicine technology and how their treatment is organized to best serve their patients' needs as well as theirs. Ordering tests can be challenging in health systems where personalized medicine is not completely incorporated into the clinical process [71]. Depending on variables including whether the test is publicly sponsored or reimbursed, ordering procedures for tests might vary between institutions and geographical areas. To further complicate the interpretation and delivery of results, the healthcare provider ordering the test might not be the same as one who interprets the results or notifies the patient of any necessary follow-up [75].

To address the complexity of interpreting personalized medicine test results, several strategies can be implemented. Building patient-centered care models ensures that patient experiences shape care pathways, including deciding which professionals assist patients throughout their testing journey and allowing extra time during consultations to discuss test ordering and results [71]. Other approaches involve creating shared decision-making models and developing tools that align with technological advances and clinical practices to aid in ordering and interpreting tests, as well as assessing their impact on patient outcomes. Additionally, establishing clear processes for managing incidental and secondary findings is crucial, such as obtaining informed consent from patients on whether they wish to receive these results and providing guidance if they are medically actionable [71]. This may also include using e-consultations and telehealth to facilitate specialized support when needed. Furthermore, enhancing equity through targeted training and workforce initiatives is essential, such as increasing education on personalized medicine for healthcare professionals, especially to address the needs of underserved or racialized populations, and creating resources to support consistent interpretation of results [71].

12.7 Future Prospects of Diagnostics in Personalized Medicine

As the field of medicine advances, diagnostics will continue to play a pivotal role, particularly in emerging therapies such as immunotherapy and regenerative medicine. These cutting-edge treatments rely on sophisticated diagnostic tools to enhance their effectiveness and ensure their safe application.

Immunotherapy, for example, heavily relies on diagnostics for patient selection and monitoring treatment progress. Biomarker tests, such as those measuring PD-L1 expression, are crucial for identifying patients who are likely to respond to checkpoint inhibitors, helping to determine the best candidates and guiding the administration of immunotherapy. Additionally, diagnostics are essential for tracking immune-related side effects, ensuring the safety and effectiveness of these treatments. Similarly, in regenerative medicine, which includes stem cell therapies and tissue engineering, diagnostics are vital for assessing the quality and functionality of stem cells before therapeutic use. Diagnostic tests also play a key role in monitoring the integration and performance of engineered tissues after implantation, providing ongoing evaluation that helps improve these advanced treatments and ensure their effectiveness and safety.

Successfully integrating validated precision and personalized medicine into clinical practice will require more than just technological advancements. Challenges related to healthcare economics, ethics, and data privacy must be addressed after technology validation. Rising global healthcare costs create both barriers and opportunities for new technologies, making innovation from the perspectives of payers and policymakers crucial. Demonstrating value will necessitate improved treatment outcomes, fewer complications, and reduced costs.

AI-based approaches in drug development hold promise for addressing these needs by lowering development costs, enhancing drug accessibility, and improving cost-effectiveness. As drug prices increase, implementation of precision medicine will be essential in reducing costs and increasing accessibility. To effectively implement personalized medicine on a global scale, a convergence of enabling technologies, regulatory frameworks, public policy, education, and funding is necessary. Biomedical engineering will play a key role in driving breakthroughs that enhance individual patient outcomes. With better regulatory and pairing strategies, we can anticipate further advancements in personalized medicine across diverse populations.

12.8 Conclusion

Diagnostics are foundational to the innovation seen in biomarker-based personalized medicine, and cell and gene therapy. Additionally, diagnostics are critical in post-market care, where they help ensure the continued safety and success of treatments, ultimately leading to better health outcomes for patients. As diagnostic technologies continue to evolve, they will unlock new possibilities in personalized medicine, revolutionizing the future of healthcare. The integration of AI and machine learning, combined with advancements in immunotherapy and regenerative medicine, will further expand the potential of diagnostics, ushering in a new era of medical excellence. Moreover, accelerating in vitro diagnostic trials will be essential for making these advanced diagnostic tools more readily available.

REFERENCES

1. Chan IS, Ginsburg GS. Personalized medicine: progress and promise. *Annu Rev Genomics Hum Genet.* 2011;12:217–44.
2. Hassan M, Awan FM, Naz A, deAndrés-Galiana EJ, Alvarez O, Cernea A, et al. Innovations in genomics and big data analytics for personalized medicine and health care: a review. *Int J Mol Sci.* 2022;23(9).
3. Iriart JAB. Precision medicine/personalized medicine: a critical analysis of movements in the transformation of biomedicine in the early 21st century. *Cad Saude Publica.* 2019;35(3):e00153118.
4. Cirillo D, Valencia A. Big data analytics for personalized medicine. *Curr Opin Biotechnol.* 2019;58:161–7.
5. Ginsburg GS, Willard HF. Genomic and personalized medicine: foundations and applications. *Transl Res.* 2009;154(6):277–87.
6. Schaefer GO, Tai ES, Sun S. Precision medicine and big data: the application of an ethics framework for big data in health and research. *Asian Bioeth Rev.* 2019;11(3):275–88.
7. V HL. *Research developments accelerate discovery, application of personalized medicine.* Healio; 2011. Available from: https://www.healio.com/news/optometry/20120413/research-developments-accelerate-discovery-application-of-personalized-medicine?gclid=CjwKCAjwlbu2BhA3EiwA3yXyuxOjAhX06S9mGrgIOwJg55qNKpIqnO69scwyvxFTAzze-9lqmwtQqRoCMNoQAvD_BwE.
8. Institute NC. BRCA1 and BRCA2: Cancer risk and genetic testing. 2001. Available from: http://www.cancer.gov/cancertopics/factsheet/risk/brca.
9. Romond EH, Perez EA, Bryant J, Suman VJ, Geyer CE Jr., Davidson NE, et al. Trastuzumab plus adjuvant chemotherapy for operable HER2-positive breast cancer. *N Engl J Med.* 2005;353(16):1673–84.
10. Masoudi-Nejad A, Wang E. Cancer modeling and network biology: accelerating toward personalized medicine. *Semin Cancer Biol.* 2015;30:1–3.
11. Meyer UA. Pharmacogenetics - five decades of therapeutic lessons from genetic diversity. *Nat Rev Genet.* 2004;5(9):669–76.
12. Tuena C, Semonella M, Fernández-Álvarez J, Colombo D, Cipresso P. Predictive Precision Medicine: Towards the Computational Challenge. In: Pravettoni, G., Triberti, S. (eds) P5 eHealth: *An Agenda for the Health Technologies of the Future.* Springer, Cham. 2020. p. 71–86.
13. Collin CB, Gebhardt T, Golebiewski M, Karaderi T, Hillemanns M, Khan FM, et al. Computational models for clinical applications in personalized medicine—guidelines and recommendations for data integration and model validation. *J Pers Med.* 2022;12(2):166.
14. Apweiler R, Beissbarth T, Berthold MR, Blüthgen N, Burmeister Y, Dammann O, et al. Whither systems medicine? *Exp Mol Med.* 2018;50(3):e453.
15. Musuamba FT, Skottheim Rusten I, Lesage R, Russo G, Bursi R, Emili L, et al. Scientific and regulatory evaluation of mechanistic in silico drug and disease models in drug development: building model credibility. *CPT Pharmacometrics Syst Pharmacol.* 2021;10(8):804–25.
16. Barredo Arrieta A, Díaz-Rodríguez N, Del Ser J, Bennetot A, Tabik S, Barbado A, et al. Explainable artificial intelligence (XAI): concepts, taxonomies, opportunities, and challenges toward responsible AI. *Inf Fusion.* 2020;58:82–115.

17. Dimiduk DM, Holm EA, Niezgoda SR. Perspectives on the impact of machine learning, deep learning, and artificial intelligence on materials, processes, and structures engineering. *Integr Mater Manuf Innov.* 2018;7(3):157–72.
18. Kitano H, Funahashi A, Matsuoka Y, Oda K. Using process diagrams for the graphical representation of biological networks. *Nat Biotechnol.* 2005;23(8):961–6.
19. Fujita KA, Ostaszewski M, Matsuoka Y, Ghosh S, Glaab E, Trefois C, et al. Integrating pathways of Parkinson's disease in a molecular interaction map. *Mol Neurobiol.* 2014;49(1):88–102.
20. Kuperstein I, Bonnet E, Nguyen HA, Cohen D, Viara E, Grieco L, et al. Atlas of cancer signalling network: a systems biology resource for integrative analysis of cancer data with Google Maps. *Oncogenesis.* 2015;4(7):e160.
21. Thiele I, Palsson B. A protocol for generating a high-quality genome-scale metabolic reconstruction. *Nat Protoc.* 2010;5(1):93–121.
22. Eduati F, Jaaks P, Wappler J, Cramer T, Merten CA, Garnett MJ, et al. Patient-specific logic models of signaling pathways from screenings on cancer biopsies to prioritize personalized combination therapies. *Mol Syst Biol.* 2020;16(2):e8664.
23. Malik-Sheriff RS, Glont M, Nguyen TVN, Tiwari K, Roberts MG, Xavier A, et al. BioModels-15 years of sharing computational models in life science. *Nucleic Acids Res.* 2020;48(D1):D407–d15.
24. Kolch W, Fey D. Personalized computational models as biomarkers. *J Pers Med.* 2017;7(3).
25. Hastings J, O'Donnell Y, Fey D, Croucher D. Applications of personalised signalling network models in precision oncology. *Pharmacol Ther.* 2020;212:107555.
26. Pérez-Urizar J, Granados-Soto V, Flores-Murrieta FJ, Castañeda-Hernández G. Pharmacokinetic-pharmacodynamic modeling: why? *Arch Med Res.* 2000;31(6):539–45.
27. Edginton A, Willmann S. Physiology-based simulations of a pathological condition. *Clin Pharmacokinet.* 2008;47:743–52.
28. Mamoshina P, Vieira A, Putin E, Zhavoronkov A. Applications of deep learning in biomedicine. *Mol Pharm.* 2016;13(5):1445–54.
29. Fröhlich H, Balling R, Beerenwinkel N, Kohlbacher O, Kumar S, Lengauer T, et al. From hype to reality: data science enabling personalized medicine. *BMC Med.* 2018;16(1):150.
30. Cardoso F, van't Veer LJ, Bogaerts J, Slaets L, Viale G, Delaloge S, et al. 70-gene signature as an aid to treatment decisions in early-stage breast cancer. *N Engl J Med.* 2016;375(8):717–29.
31. Marchio C, Balmativola D, Castiglione R, Annaratone L, Sapino A. Predictive diagnostic pathology in the target therapy era in breast cancer. *Curr Drug Targets.* 2017;18(1):4–12.
32. Viale G, de Snoo FA, Slaets L, Bogaerts J, van't Veer L, Rutgers EJ, et al. Immunohistochemical versus molecular (BluePrint and MammaPrint) subtyping of breast carcinoma: Outcome results from the EORTC 10041/BIG 3-04 MINDACT trial. *Breast Cancer Res Treat.* 2018;167(1):123–31.
33. van't Veer LJ, Dai H, van de Vijver MJ, He YD, Hart AA, Mao M, et al. Gene expression profiling predicts clinical outcome of breast cancer. *Nature.* 2002;415(6871):530–6.
34. Cernea A, Fernández-Martínez JL, deAndrés-Galiana EJ, Fernández-Ovies FJ, Alvarez-Machancoses O, Fernández-Muñiz Z, et al. Robust pathway sampling in phenotype prediction. Application to triple negative breast cancer. *BMC Bioinformatics.* 2020;21(Suppl 2):89.
35. Huang Z, Shao G, Li L. Micro/nano functional devices fabricated by additive manufacturing. *Prog Mater Sci.* 2023;131:101020.
36. Yu Y, Zhang Y, Martin JA, Ozbolat IT. Evaluation of cell viability and functionality in vessel-like bioprintable cell-laden tubular channels. *J Biomech Eng.* 2013;135(9):91011.
37. Wei Long N. Controlling droplet impact velocity and droplet volume: Key factors to achieving high cell viability in sub-nanoliter droplet-based bioprinting. *IJB.* 2021;8(1):424.
38. Cui X, Gao G, Qiu Y. Accelerated myotube formation using bioprinting technology for biosensor applications. *Biotechnol Lett.* 2013;35(3):315–21.
39. Jammalamadaka U, Tappa K. Recent advances in biomaterials for 3D printing and tissue engineering. *J Funct Biomater.* 2018;9(1):22.
40. Leberfinger AN, Ravnic DJ, Dhawan A, Ozbolat IT. Concise review: Bioprinting of stem cells for transplantable tissue fabrication. *Stem Cells Transl Med.* 2017;6(10):1940–8.
41. Duong VT, Dang TT, Hwang CH, Back SH, Koo KI. Coaxial printing of double-layered and free-standing blood vessel analogues without ultraviolet illumination for high-volume vascularized tissue. *Biofabrication.* 2020;12(4):045033.

42. Mandrycky C, Wang Z, Kim K, Kim DH. 3D bioprinting for engineering complex tissues. *Biotechnol Adv.* 2016;34(4):422–34.
43. Lam EHY, Yu F, Zhu S, Wang Z. 3D bioprinting for next-generation personalized medicine. *Int J Mol Sci.* 2023;24(7).
44. Kačarević ŽP, Rider PM, Alkildani S, Retnasingh S, Smeets R, Jung O, et al. An introduction to 3D bioprinting: possibilities, challenges and future aspects. *Materials.* 2018;11(11):2199.
45. Wang DZ, Jin X, Dai R, Holzman J, Kim K. An ultrafast hydrogel photocrosslinking method for direct laser bioprinting. *RSC Adv.* 2016;6:21099–104.
46. Gauvin R, Chen YC, Lee JW, Soman P, Zorlutuna P, Nichol JW, et al. Microfabrication of complex porous tissue engineering scaffolds using 3D projection stereolithography. *Biomaterials.* 2012;33(15):3824–34.
47. Hoffmann A, Leonards H, Tobies N, Pongratz L, Kreuels K, Kreimendahl F, et al. New stereolithographic resin providing functional surfaces for biocompatible three-dimensional printing. *J Tissue Eng.* 2017;8:2041731417744485.
48. Knott GJ, Doudna JA. CRISPR-Cas guides the future of genetic engineering. *Science.* 2018;361(6405):866–9.
49. Pardee K, Green AA, Takahashi MK, Braff D, Lambert G, Lee JW, et al. Rapid, low-cost detection of Zika virus using programmable biomolecular components. *Cell.* 2016;165(5):1255–66.
50. Patchsung M, Jantarug K, Pattama A, Aphicho K, Suraritdechachai S, Meesawat P, et al. Clinical validation of a Cas13-based assay for the detection of SARS-CoV-2 RNA. *Nat Biomed Eng.* 2020;4(12):1140–9.
51. Harrington LB, Burstein D, Chen JS, Paez-Espino D, Ma E, Witte IP, et al. Programmed DNA destruction by miniature CRISPR-Cas14 enzymes. *Science.* 2018;362(6416):839–42.
52. Austin-Tse CA, Jobanputra V, Perry DL, Bick D, Taft RJ, Venner E, et al. Best practices for the interpretation and reporting of clinical whole genome sequencing. *NPJ Genom Med.* 2022;7(1):27.
53. Korf BR, Rehm HL. New approaches to molecular diagnosis. *Jama.* 2013;309(14):1511–21.
54. Johnson KB, Wei WQ, Weeraratne D, et al. Precision Medicine, AI, and the Future of Personalized Health Care. *Clin Transl Sci.* 2021;14(1):86–93.
55. Bombard Y, Hayeems RZ. How digital tools can advance quality and equity in genomic medicine. *Nat Rev Genet.* 2020;21(9):505–6.
56. Alturkistani A, Greenfield G, Greaves F, Aliabadi S, Jenkins RH, Costelloe C. Patient Portal Functionalities and Uptake: Systematic Review Protocol. *JMIR Res Protoc.* 2020;9(7):e14975.
57. Shickh S, Rafferty SA, Clausen M, Kodida R, Mighton C, Panchal S, et al. The role of digital tools in the delivery of genomic medicine: enhancing patient-centered care. *Genet Med.* 2021;23(6):1086–94.
58. Whiwon L, Salma S, Daniel A, Stephanie L, Marc C, Cherith S, et al. Patient-facing digital tools for delivering genetic services: A systematic review. *J Med Genet.* 2023;60(1):1–10.
59. Husereau D, Steuten L, Muthu V, Thomas DM, Spinner DS, Ivany C, et al. Effective and efficient delivery of genome-based testing—What conditions are necessary for health system readiness? *Healthcare (Basel).* 2022;10(10).
60. Washington Uo. The ShareDNA App. 2023.
61. Jujjavarapu C, Anandasakaran J, Amendola LM, Haas C, Zampino E, Henrikson NB, et al. ShareDNA: a smartphone app to facilitate family communication of genetic results. *BMC Med Genomics.* 2021;14(1):10.
62. Hasin Y, Seldin M, Lusis A. Multi-omics approaches to disease. *Genome Biol.* 2017;18(1):83.
63. Lalonde E, Rentas S, Lin F, Dulik MC, Skraban CM, Spinner NB. Genomic diagnosis for pediatric disorders: revolution and evolution. *Front Pediatr.* 2020;8:373.
64. Cuppen E, Elemento O, Rosenquist R, Nikic S, M IJ, Zaleski ID, et al. Implementation of whole-genome and transcriptome sequencing into clinical cancer care. *JCO Precis Oncol.* 2022;6:e2200245.
65. Krantz ID, Medne L, Weatherly JM, Wild KT, Biswas S, Devkota B, et al. Effect of whole-genome sequencing on the clinical management of acutely ill infants with suspected genetic disease: A randomized clinical trial. *JAMA Pediatr.* 2021;175(12):1218–26.
66. Horak P, Heining C, Kreutzfeldt S, Hutter B, Mock A, Hüllein J, et al. Comprehensive genomic and transcriptomic analysis for guiding therapeutic decisions in patients with rare cancers. *Cancer Discov.* 2021;11(11):2780–95.
67. Gorzynski JE, Goenka SD, Shafin K, Jensen TD, Fisk DG, Grove ME, et al. Ultrarapid nanopore genome sequencing in a critical care setting. *N Engl J Med.* 2022;386(7):700–2.

68. Fairclough L, Hill J, Bryant H, Kitchen-Clarke L. Accelerating knowledge to action: the pan-Canadian cancer control strategy. *Curr Oncol.* 2012;19(2):70–7.
69. Lone SN, Nisar S, Masoodi T, Singh M, Rizwan A, Hashem S, et al. Liquid biopsy: A step closer to transform diagnosis, prognosis and future of cancer treatments. *Mol Cancer.* 2022;21(1):79.
70. Ignatiadis M, Sledge GW, Jeffrey SS. Liquid biopsy enters the clinic - implementation issues and future challenges. *Nat Rev Clin Oncol.* 2021;18(5):297–312.
71. Basharat S, Smith A, Nazia D, Rader T. *Watch List: Top 10 precision medicine technologies and issues.* Ontario: Canadian Agency for Drugs and Technologies in Health; 2023.
72. Mapes BM, Foster CS, Kusnoor SV, Epelbaum MI, AuYoung M, Jenkins G, et al. Diversity and inclusion for the All of Us research program: A scoping review. *PLoS One.* 2020;15(7):e0234962.
73. Sharma Y, Cox L, Kruger L, Channamsetty V, Haga SB. Evaluating primary care providers' readiness for delivering genetic and genomic services to underserved populations. *Public Health Genomics.* 2021;7:1–10.
74. Erdmann A, Rehmann-Sutter C, Bozzaro C. Patients' and professionals' views related to ethical issues in precision medicine: A mixed research synthesis. *BMC Med Ethics.* 2021;22(1):116.
75. Smith A, Loshak H. *CADTH rapid response reports: pharmacogenomic testing for medication selection: a rapid qualitative review.* Ottawa, ON: Canadian Agency for Drugs and Technologies in Health; 2020.

13

Emerging Technologies in Cancer Diagnosis

Sheila A. Santa and Emmanuel A. Tagoe

13.1 Introduction

Cancer, also termed malignancy or neoplasm, generally refers to a group of diseases capable of affecting any part of the body [1]. Cancers are grouped according to their organ or tissue of origin but also based on the molecular characteristics of their respective cell [2]. Generally, cancers are characterized by the rapid growth of abnormal cells which extend beyond their boundaries, with the potential to invade neighboring tissues; this process is termed metastasis and is mostly the primary cause of death from cancers [1]. Additionally, cancer cells are able to reprogram several metabolic pathways to meet their needs for bio energy, biosynthesis, and redox control [3]. Changes in the metabolism of nutrients such as glucose, amino acid, and fatty acid are associated with cancer risk and can be regulated with healthy lifestyles including healthy diet, calorie restriction, and regular physical activity [4]. Aside from changes in metabolism, many other factors including radiation, chemicals, and viruses have been implicated in the etiology and pathogenesis of the disease [5].

Understanding the location, size, stage, and molecular characteristics of cancer is very essential for cancer diagnosis and management. Diagnostic tools play a crucial role in the detection, characterization, and monitoring of tumors leading to better disease outcomes [6]. Cancer detection focuses on identifying symptomatic patients as early as possible and may also involve screening healthy individuals to identify those having cancers before symptoms appear. Characterization however refers to determining the stage and prognosis of the tumor, while monitoring focuses on observing the progression of the tumor, its response to treatment, and how it impacts the rest of the body over time [7, 8]. Early diagnosis has been shown to improve the effectiveness of various therapies and significantly reduce the adverse effects of these therapies [9].

Currently, traditional diagnostic approaches such as: physical examination, laboratory investigations to detect biomarkers, combination of radiologic and nuclear medicine-based non-invasive imaging modalities like; computerized X-ray scan (computed tomography (CT) scan), ultrasonography (US), magnetic resonance imaging (MRI), bone scan, positron emission tomography; histopathological examination of biopsies and immunological probes coupled with flow cytometric analysis have all played a significant role in the diagnosis of cancer [10]. Among these diagnostic methods, imaging is widely used for the purposes of screening, staging, and monitoring tumor progression, and is able to identify a diverse category of cancers [11].

Over the past decades, these diagnostic techniques have played a central role in reducing cancer-related morbidities and mortalities. However, most of them lack clinical and cost-effectiveness and have inherent limitations of non-specificity and poor efficiency especially, in cases of early-stage malignancies [10]. Based on the limitation of these traditional methods, highly advanced strategies are essential to track disease onset and analyze response to treatment to improve prognosis, enhance quality of life, and

DOI: 10.1201/9781003486909-13

improve the recovery rate in patients. Thus, emerging diagnostic biomarkers and approaches are being optimized to effectively track disease onset and monitor therapy efficiency to improve disease outcomes.

Emerging diagnostic approaches such as nanoparticles, extracellular vesicles, targeted therapy, gene therapy, cell-free DNA, microRNAs, OMICS (molecular omics – genomics, transcriptomics, proteomics, metabolomics; and structural omics – radiomics, pathomics), and artificial intelligence are being optimized to detect cancer-specific signals in real time to improve cancer management [12–14]. Compared to the traditional methods, these emerging strategies hold great promise in providing a high degree of accuracy, sensitivity, and specificity for the efficient and early detection of cancers. Additionally, most of these methods are non-invasive, thus posing minimal or no injury to patients during the process of diagnosis. Similarly, some of these techniques are able to predict appropriate and specific treatment plans hence enhancing treatment outcomes.

The subsequent sections of this chapter will elaborate on the burden of cancer, the various traditional methods of cancer diagnosis with their accompanying strengths and limitations, the emerging methods of cancer diagnosis with their strength and limitations, and a future perspective.

13.2 Burden of Cancer

The incidence and mortality rates of cancer have been on the rise globally making cancer one of the leading causes of premature death. In the year 2020, an estimated 19.3 million new cancer cases and almost 10.0 million cancer deaths were recorded globally [15]. Figure 13.1 depicts the most common cancers diagnosed in men and women globally in 2020. Female breast cancer was the most diagnosed cancer (11.7%), followed by lung (11.4%), colorectal (10.0 %), prostate (7.3%), and stomach (5.6%) cancers respectively [15]. Lung cancer however recorded the most deaths (18%), followed by colorectal (9.4%), liver (8.3%), stomach (7.7%), and female breast (6.9%) cancers [15] (Figure 13.1).

In the United States, mortality rates for prostate, stomach, and uterine corpus cancers are reported to be two-fold higher in black people compared to White people. Similarly, liver, stomach, and kidney cancers are reported to be two-fold higher in Native American people compared to White people showing some disparity in cancer incidence and mortality in this region [16]. Overall, an estimated 2,001,140 new cancer cases and 611,720 cancer deaths are estimated to occur in the United States in the year 2024 [16].

Similarly in sub-Saharan Africa in the year 2020, an estimated 801,392 new cancer cases and 520,158 cancer deaths were reported [17]. In women, breast and cervical cancers are the two most common cancers with breast cancer emerging as the leading cancer in 28 countries, followed by cervical cancer as the leading cancer in 19 countries [17]. In men, prostate cancer reported the highest incidence in 40 countries, followed by liver cancer and colorectal cancer [17]. Although cancer incidence appears lower

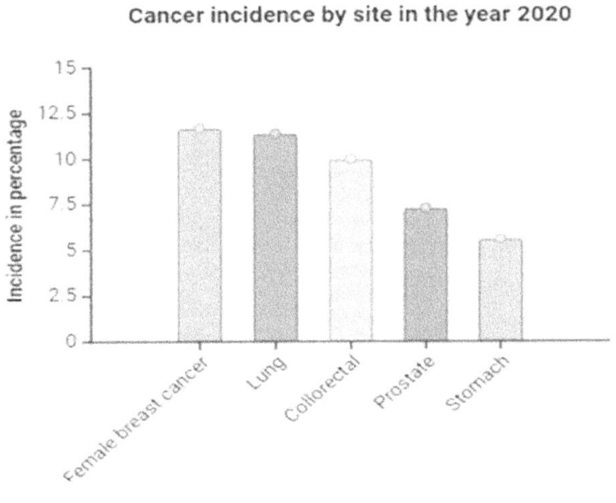

FIGURE 13.1 Cancer incidence in 2020.

in countries with lower Human Development Index (HDI) – that is countries with lower life expectancy, education, and per capita income indicators – cancer deaths are generally higher [18]. For example, breast cancer incidences in countries with high HDI is reported to be about 1 in 12 women in their lifetime, and death is about 1 in 71 women while incidence in countries with low HDI is reported to be 1 in 27 women in their lifetime, and deaths, 1 in 48 women [18].

Globally, an estimated 35 million new cancer cases are expected to occur in the year 2050, a staggering 77% increase from the estimated 20 million cases in 2022 [18]. The greatest increase in incidence is expected to occur in high HDI countries with an additional 4.8 million new cases [18]. Yet the most striking increase in incidence is projected to occur in low (142%) and medium (99%) HDI countries; cancer mortalities are expected to double in these countries by the year 2050 [18]. These increasing cancer burdens reflect increasing population aging and growth, as well as increasing risk factors such as tobacco, alcohol, obesity, exposure to carcinogenic substances, and more [18].

Though significant progress has been made in the early detection, treatment, and care of cancer patients, disparities in cancer outcomes exist between high and low-income regions and also within countries [19]. Hence the need for efficient and affordable diagnostic and treatment options to bridge the gap of inequalities in cancer management and outcomes.

13.3 Traditional Approaches to Cancer Diagnosis

Traditionally, cancer diagnosis methods comprise various techniques to detect the presence and type of cancers. Typically, patients are physically examined for lumps or irregularities in the body as well as any noticeable changes in the skin or mucous membranes. Imaging may also be carried out to detect tumors in bones and certain organs. Sometimes examination of blood, urine, and biopsies are carried out to identify tumor markers and cancer cells or unusual substance levels in the body. Figure 13.2 summarizes the traditional approaches to cancer diagnosis

Physical examination is usually the first step in cancer diagnosis and has a great clinical utility. Suspicion of cancer is typically followed by clinical history and a methodical, comprehensive physical examination to detect a possible primary area of the cancer and map out the extent of disease [20]. Lymph node examination for example helps to clinically differentiate benign from malignant nodes, determine disease stage, or discover unknown primary cancer location [20]. A comprehensive physical examination is very useful in identifying features such as masses, jaundice, pleural effusions, hepatomegaly, ascites, and raised intracranial pressure, all suggestive of metastatic disease [20]. Physical examination is usually followed by a battery of laboratory tests including complete blood count, creatinine level, electrolyte level, calcium, magnesium, and phosphate levels; liver function test, including albumin level test, international normalized ratio test, lactate dehydrogenase level, serum protein electrophoresis, and tumor markers; with a combination of radiologic and nuclear medicine-based non-invasive imaging modalities as appropriate [11]. In spite of the great clinical utility of physical examination, it has long

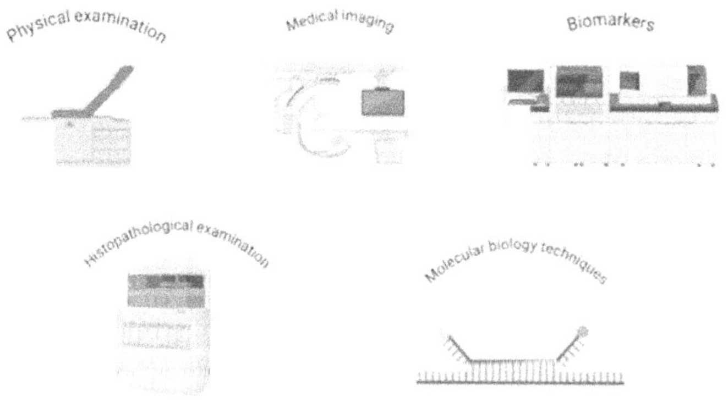

FIGURE 13.2 Traditional approach to cancer diagnosis.

been plagued with limitations such as; differences in the skill and experience of the examiner, variations in the definition of outline and in the texture of the cancer, variations in the texture of the normal surrounding tissue, and biologic variations in the threshold size of a cancer before distant metastases occur [21]. These limitations have been shown to contribute to inadequacies and errors in the outcome of a physical examination leading to delayed diagnosis, incorrect diagnosis, unnecessary treatment, no or delayed treatment, unnecessary diagnostic cost, unnecessary exposure to radiation or contrast, and complications caused by treatments [21].

13.3.1 Biomarkers

Biomarkers are biological molecules, structures or activities present in the body that can be used to predict the occurrence of any disease [22]. Biomarkers have been used for decades in oncology and can be found in blood, urine, cerebrospinal fluid, or other body tissues and are mostly elevated in association with cancer [23]. Tumor markers on the other hand are a subset of biomarkers and include heterogeneous group of molecules including; hormones (β-human chorionic gonadotropin), enzymes (prostate-specific antigen), glycoproteins (cancer antigen 125], and oncofetal antigens (carcinoembryonic antigen and α-fetoprotein) which indicate the presence of cancer or provide information about the likely future behavior of a cancer [24]. In clinical practice, tumor markers are frequently examined as non-invasive indicators to diagnose cancer, evaluate tumor progression, and predict prognosis [25]. For example carcinoembryonic antigen (CEA) is used in the diagnosis of colon and hepatocellular cancers; carbohydrate antigen 19-9 is used to predict pancreatic and bile duct cancer; Urinary 5-HIAA is used for neuroendocrine cancer; cancer antigen 15-3 is used for breast cancer; cancer antigen 125 for ovarian cancer; prostate-specific antigen (PSA) for prostate cancer; Alpha-Fetoprotein (αFP) for hepatocellular cancer and germ cell cancers; Beta-Human Chorionic Gonadotropin (βHCG) for germ cell and gestational trophoblastic cancer; thyroglobulin for thyroid cancers; Fecal Occult Blood Test (FOBT) for colorectal cancer; Vanillylmandelic Acid and Homovanillic Acid (VMA/HVA) for neuroblastoma; pepsinogen for gastric cancer; and Ki-67 proliferation index in breast cancer and microsatellite instability (MSI) status in colorectal cancer used to determine prognosis [20, 25, 26].

Generally, an ideal tumor marker is expected to have a high positive and negative predictive value, be inexpensive, have a simple, standardized, and automated assay with clearly defined reference limits, be acceptable to subjects undergoing the test, have its clinical value validated in a large prospective trial, be highly specific to a given tumor type, provide a lead-time over clinical diagnosis and have levels that correlate reliably with the tumor burden [27]. Table 13.1 outlines the currently used tumor markers in clinical practice and their associated malignancies.

Currently, the ideal tumor marker does not exist. Available markers routinely used in clinical practice lack sufficiently high specificity and sensitivity and are mainly used as laboratory tests to support diagnosis or in monitoring disease progression [43]. Assays such as high-performance liquid chromatography (HPLC), polymerase chain reaction (PCR), Western blotting, radioimmunoassay (RIA), enzyme-linked immunosorbent assay (ELISA), and immunohistochemistry (IHC) are mostly used for tumor marker analysis. These assays are however limited in terms of sensitivity, specificity, and stability further reducing the overall efficiency of tumor markers in cancer diagnosis [25].

13.3.2 Medical Imaging Techniques

Medical imaging is one of the most widely applied techniques in medical practice to assist with cancer diagnosis, staging, surgery, radiotherapy and to monitor a patient's response to treatment [44]. Medical imaging creates images of the human body by incorporating radiology, endoscopy, thermography, medical photography, and microscopy [45]. Tools such as X-ray, Computed Tomography, Ultra Sonography (US), Magnetic Resonance Imaging, and Positron Emission Tomography (PET), are mostly employed to shed light on the physical structure, metabolic activity, and functional status of the cancer tissue [45].

TABLE 13.1

Tumor markers used in clinical practice

Tumor marker	Cancer type	Reference
Steroids, Catecholamines	Adrenal cancer	
CA 15-3, 27.29; ER/PR/ HEGFR-2	Breast cancer	[28]
FDP, NMP/22, BTA, CEA	Bladder cancer	[10]
CEA, FOBT	Colorectal cancer	[29]
Pepsinogen,	Gastric cancer	[30]
CA 19-9	Pancreatic, bile duct cancers	[31]
KIT	Gastrointestinal cancer	[10]
5-HIAA	Neuroendocrine, Carcinoid cancers	[32, 33]
CA 125, HE4	Ovarian cancers	[34]
PSA	Prostate cancers	[35]
αFP, CEA	Hepatocellular cancer	[36]
αFP, βHCG	Germ cell cancer	[37]
βHCG	Gestational trophoblastic cancer	[38]
TG, Calcitonin	Thyroid cancer	[39, 40]
LDH, Cytogenetic alterations	Lymphomas	[26]
Tyrosinase	Melanoma	[41]
HVA and VMA	Neuroblastoma	[42]

CA 15-3, 27.29: Cancer antigen 15-3, 27.29; **CA 19-9**: Carbohydrate antigen 19-9; **ER**: Estrogen receptor; **PR**: Progesterone receptor; **HEGFR**: Human epidermal growth factor receptor 2; **HE4**: human epididymis protein 4; **EGFR**: Epidermal growth factor receptor; **FDP**: Fibrinogen degradation product; **NMP/22**: Nuclear Matrix Protein 22; **BTA**: Bladder tumor antigen; **CEA**: Carcinoembryonic antigen; **FOBT**: Fecal Occult Blood Test; **KIT**: tyrosine kinase; **5-HIAA**: 5-hydroxyindoleacetic acid; **PSA**: Prostate-specific antigen; **αFP**: Alpha-Fetoprotein; **βHCG**: Beta-Human Chorionic Gonadotropin; **TG**: thyroglobulin; **VMA and HVA**: Vanillylmandelic acid and Homovanillic acid.

13.3.2.1 X-Rays

X-rays are high-energy electromagnetic radiation with short wavelengths and one of the most widely used electromagnetic waves in clinical practice able to penetrate solids and ionizing gases [46]. X-ray images (radiographs) are obtained by positioning the patient in such a way that the part of the body being imaged is located between an X-ray source (X-ray machine) and an X-ray detector. X-rays are then released from the machine and projected toward the image detector placed behind the patient's body causing darkening of the X-ray plate [47]. X-rays are partly hindered by soft tissues, showing up as gray on the X-ray plate; while bone and other hard tissues massively block the rays, resulting in a light-toned shadow. X-rays are therefore more appropriate for visualizing hard body structures such as teeth and bones [47]. Excessive exposure to high-energy radiations such as X-rays has the potential to damage cells and cause changes that can lead to cancer hence more sophisticated and safer imaging techniques are currently in use; nonetheless, X-ray is still utilized in medical imaging, especially for bone and teeth [47]. The hazards of X-rays to the patient and the operator are managed by proper shielding and limiting exposure [47]. Typically, conventional X-ray is only able to capture two-dimensional images of the body from a single angle; current imaging techniques however are able to produce three-dimensional images revealing aspects of the body functioning [48].

13.3.2.2 Computed Tomography

Computed tomography is a non-invasive computerized X-ray imaging technique which utilizes computers to analyze multiple cross-sectional X-ray images (slices) [49]. During CT scans, the patient is placed on a motorized platform and the computerized axial tomography (CAT) scanner moves quickly to rotate at 360 degrees about the patient, taking images in the process [50]. The computer then combines these slices into a two-dimensional view of the scanned area revealing in-depth details about structures in the body [50]. CT images are called tomographic images and contain more detailed information such as the size of a mass down to a millimeter, than conventional X-rays [50].

Technological advancements have improved both the hardwares and softwares used for CT scanning, enabling the capture of exquisite soft tissue detail in a non-invasive fashion within a short period of time [51]. Tomographic images are more desirable for evaluating soft tissue masses such as brain, thoracic and abdominal viscera, and lungs, due to their higher contrast sensitivity than conventional radiography [47]. However, CT scanning exposes patients to a higher dose of radiation compared to X-rays predisposing patients to an increased risk of developing cancer [52].

13.3.2.3 Magnetic Resonance Imaging

Magnetic Resonance Imaging is a non-invasive medical imaging technique that relies on the principle that matter emits radio signals when exposed to magnetic fields and radio waves [53]. The application of MRI in detecting morphological changes is grounded in its capacity to identify variations in proton density and the relaxation times of magnetic spins [54]. An MRI scanner is typically composed of a primary magnet, a radio frequency (RF) component, and a magnetic field gradient system [55]. The main magnet produces a consistent magnetic field, and the system's three perpendicular gradient coils help to localize signals. Additionally, the RF component which consists of a transmitter coil creates a rotating magnetic field to stimulate the spin system, and a receiver coil, which converts the resulting magnetization into electrical impulses. Subsequently, the MRI scanner picks up signals that are then reconstructed into images by a digital computer [55]. A significant benefit of MRI is that it does not expose patients to radiation; however, it is highly expensive and associated with significant discomfort [56]. Additionally, individuals with iron-containing metallic implants, such as internal sutures or certain prosthetic devices cannot undergo MRI scanning due to the risk of dislodging these implants [57].

13.3.2.4 Positron Emission Tomography

Positron emission tomography is a non-invasive imaging technique that provides physiological information through the injection of radioactive compounds known as radiotracers, the detection of emitted radiation, and the reconstruction of the radiotracer's distribution [58]. The radiation emitted by PET scans is short-lived, making it relatively safe for administration to the body [59]. PET scans are instrumental in depicting various physiological activities, including nutrient metabolism and blood flow within organs, and are extensively utilized in diagnosing a multitude of conditions such as cancer, brain and heart diseases [60]. The type of information provided by PET is based on the imaging agent and the disease present and may include detection, classification, staging, prognosis, treatment planning, assessing response to therapy, and surveillance [61].

13.3.2.5 Ultrasonography

Ultrasonography is a well-established clinical imaging technique that uses high-frequency sound waves transmitted into the body to create an echo signal, which is then converted by a computer into a real-time image [62]. Ultrasonography is used in sensitive situations such as pregnancy because it is safe and the least invasive of all imaging techniques [63]. It also provides real-time, quantitative, anatomical, and physiological information in humans and is mostly applied in the study of heart function, blood flow in the neck or extremities, gallbladder disease, and fetal growth and development [64]. Ultrasonography is frequently used for guiding interventional clinical procedures because it lacks ionizing radiation and has relatively low purchase and maintenance costs [65]. Nevertheless, ultrasonography is unable to penetrate bone and gas and the image quality is heavily dependent on the operator. Also, it has inherent limitations in resolution, sensitivity, and contrast generation thus hindering its ability to effectively detect, characterize, and monitor cancer growth and progression [45]

13.3.3 Histopathological Techniques for Cancer Diagnosis

Histopathological techniques are widely regarded as the gold standard for diagnosing and grading cancers [66]. The technique employs the use of dyes such as Hematoxylin and Eosin (H and E) stains to enhance the visualization of tissue structures obtained from patients through biopsies, surgical resection, fine needle aspiration, and autopsy with the aid of a microscope [67]. During the process of H and E staining, hematoxylin complexes with aluminum to become positively charged thus acting as a basic dye [68]. The positive charge permits it to bind to the acidic structures of tissues and cells (basophilic cell components) such as chromatin, ribosomes, and RNA-rich cytoplasmic areas, thus imparting a blue or purple color as a result [68]. In reverse, Eosin is anionic and acts as an acidic dye. It is negatively charged and binds to the basic structures of the cell (acidophilic components), such as amino groups on proteins in the cytoplasm imparting various shades of pink [69]. Images generated from histopathological staining are freely scalable, which enhances the visualization of microscopic details in tissues, thereby improving detection and accuracy [70]. Pathologists typically use a microscope to directly observe, analyze, and grade tissues to diagnose cancer. However, this process is cumbersome and can lead to dizziness and cervical fatigue for the pathologist [71].

13.3.4 Immunological Probes and Molecular Biology Techniques for Cancer Diagnosis

13.3.4.1 Immunological Probes

Immunological probes play a crucial role in cancer diagnosis due to their ability to detect specific antigens that are associated with cancer [72]. These probes leverage on the body's immune system or synthetic antibodies to recognize and bind to antigens, enabling the identification and characterization of cancerous cells or tissues [73]. Monoclonal or polyclonal antibodies are mostly designed to target-specific antigens that are over expressed or uniquely expressed on cancer cells, allowing for precise detection to distinguish cancerous cells from healthy ones [74]. Immunological probes are utilized in assays such as immunostaining, ELISA, flow cytometry, and DNA and RNA-based hybridization for the diagnosis of cancers [75].

Immunostaining, also called immunolabeling or immunolocalization, uses antibodies to assess antigen distribution in healthy and diseased tissues, relying on tumor antigen expression in cancer cells for diagnosis [76]. The technique is widely used in medical research and clinical practice because it is easy to perform, provides quick and cost-efficient results, and enables evaluation of protein localization in tumor structures. It can be applied to both cells (immunocytostaining) and tissues (immunohistostaining) [76]. During the process of immunostaining, monoclonal or polyclonal antibodies are labeled with a fluorochrome (fluorescent dye), enzyme, and so on. When a fluorescent dye is used to label the antibody, the technique is termed immunofluorescence, similarly, the term immunoenzyme/immunochemistry is used when an enzyme is used to label the antibody [77].

Based on these factors, techniques such as immunohistochemistry (IHC), immunocytochemistry (ICC), immunocytofluorescence (ICF), and immunohistofluorence (IHF) have emerged in the pathology lab [77]. The labeled antibody is usually incubated with the sample of choice containing the target antigen and the resulting bound antigen-antibody complex is visualized under a light or fluorescent microscope to identify the areas marked by the fluorescence or the chromogen [78]. In IHC, various enzymatic labels such as horseradish peroxidase (HRP) or alkaline phosphatase (AP) are used, along with chromogens like 3-Amino-9-Ethylcarbazole (AEC), 3,3′,5,5′-Tetramethylbenzidine (TMB), and 3,3′-Diaminobenzidine (DAB) to produce different colors for detecting the antigens of interest. On the other hand, IF relies on fluorescent signals from fluorophores such as Fluorescein isothiocyanate (FITC), Texas Red, Cyanine5 (Cy5), and Alexa Fluors, combined with a nuclear label, typically 4′,6-diamidino-2-phenylindole (DAPI) or Hoechst[77]. The brightness of the fluorescence or the intensity of the color is used to gauge the proportion of the tumor cells harboring the antigen of interest. These techniques are extensively applied to target antigens expressed by very specific forms of cancers, thus useful for diagnosing specific cancers [79].

TABLE 13.2
Strengths and weaknesses of immunostaining methods

Immunostaining methods	Strengths	Weaknesses
Immunohistochemistry (IHC)	Provides permanent labeling of antigens in tissues	Have a lower range of targets
	Tissue architecture can be clearly visualized	Not convenient for multiplexing
	It has a stronger sensitivity	Not appropriate for co-localization studies
Immunofluorescence (IF)	Appropriate for co-localization studies	Provides a non-permanent labeling of target
	Convenient for multiplexing and simpler to perform	Prone to autofluorescence
	Has a higher range of target	Has a lower sensitivity

Immunohistochemistry and immunofluorescence both aim to visualize protein expression patterns, yet they differ in detection methods, visualization techniques, multiplexing capabilities, and their various applications [80]. Immunohistochemistry is well-suited for tissue-based analysis and clinical diagnostics, whereas immunofluorescence is valuable for high-resolution imaging and multiplexed protein detection in experimental settings [80]. Table 13.2 summarizes the strengths and weaknesses of each method.

There are currently two immune-staining methods in use regardless of the enzyme or fluorochrome used: direct and indirect [76]. Direct immunostaining involves a primary antibody directly linked to a label, known as a conjugate antibody. On the other hand, the indirect method uses an unconjugated primary antibody specific to the target antigen, followed by a labeled secondary antibody that binds to the primary antibody [76]. The direct method is often the preferred choice when a large amount of conjugated primary antibody is available. Additionally, it involves fewer steps with a large signal-to-noise ratio resulting from the reduced number of non-specific sites to which secondary antibodies bind. However, this method is associated with reduced sensitivity hence a large amount of antibody is mostly utilized to improve the sensitivity [76]. Some researchers prefer the indirect method because the primary antibody is relatively stable and the method provides enhanced signal strength through the binding of one or more secondary antibodies to the primary antibody; however, it is time-consuming [81].

13.3.4.2 Molecular Biology Techniques

Polymerase Chain Reaction is a fundamental technique in molecular biology revolutionizing cancer diagnosis and research [82]. PCR is utilized to amplify specific DNA sequences, enabling the detection of genetic alterations associated with cancer [82]. Usually, specific primers to known mutation sites such as oncogenes and tumor suppressor genes are designed to identify mutations that drive cancer development [83].

PCR-based methods are utilized for the detection of mutations in frequently mutated genes [84]. For example, quantitative PCR (qPCR) is used to measure the amount of DNA in a sample, thereby providing quantitative data about gene expression levels, gene copy number variations, or the prevalence of specific mutations [84]. Similarly, reverse transcription PCR (RT-PCR) or nested PCR are useful in detecting fusion genes resulting from chromosomal translocations, which are hallmark events in certain types of cancer [85]. Digital PCR (dPCR) and single-cell PCR are advanced techniques used to detect rare mutant alleles associated with diseases and analyze genetic alterations at the single-cell level to understand tumor heterogeneity and clonal evolution [86]. Methylation-specific PCR (MSP) however is employed to detect DNA methylation patterns associated with cancer development, serving as a potential biomarker for early cancer detection and prognosis [87]. PCR-based methods are also useful in detecting viral

DNA or RNA sequences in cancer tissues, aiding in the diagnosis and management of virus-associated cancers [88].

Aside from PCR-based methods, in situ hybridization is another molecular diagnostic technique that uses labeled DNA probes to detect chromosomal abnormalities in cancer [89]. Fluorescence in Situ Hybridization (FISH) and Chromogenic in Situ Hybridization (CISH) are used in the field of molecular pathology and molecular oncology to identify chromosomal aberrations such as rearrangements resulting from translocations, insertions or inversions, and losses (deletions) and gains aiding in tumor classification [90]. Both methods of in situ hybridization are based on the same principle of attaching to the region of interest, detecting genetic markers that are crucial in patient risk stratification, and evaluating treatment decisions [90]. CISH has been reported to have a sensitivity of 97.5% and a specificity of 94% for detecting HER-2/neu gene amplification, making it comparable to FISH [91].

Despite the significant clinical benefits of traditional diagnostic methods in cancer management, some, like biopsies, are invasive and can cause discomfort, pain, and potential complications [92]. Early-stage cancers, often asymptomatic, may not be visible or detectable by many traditional techniques. For example, histopathological examinations depend on pathologists' expertise, introducing subjectivity; different pathologists may interpret the same sample differently, leading to inconsistent results [93]. Moreover, traditional methods can be time-consuming, potentially delaying treatment initiation and worsening prognosis [94]. Repeated imaging tests, such as CT scans, expose patients to ionizing radiation, increasing the risk of secondary cancers [52]. Additionally, diagnostic imaging and biopsy procedures can be costly, adding to the overall expense of cancer care [95]. Consequently, there is a need for advanced diagnostic technologies like liquid biopsies, molecular imaging, and advanced genomic techniques, which aim to overcome these challenges by offering less invasive, more precise, and quicker diagnostic alternatives.

13.4 Emerging Technologies in Cancer Diagnosis

Emerging diagnostic approaches are being optimized to detect cancer-specific signals in real time [12–14]. Figure 13.3 gives a summary of some emerging approaches in cancer diagnosis.

13.4.1 Nanoparticles

Nanoparticles are becoming increasingly important in the field of cancer diagnosis due to their unique characteristics and diverse functionalities [96]. They enhance the sensitivity and specificity of various imaging technologies including MRI, CT, and PET [96]. They can also be tailored to specifically target cancer cells, resulting in clearer and more precise images [96]. Nanoparticles are adopted for use as contrast agents that selectively accumulate in cancerous tissues, thereby improving the differentiation between healthy and diseased tissues in imaging procedures thus enabling better visualization and delineation of tumors [97].

Furthermore, nanoparticles are being linked to specific biomarkers or ligands that bind to cancer-specific molecules, facilitating molecular imaging [98]. This allows for the detection of cancer at early stages by identifying molecular changes before structural changes occur [98]. Most importantly, nanoparticles enable less invasive diagnostic procedures compared to traditional biopsy methods [99]. For example, liquid biopsies using nanoparticle-based assays can detect cancer-related biomarkers in bodily fluids such as blood, reducing the necessity for surgical tissue samples [99].

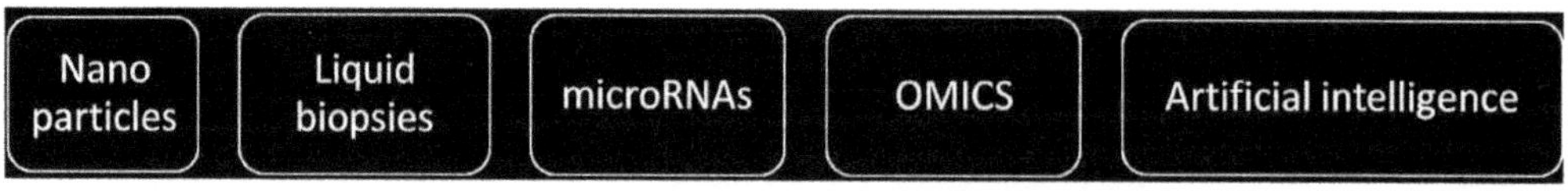

FIGURE 13.3 Emerging technologies in cancer diagnosis.

In summary, nanoparticles are a potent and adaptable tool in cancer diagnosis, offering improved imaging capabilities, targeted delivery, and real-time monitoring, all of which contribute to more accurate, early, and minimally invasive cancer detection and management.

13.4.2 Liquid Biopsies

Liquid biopsies are a minimally invasive diagnostic method used to detect cancer and other diseases through a blood sample [100]. Unlike traditional tissue biopsies that require surgical procedures to extract tissue samples, liquid biopsies analyze extracellular vesicles, cell-free DNA (cfDNA), circulating tumor DNA (ctDNA), circulating tumor cells (CTCs), and other biomarkers in the blood [100]. This technique is non-invasive allowing for more frequent monitoring of the disease, helping in the detection of recurrence or progression, and evaluating the effectiveness of treatments [101]. Liquid biopsies are able to detect cancer at an early stage with the potential to provide a more comprehensive view of the genetic landscape of a tumor, thus capturing heterogeneity that might be missed with a single tissue biopsy [102]. Research and development are ongoing to improve the sensitivity, specificity, and clinical utility of liquid biopsies.

13.4.2.1 Extracellular Vesicles

Extracellular vesicles (EVs) are tiny membrane-bound particles released by cells, and play a significant role in intercellular communication [103]. EVs carry various biomolecules, including proteins, lipids, RNA, and DNA, which reflect the state of their parent cells [104]. Tumor-derived EVs are employed as biomarkers for different cancer types and can be isolated from bodily fluids such as blood, urine, and saliva, making them accessible through non-invasive or minimally invasive methods, unlike traditional biopsy [105].

Changes in the composition and abundance of EVs can occur early in cancer development, potentially enabling earlier diagnosis compared to traditional methods [106]. Thus monitoring EVs can offer insights into tumor dynamics and response to treatment, aiding in personalized therapy and real-time monitoring of disease progression [106].

Recent advances in isolation and characterization techniques, such as ultracentrifugation, microfluidics, and high-throughput sequencing, have improved the sensitivity and specificity of EV-based diagnostics; and represent a promising, non-invasive diagnostic tool with the potential to revolutionize cancer detection and management (Havers et al., 2023).

13.4.3 Cell-Free DNA

Cell-free DNA (cfDNA) is another promising technique for cancer diagnosis. It involves analyzing DNA fragments found in the blood plasma, originating from normal or cancer cells [107]. cfDNA is obtained through a simple blood draw, making it a non-invasive alternative to traditional biopsy methods that require tissue samples [108]. It can detect cancer at an early stage by identifying specific genetic mutations, chromosomal abnormalities, and epigenetic changes associated with cancers [108]. It is applicable to various cancer types and useful for cancers that are difficult to biopsy [108]. Advances in next-generation sequencing (NGS) and digital PCR have improved the sensitivity and specificity of cfDNA analysis, allowing for the detection of low levels of tumor DNA [109].

Though cfDNA can provide a comprehensive overview of the genetic landscape of tumors, including mutations, copy number variations, and methylation patterns; its low concentrations in early-stage cancers make detection challenging, requiring standardized protocols and guidelines for consistent and accurate results across different laboratories [110]. Also, distinguishing between cfDNA from tumor cells and normal cells requires sophisticated bioinformatics tools and expertise making the procedure cumbersome [111]. In summary, cell-free DNA offers a non-invasive, sensitive, and personalized approach to detecting and monitoring cancer. However, further research and standardization are needed to fully realize its potential in clinical practice [112].

13.4.4 Circulating Tumor DNA

Circulating tumor DNA (ctDNA) is a promising biomarker for cancer diagnosis and monitoring. ctDNA refers to small fragments of DNA released into the bloodstream by tumor cells [113]. These fragments can provide valuable information about the genetic makeup of tumors, making them useful for various applications in oncology [113]. Detecting ctDNA in blood samples can help identify the presence of cancer at an early stage, often before symptoms appear offering a non-invasive alternative to traditional tissue biopsies. ctDNA is useful in determining the type of cancer and its genetic mutations, aiding in accurate diagnosis and personalized treatment planning [114]. The quantity and genetic characteristics of ctDNA can provide prognostic information, helping to predict the likely course and outcome of the disease. Techniques such as NGS, Digital PCR, and BEAMing (Beads, Emulsion, Amplification, and Magnetics) are very useful for the comprehensive analysis of genetic mutations in ctDNA [115].

13.4.5 Circulating Tumor Cells

Circulating tumor cells are cancer cells that have detached from a primary tumor and are found in the bloodstream. They are a key area of research and clinical interest owing to their utility in early cancer detection and diagnosis [116]. These cells are shed by tumors into the bloodstream, identifying them can indicate the presence of cancer before it is detectable by imaging or other methods [117]. The number and characteristics of CTCs can provide important prognostic information; for example, higher counts of CTCs are often associated with a poorer prognosis and can indicate more aggressive disease. A decrease in the number of CTCs during treatment often correlates with a positive response, while an increase may indicate treatment resistance or disease progression [118]. Studying and characterizing CTCs can help researchers understand the process of metastasis and potential ways to intervene as these cells are responsible for spreading cancer to distant organs [119]. By understanding the specific mutations and pathways active in CTCs, therapies can be tailored to target those mechanisms [120].

Currently, the only FDA-approved method for CTC detection in clinical settings is CellSearch System which uses immunomagnetic separation and immunofluorescent labeling to identify and count CTCs [121]. However, microfluidic devices are able to capture CTCs based on size or other physical properties and are designed to process blood samples and isolate CTCs with high efficiency [122]. PCR and NGS can be used to detect specific genetic markers and detailed genetic analysis of CTCs, providing a sensitive and specific approach to identification and revealing mutations, gene expression profiles, and other molecular features [123]. Ensuring that CTC detection methods are both sensitive (able to detect low levels of CTCs) and specific (accurately distinguishing CTCs from other cells) is critical. More research is needed to integrate CTC analysis into routine clinical practice, including standardizing methods and demonstrating clear clinical benefits. Research into CTCs holds promise for improving cancer diagnosis, treatment, and understanding of metastasis, potentially leading to better outcomes for patients

13.5 MicroRNAs

MicroRNAs (miRNAs) on the other hand are small, noncoding RNA molecules that play a critical role in gene regulation [124]. They exhibit distinct expression patterns in different types of cancers, allowing for accurate identification and classification of cancer types [124]. miRNAs serve as biomarkers for early cancer detection and prognosis and levels can be detected in body fluids such as blood, urine, and saliva, making them accessible and minimally invasive diagnostic tools [125]. Also, they provide high specificity and sensitivity in cancer detection, even in the early stages, thus improving the chances of successful treatment [126]. Similarly, circulating miRNAs found in blood allow for non-invasive diagnostic tests, which are less painful and risky compared to traditional biopsy methods and profiles can aid in the development of personalized medicine approaches by tailoring treatments based on individual miRNA expression patterns [127].

In summary, miRNAs are valuable in cancer diagnosis due to their distinct expression in various cancers, ease of detection in body fluids, and potential to guide personalized treatment strategies [128].

13.6 OMICS

OMICS refers to the collective technologies used to explore the roles, relationships, and actions of the various types of molecules that make up the cells of an organism [129]. The major types of omics include genomics, transcriptomics, proteomics, and metabolomics, and are emerging as powerful tools in cancer diagnosis due to their ability to provide comprehensive and detailed insights into the molecular mechanisms underlying cancer [129]. Genomics, the study of the entire genome including the complete set of DNA in an organism is able to identify genetic mutations, alterations, and variations associated with cancer [130]. Techniques such as NGS allow for the detection of mutations in cancer-related genes, helping to diagnose specific types of cancer and predict patient outcomes [131]. Alternatively, transcriptomics involves the study of the transcriptome, the complete set of RNA transcripts produced by the genome [132]. This provides insights into gene expression profiles and how they differ in cancerous cells compared to normal cells [132]. RNA sequencing (RNA-seq) can identify upregulated or downregulated genes, contributing to the understanding of cancer biology and aiding in the identification of biomarkers for early diagnosis [133].

Similarly, proteomics involves the study of the proteome, the entire set of proteins expressed by a genome, cell, tissue, or organism, and examines protein expression, modifications, and interactions [134]. Mass spectrometry and protein microarrays are used to identify protein biomarkers and signaling pathways involved in cancer, offering potential targets for diagnosis and therapy [133].

Finally, metabolomics examines the metabolome, the complete set of small-molecule metabolites found within a biological sample [135]. It analyzes metabolic changes in cancer cells. Techniques like nuclear magnetic resonance (NMR) spectroscopy and mass spectrometry detect alterations in metabolites that can serve as biomarkers for cancer detection and provide insights into the metabolic pathways altered in cancer [136].

Combining data from genomics, transcriptomics, proteomics, and metabolomics provides a holistic view of cancer biology. Integrated omics approaches can identify complex molecular signatures and pathways involved in cancer, improving the accuracy of diagnosis and allowing for personalized treatment strategies [137]. Additionally, OMICS technologies are instrumental in discovering new biomarkers for various types of cancer, enhancing the specificity and sensitivity of diagnostic tests [138]. Managing and interpreting the vast amount of data generated by omics technologies is complex and requires advanced bioinformatics tools [139]. However, translating OMICS research findings into clinical practice involves rigorous validation and standardization of methods, and the high costs and the need for specialized equipment and expertise can limit the widespread adoption of OMICS technologies in routine clinical settings [140]. In summary, OMICS technologies are transforming cancer diagnosis by providing detailed molecular insights, enabling early detection, and paving the way for personalized medicine. Despite challenges, ongoing advancements in omics and bioinformatics are likely to enhance their clinical utility and accessibility [140].

13.7 Artificial Intelligence

Artificial intelligence (AI) in medicine involves using algorithms and software to emulate human cognitive processes for analyzing, interpreting, and understanding complex medical and healthcare data [141]. Within this domain, AI encompasses various subfields such as machine learning, natural language processing, robotics, and computer vision [141].

In oncology, AI encompasses the deployment of sophisticated computational algorithms and machine learning methods to improve cancer diagnosis, treatment, and research (Kourou et al., 2021). Artificial intelligence is playing a crucial role in the early detection and diagnosis of cancers [142]. AI algorithms, particularly those based on deep learning, a subfield of machine learning, can analyze medical images such as X-rays, CT scans, MRI scans, and mammograms with high accuracy, and identify patterns and anomalies that might be missed by human eyes [142]. AI systems can assist pathologists by analyzing tissue samples and processing large volumes of data quickly, thus helping to identify cancer at a microscopic level with greater precision [143]. In genetics, AI tools are being optimized to analyze genetic information to identify mutations and other genetic markers associated with different types of cancers; thus enhancing the understanding of the genetic basis of cancer, predicting cancer risk, and aiding in personalizing treatment plans based on an individual's genetic profile [144]. Furthermore, AI models are being employed to assess an individual's risk of developing cancer by analyzing various factors including family history, lifestyle, and environmental exposures; these models can provide personalized risk scores, enabling proactive monitoring and preventive measures [144]. AI models are also useful in streamlining the process of matching patients with appropriate clinical trials based on their unique cancer profiles, thus facilitating access to cutting-edge treatments and accelerating the development of new cancer therapies [145]. Overall, AI enhances the accuracy, efficiency, and personalization of cancer diagnosis and treatment, offering significant potential to improve patient outcomes and revolutionize oncology [146]. Though these emerging technologies of cancer diagnosis hold great promise, they are still being optimized and are associated with limitations of cost, accessibility, technical complexity, ethical, and privacy concerns [147].

13.8 Future Direction

The future of emerging technologies in cancer diagnosis is promising, driven by rapid advancements in various fields such as genomics, AI, imaging technologies, and liquid biopsies. These innovations are expected to enhance early detection, accuracy, and personalized treatment of cancer [148]. Next-generation sequencing allows for comprehensive genomic profiling of tumors, enabling the identification of specific genetic mutations and alterations. This facilitates the development of targeted therapies tailored to an individual's genetic profile (Mahmood et al., 2024). CRISPR technology is being explored for its potential in identifying and validating new cancer biomarkers, which can improve early detection and treatment strategies [149].

AI algorithms are also being developed to enhance the accuracy of imaging techniques like MRI, CT, and PET scans to assist radiologists in identifying subtle patterns and anomalies that may indicate early-stage cancer [150]. Machine learning models for instance can analyze large datasets to predict cancer risk and outcomes, aiding in early diagnosis and personalized treatment plans [146]. Advanced imaging techniques such as molecular imaging and hyperpolarized MRI have great potential to provide detailed images at the molecular level and to enhance the visibility of metabolic changes in tissues, potentially allowing for the early detection and characterization of cancerous changes [151]. Currently, research is uncovering links between the microbiome and cancer to discover new biomarkers for early cancer detection [152].

Embracing emerging technologies has the potential to revolutionize cancer diagnosis. By combining expertise from genomics, bioinformatics, engineering, and clinical practice, comprehensive diagnostic solutions to harness big data and cloud computing can be developed. This integration and analysis of diverse datasets can provide better diagnostic insights, ultimately facilitating more individualized diagnostic and treatment approaches based on a patient's unique biological profile. Overall, these advancements aim to enhance early cancer detection and improve accurate diagnosis, leading to better patient outcomes and more effective treatment strategies.

REFERENCES

1. World Health Organization (WHO). Cancer [Internet]. 2022 [cited 2024 Jan 26]. Available from: https://www.who.int/news-room/fact-sheets/detail/cancer
2. Krieghoff-Henning E, Folkerts J, Penzkofer A, Weg-Remers S. Cancer – an overview. *Med Monatsschr Pharm.* 2017 Feb;40(2):48–54.
3. Martínez-Reyes I, Chandel NS. Cancer metabolism: looking forward. *Nat Rev Cancer.* 2021 Oct;21(10):669–80.
4. Choi JW, Hua TNM. Impact of lifestyle behaviors on cancer risk and prevention. *J Lifestyle Med.* 2021 Jan 31;11(1):1–7.

5. Cooper GM. The development and causes of cancer. In: *The cell: a molecular approach*, 2nd ed. [Internet]. Sinauer Associates; 2024 [cited 2024 Jan 30]. Available from: https://www.ncbi.nlm.nih.gov/books/NBK9963/
6. Kamali H, Golmohammadzadeh S, Zare H, Nosrati R, Fereidouni M, Safarpour H. The recent advancements in the early detection of cancer biomarkers by DNAzyme-assisted aptasensors. *J Nanobiotechnology*. 2022 Oct 4;20(1):438.
7. Loud J, Murphy J. Cancer screening and early detection in the 21st century. *Semin Oncol Nurs*. 2017 May;33(2):121–8.
8. World Health Organization (WHO). Cancer - Screening and early detection [Internet]. 2010 [cited 2024 Mar 13]. Available from: https://www.who.int/europe/news-room/fact-sheets/item/cancer-screening-and-early-detection-of-cancer
9. Debela DT, Muzazu SG, Heraro KD, Ndalama MT, Mesele BW, Haile DC, et al. New approaches and procedures for cancer treatment: current perspectives. *SAGE Open Med*. 2021 Aug 12;9:20503121211034366.
10. Thenrajan T, Alwarappan S, Wilson J. Molecular diagnosis and cancer prognosis—a concise review. *Diagnostics*. 2023 Feb 17;13(4):766.
11. Pulumati A, Pulumati A, Dwarakanath BS, Verma A, Papineni RVL. Technological advancements in cancer diagnostics: improvements and limitations. *Cancer Rep*. 2023 Jan 6;6(2):e1764.
12. Berger MF, Mardis ER. The emerging clinical relevance of genomics in cancer medicine. *Nat Rev Clin Oncol*. 2018 Jun;15(6):353–65.
13. Cisneros-Villanueva M, Hidalgo-Pérez L, Rios-Romero M, Cedro-Tanda A, Ruiz-Villavicencio CA, Page K, et al. Cell-free DNA analysis in current cancer clinical trials: a review. *Br J Cancer*. 2022 Feb;126(3):391–400.
14. Kim T, Croce CM. MicroRNA: trends in clinical trials of cancer diagnosis and therapy strategies. *Exp Mol Med*. 2023 Jul;55(7):1314–21.
15. Ferlay J, Colombet M, Soerjomataram I, Parkin DM, Piñeros M, Znaor A, et al. Cancer statistics for the year 2020: an overview. *Int J Cancer*. 2021 Apr 5. doi: 10.1002/ijc.33588.
16. Siegel RL, Giaquinto AN, Jemal A. Cancer statistics, 2024. *CA Cancer J Clin*. 2024 Jan 1;74(1):12–49.
17. Bray F, Parkin DM, African Cancer Registry Network. Cancer in sub-Saharan Africa in 2020: a review of current estimates of the national burden, data gaps, and future needs. *Lancet Oncol*. 2022 Jun;23(6):719–28.
18. World Health Organization (WHO). Global cancer burden growing, amidst mounting need for services [Internet]. 2024 [cited 2024 Mar 13]. Available from: https://www.who.int/news/item/01-02-2024-global-cancer-burden-growing--amidst-mounting-need-for-services
19. dos-Santos-Silva I, Gupta S, Orem J, Shulman LN. Global disparities in access to cancer care. *Commun Med*. 2022 Apr 7;2(1):1–4.
20. Wilkinson AN. Cancer diagnosis in primary care. *Can Fam Physician*. 2021 Apr;67(4):265–8.
21. Verghese A, Charlton B, Kassirer JP, Ramsey M, Ioannidis JPA. Inadequacies of physical examination as a cause of medical errors and adverse events: a collection of vignettes. *Am J Med*. 2015 Dec 1;128(12):1322–1324.e3.
22. Sung H, Ferlay J, Siegel RL, Laversanne M, Soerjomataram I, Jemal A, et al. Global cancer statistics 2020: GLOBOCAN estimates of incidence and mortality worldwide for 36 cancers in 185 countries. *CA Cancer J Clin*. 2021;71(3):209–49.
23. Schiffman JD, Fisher PG, Gibbs P. Early detection of cancer: past, present, and future. *Am Soc Clin Oncol Educ Book*. 2015 May;(35):57–65.
24. Kamada T, Ohdaira H, Takahashi J, Aida T, Nakashima K, Ito E, et al. Novel tumor marker index using carcinoembryonic antigen and carbohydrate antigen 19-9 is a significant prognostic factor for resectable colorectal cancer. *Sci Rep*. 2024 Feb 20;14(1):4192.
25. Kaushal A, Kaur N, Sharma S, Sharma AK, Kala D, Prakash H, et al. Current update on biomarkers for detection of cancer: comprehensive analysis. *Vaccines*. 2022 Dec 13;10(12):2138.
26. Duffy MJ. Tumor markers in clinical practice: a review focusing on common solid cancers. *Med Princ Pract*. 2012 Dec;22(1):4–11.
27. Bodaghi A, Fattahi N, Ramazani A. Biomarkers: promising and valuable tools towards diagnosis, prognosis and treatment of Covid-19 and other diseases. *Heliyon*. 2023 Jan 30;9(2):e13323.
28. Kabel AM. Tumor markers of breast cancer: new perspectives. *J Oncol Sci*. 2017 Apr 1;3(1):5–11.

29. Lakemeyer L, Sander S, Wittau M, Henne-Bruns D, Kornmann M, Lemke J. Diagnostic and prognostic value of CEA and CA19-9 in colorectal cancer. *Diseases.* 2021 Mar 17;9(1):21.
30. Qin Y, Geng JX, Huang B. Clinical value of serum pepsinogen in the diagnosis and treatment of gastric diseases. *World J Gastrointest Oncol.* 2023 Jul 15;15(7):1174–81.
31. Boyd LNC, Ali M, Kam L, Puik JR, Rodrigues SMF, Zwart ES, et al. The diagnostic value of the CA19-9 and bilirubin ratio in patients with pancreatic cancer, distal bile duct cancer and benign periampullary diseases, a novel approach. *Cancers.* 2022 Jan 11;14(2):344.
32. Carling RS, Degg TJ, Allen KR, Bax NDS, Barth JH. Evaluation of whole blood serotonin and plasma and urine 5-hydroxyindole acetic acid in diagnosis of carcinoid disease. *Ann Clin Biochem.* 2002 Nov;39(Pt 6):577–82.
33. Wedin M, Mehta S, Angerås-Kraftling J, Wallin G, Daskalakis K. The role of serum 5-HIAA as a predictor of progression and an alternative to 24-h urine 5-HIAA in well-differentiated neuroendocrine neoplasms. *Biology.* 2021 Jan 21;10(2):76.
34. Fabbro M, Lamy PJ, Touraine C, Floquet A, Ray-Coquard I, Mollevi C. HE4 and CA-125 kinetics to predict outcome in patients with recurrent epithelial ovarian carcinoma: the META4 clinical trial. *Front Oncol* [Internet]. 2024 Jan 11;13. [cited 2024 Mar 21]. Available from: https://www.frontiersin.org/journals/oncology/articles/10.3389/fonc.2023.1308630/full
35. Whiting D, Bott SR. Current diagnostics for prostate cancer. In: Bott SR, Ng KL, editors. *Prostate cancer* [Internet]. Brisbane (AU): Exon Publications; 2021 [cited 2024 Mar 21]. Available from: http://www.ncbi.nlm.nih.gov/books/NBK571327/
36. EDOO MIA, Chutturghoon VK, WUSU-ANSAH GK, ZHU H, ZHEN TY, XIE HY, et al. Serum biomarkers AFP, CEA and CA19-9 combined detection for early diagnosis of hepatocellular carcinoma. *Iran J Public Health.* 2019 Feb;48(2):314–22.
37. Pedrazzoli P, Rosti G, Soresini E, Ciani S, Secondino S. Serum tumour markers in germ cell tumours: From diagnosis to cure. *Crit Rev Oncol Hematol.* 2021 Mar 1;159:103224.
38. Moghadam M, Nourkhomami S, Mousavi Seresht L, Azimi H, Bolandi S, Zavari T, et al. B-hCG and H-hCG levels in patients with gestational trophoblastic neoplasia. *Curr Gynecol Oncol.* 2020 Dec 31;18:e34–8.
39. Prpić M, Franceschi M, Romić M, Jukić T, Kusić Z. Thyroglobulin as a tumor marker in differentiated thyroid cancer – clinical considerations. *Acta Clin Croat.* 2018 Sep;57(3):518–27.
40. Verbeek HH, de Groot JWB, Sluiter WJ, Muller Kobold AC, van den Heuvel ER, Plukker JT, et al. Calcitonin testing for detection of medullary thyroid cancer in people with thyroid nodules. *Cochrane Database Syst Rev.* 2020 Mar 16;2020(3):CD010159.
41. Weinstein D, Leininger J, Hamby C, Safai B. Diagnostic and prognostic biomarkers in melanoma. *J Clin Aesthetic Dermatol.* 2014 Jun;7(6):13.
42. Shen Y, Li H, Lu J, Luo X, Guan Q, Cheng L. Analytical validation and clinical application of urinary vanillylmandelic acid and homovanillic acid by LC-MS/MS for diagnosis of neuroblastoma. *Biomed Chromatogr.* 2019 Jun;33(6):e4484.
43. Jain R, Mehta S, Mehta A, Mehta V. Tumor markers in clinical practice. *Panacea J Med Sci.* 2022 Apr 28;12:1–3.
44. Gerami R, Sadeghi Joni S, Akhondi N, Etemadi A, Fosouli M, Eghbal AF, et al. A literature review on the imaging methods for breast cancer. *Int J Physiol Pathophysiol Pharmacol.* 2022 Jun 15;14(3):171–6.
45. Biga LM, Bronson S, Dawson S, Harwell A, Hopkins R, Kaufmann J, et al. 1.5 Medical imaging. 2019 Sep 26 [cited 2024 Mar 26]. Available from: https://open.oregonstate.education/aandp/chapter/1-5-medical-imaging/
46. Jokar S, Khazaei S, Behnammanesh H, Laranjo M, Beiki D, Botelho MF. Chapter 5 - X-ray-based cancer diagnosis and treatment methods. In: Khafaji M, Bavi O, editors. *Electromagnetic waves-based cancer diagnosis and therapy* [Internet]. Academic Press; 2023. p. 239–94. [cited 2024 Mar 26]. Available from: https://www.sciencedirect.com/science/article/pii/B9780323996280000010
47. Nakashima J, Duong H. Radiology, Image production and evaluation. In: *StatPearls* [Internet]. Treasure Island (FL): StatPearls Publishing; 2024 [cited 2024 Mar 26]. Available from: http://www.ncbi.nlm.nih.gov/books/NBK553145/
48. Berger M, Yang Q, Maier A. X-ray imaging. In: Maier A, Steidl S, Christlein V, Hornegger J, editors. *Medical imaging systems: an introductory guide* [Internet]. Cham (CH): Springer; 2018 [cited 2024 Jun 28]. Available from: http://www.ncbi.nlm.nih.gov/books/NBK546155/

49. Hussain S, Mubeen I, Ullah N, Shah SSUD, Khan BA, Zahoor M, et al. Modern diagnostic imaging technique applications and risk factors in the medical field: A review. *BioMed Res Int.* 2022 Jun 6;2022:5164970.
50. Patel PR, De Jesus O. CT scan. In: *StatPearls* [Internet]. Treasure Island (FL): StatPearls Publishing; 2024 [cited 2024 Mar 28]. Available from: http://www.ncbi.nlm.nih.gov/books/NBK567796/
51. Hsieh J, Flohr T. Computed tomography recent history and future perspectives. *J Med Imaging.* 2021 Sep;8(5):052109.
52. Cao CF, Ma KL, Shan H, Liu TF, Zhao SQ, Wan Y, et al. CT scans and cancer risks: A systematic review and dose-response meta-analysis. *BMC Cancer.* 2022 Nov 30;22:1238.
53. Messiou C, Hillengass J, Delorme S, Lecouvet FE, Moulopoulos LA, Collins DJ, et al. Guidelines for acquisition, interpretation, and reporting of whole-body MRI in myeloma: Myeloma response assessment and diagnosis system (MY-RADS). *Radiology.* 2019 Apr;291(1):5–13.
54. Rajpal S, Tong MS, Borchers J, Zareba KM, Obarski TP, Simonetti OP, et al. Cardiovascular magnetic resonance findings in competitive athletes recovering from COVID-19 infection. *JAMA Cardiol* [Internet]. 2020 Sep 11 [cited 2024 May 20]. Available from: https://jamanetwork.com/journals/jamacardiology/fullarticle/2770645
55. Fallegger F, Schiavone G, Pirondini E, Wagner FB, Vachicouras N, Serex L, et al. MRI-compatible and conformal electrocorticography grids for translational research. *Adv Sci.* 2021;8(9):2003761.
56. Hemond CC, Bakshi R. Magnetic resonance imaging in multiple sclerosis. *Cold Spring Harb Perspect Med.* 2018 May 1;8(5):a028969.
57. Hasan AM, Jalab HA, Meziane F, Kahtan H, Al-Ahmad AS. Combining deep and handcrafted image features for MRI brain scan classification. *IEEE Access.* 2019;7:79959–67.
58. Chen KT, Gong E, de Carvalho Macruz FB, Xu J, Boumis A, Khalighi M, et al. Ultra-low-dose 18F-florbetaben amyloid PET imaging using deep learning with multi-contrast MRI inputs. *Radiology.* 2020 Sep;296(3):E195.
59. Baumann M, Krause M, Overgaard J, Debus J, Bentzen SM, Daartz J, et al. Radiation oncology in the era of precision medicine. *Nat Rev Cancer.* 2016 Apr;16(4):234–49.
60. Eskian M, Alavi A, Khorasanizadeh M, Viglianti BL, Jacobsson H, Barwick TD, et al. Effect of blood glucose level on standardized uptake value (SUV) in 18F- FDG PET-scan: a systematic review and meta-analysis of 20,807 individual SUV measurements. *Eur J Nucl Med Mol Imaging.* 2019 Jan 1;46(1):224–37.
61. Vandenberghe S, Moskal P, Karp JS. State of the art in total body PET. *EJNMMI Phys.* 2020 May 25;7(1):35.
62. Liu J, Chen SW, Liu F, Li QP, Kong XY, Feng ZC. The diagnosis of neonatal pulmonary atelectasis using lung ultrasonography. *Chest.* 2015 Apr;147(4):1013–9.
63. Whitson MR, Mayo PH. Ultrasonography in the emergency department. *Crit Care Lond Engl.* 2016 Aug 15;20(1):227.
64. Shamshad F, Khan S, Zamir SW, Khan MH, Hayat M, Khan FS, et al. Transformers in medical imaging: A survey. *Med Image Anal.* 2023 Aug 1;88:102802.
65. Rafailidis V, Huang DY, Yusuf GT, Sidhu PS. General principles and overview of vascular contrast-enhanced ultrasonography. *Ultrason Seoul Korea.* 2020 Jan;39(1):22–42.
66. Xue D, Zhou X, Li C, Yao Y, Rahaman M, Zhang J, et al. An application of transfer learning and ensemble learning techniques for cervical histopathology image classification. *IEEE Access* [Internet]. 2020 [cited 2024 May 28]. Available from: https://www.semanticscholar.org/paper/An-Application-of-Transfer-Learning-and-Ensemble-Xue-Zhou/193ac0bb754c4b2c1e80829db9e51a45c3819eab
67. Li D, Hui H, Zhang Y, Tong W, Tian F, Yang X, et al. Deep learning for virtual histological staining of bright-field microscopic images of unlabeled carotid artery tissue. *Mol Imaging Biol.* 2020 Oct 1;22(5):1301–9.
68. Mercan C, Mooij GCAM, Tellez D, Lotz J, Weiss N, Gerven M, et al. *Virtual staining for mitosis detection in breast histopathology.*2020 IEEE 17th International Symposium on Biomedical Imaging (ISBI). 1770 p.
69. Bancroft J, Layton C. The hematoxylins and eosin. In: Bancroft J, Layton C, editors. *The theory and practice of histological techniques.* 7th ed. Elsevier, Amsterdam; 2013. p. 173–86.
70. Ueno H, Kajiwara Y, Ajioka Y, Sugai T, Sekine S, Ishiguro M, et al. Histopathological atlas of desmoplastic reaction characterization in colorectal cancer. *Jpn J Clin Oncol.* 2021 May 28;51(6):1004–12.

71. Wei JW, Tafe LJ, Linnik YA, Vaickus LJ, Tomita N, Hassanpour S. Pathologist-level classification of histologic patterns on resected lung adenocarcinoma slides with deep neural networks. *Sci Rep.* 2019 Mar 4;9(1):3358.
72. Kurki P, Ogata K, Tan EM. Monoclonal antibodies to proliferating cell nuclear antigen (PCNA)/cyclin as probes for proliferating cells by immunofluorescence microscopy and flow cytometry. *J Immunol Methods.* 1988 Apr 22;109(1):49–59.
73. Zhang L, Du X, Chen Z, Chen C, Gong N, Song Y, et al. Instrument-free and visual detection of salmonella based on magnetic nanoparticles and an antibody probe immunosensor. *Int J Mol Sci.* 2019 Sep 19;20(18):4645.
74. Walker LM, Burton DR. Passive immunotherapy of viral infections: 'super-antibodies' enter the fray. *Nat Rev Immunol.* 2018 May;18(5):297–308.
75. Slieman TA, Leheste J. Chapter 1 - Introduction to immunological techniques in the clinical laboratory. In: Pavia CS, Gurtler V, editors. *Methods in microbiology* [Internet]. Academic Press; 2020. p. 1–16. [cited 2024 May 28] (Immunological Methods in Microbiology; vol. 47). Available from: https://www.sciencedirect.com/science/article/pii/S0580951720300015
76. Piña R, Santos-Díaz AI, Orta-Salazar E, Aguilar-Vazquez AR, Mantellero CA, Acosta-Galeana I, et al. Ten approaches that improve immunostaining: a review of the latest advances for the optimization of immunofluorescence. *Int J Mol Sci.* 2022 Jan 26;23(3):1426.
77. Hussaini HM, Seo B, Rich AM. Immunohistochemistry and immunofluorescence. In: Seymour GJ, Cullinan MP, Heng NCK, Cooper PR, editors. *Oral biology: molecular techniques and applications* [Internet]. New York, NY: Springer US; 2023. p. 439–50. [cited 2024 May 28]. Available from: https://doi.org/10.1007/978-1-0716-2780-8_26
78. Magaki S, Hojat SA, Wei B, So A, Yong WH. An introduction to the performance of immunohistochemistry. *Methods Mol Biol Clifton NJ.* 2019;1897:289–98.
79. Olson C. IFA proof of principle experiments. *IEEE Trans Nucl Sci* [Internet]. 1979 [cited 2024 May 29]. Available from: https://www.semanticscholar.org/paper/IFA-Proof-of-Principle-Experiments-Olson/b7beedc697167865df8303887c031fa9c7c6bdfd
80. Tan WCC, Nerurkar SN, Cai HY, Ng HHM, Wu D, Wee YTF, et al. Overview of multiplex immunohistochemistry/immunofluorescence techniques in the era of cancer immunotherapy. *Cancer Commun Lond Engl.* 2020 Apr;40(4):135–53.
81. Im K, Mareninov S, Diaz MFP, Yong WH. An introduction to performing immunofluorescence staining. *Methods Mol Biol Clifton NJ.* 2019;1897:299–311.
82. Ishmael FT, Stellato C. Principles and applications of polymerase chain reaction: basic science for the practicing physician. *Ann Allergy Asthma Immunol Off Publ Am Coll Allergy Asthma Immunol.* 2008 Oct;101(4):437–43.
83. Ghannam MG, Varacallo M. Biochemistry, polymerase chain reaction. In: *StatPearls* [Internet]. Treasure Island (FL): StatPearls Publishing; 2024 [cited 2024 Jun 5]. Available from: http://www.ncbi.nlm.nih.gov/books/NBK535453/
84. Artika IM, Dewi YP, Nainggolan IM, Siregar JE, Antonjaya U. Real-time polymerase chain reaction: current techniques, applications, and role in COVID-19 diagnosis. *Genes.* 2022 Dec 16;13(12):2387.
85. Bachman J. Reverse-transcription PCR (RT-PCR). *Methods Enzymol.* 2013;530:67–74.
86. Fang W, Liu X, Maiga M, Cao W, Mu Y, Yan Q, et al. Digital PCR for single-cell analysis. *Biosensors* [Internet]. 2024 Feb;14(2). [cited 2024 Jun 28]. Available from: https://www.ncbi.nlm.nih.gov/pmc/articles/PMC10886679/
87. Ku JL, Jeon YK, Park JG. Methylation-specific PCR. *Methods Mol Biol Clifton NJ.* 2011;791:23–32.
88. Artika IM, Wiyatno A, Ma'roef CN. Pathogenic viruses: molecular detection and characterization. *Infect Genet Evol.* 2020 Jul 1;81:104215.
89. Veselinyová D, Mašlanková J, Kalinová K, Mičková H, Mareková M, Rabajdová M. Selected in situ hybridization methods: principles and application. *Molecules.* 2021 Jun 24;26(13):3874.
90. Chrzanowska NM, Kowalewski J, Lewandowska MA. Use of fluorescence in situ hybridization (FISH) in diagnosis and tailored therapies in solid Tumors. *Molecules.* 2020 Apr 17;25(8):1864.
91. Sáez A, Andreu FJ, Seguí MA, Baré ML, Fernández S, Dinarés C, et al. HER-2 gene amplification by chromogenic in situ hybridisation (CISH) compared with fluorescence in situ hybridisation (FISH) in breast cancer-A study of two hundred cases. *Breast Edinb Scotl.* 2006 Aug;15(4):519–27.

92. Montagnana M, Lippi G. Cancer diagnostics: current concepts and future perspectives. *Ann Transl Med.* 2017 Jul;5(13):268.
93. Dewi A, Purwanto B, Widjiati W. *Introduction of histopathology.* London, UK: IntechOpen; 2023.
94. Dobson CM, Russell AJ, Rubin GP. Patient delay in cancer diagnosis: what do we really mean and can we be more specific? *BMC Health Serv Res.* 2014 Sep 12;14:387.
95. Hadian M, Jabbari A, Mazaheri E, Norouzi M. What is the impact of clinical guidelines on imaging costs? *J Educ Health Promot.* 2021 Jan 28;10:10.
96. Gavas S, Quazi S, Karpiński TM. Nanoparticles for cancer therapy: current progress and challenges. *Nanoscale Res Lett* [Internet]. 2021;16. [cited 2024 Jun 7]. Available from: https://www.ncbi.nlm.nih.gov/pmc/articles/PMC8645667/
97. Baranwal J, Barse B, Di Petrillo A, Gatto G, Pilia L, Kumar A. Nanoparticles in cancer diagnosis and treatment. *Materials.* 2023 Jul 30;16(15):5354.
98. Han X, Xu K, Taratula O, Farsad K. Applications of nanoparticles in biomedical imaging. *Nanoscale.* 2019 Jan 17;11(3):799–819.
99. Kalogianni DP. Nanotechnology in emerging liquid biopsy applications. *Nano Converg.* 2021 May 2;8(1):13.
100. Nikanjam M, Kato S, Kurzrock R. Liquid biopsy: current technology and clinical applications. *J Hematol Oncol.* 2022 Sep 12;15(1):131.
101. Hirahata T, Ul Quraish R, Quraish AU, Ul Quraish S, Naz M, Razzaq MA. Liquid biopsy: a distinctive approach to the diagnosis and prognosis of cancer. *Cancer Inform.* 2022;21:11769351221076062.
102. Heidrich I, Ačkar L, Mossahebi Mohammadi P, Pantel K. Liquid biopsies: Potential and challenges. *Int J Cancer.* 2021;148(3):528–45.
103. Liu YJ, Wang C. A review of the regulatory mechanisms of extracellular vesicles-mediated intercellular communication. *Cell Commun Signal.* 2023 Apr 13;21(1):77.
104. Kodam SP, Ullah M. Diagnostic and therapeutic potential of extracellular vesicles. *Technol Cancer Res Treat.* 2021 Oct 9;20:15330338211041203.
105. Tai YL, Chu PY, Lee BH, Chen KC, Yang CY, Kuo WH, et al. Basics and applications of tumor-derived extracellular vesicles. *J Biomed Sci.* 2019 May 11;26:35.
106. Kumar MA, Baba SK, Sadida HQ, Marzooqi SA, Jerobin J, Altemani FH, et al. Extracellular vesicles as tools and targets in therapy for diseases. *Signal Transduct Target Ther.* 2024 Feb 5;9(1):1–41.
107. Cisneros-Villanueva M, Hidalgo-Pérez L, Rios-Romero M, Cedro-Tanda A, Ruiz-Villavicencio CA, Page K, et al. Cell-free DNA analysis in current cancer clinical trials: a review. *Br J Cancer.* 2022 Feb;126(3):391–400.
108. Gao Q, Zeng Q, Wang Z, Li C, Xu Y, Cui P, et al. Circulating cell-free DNA for cancer early detection. *The Innovation* [Internet]. 2022 Jul 12;3(4). [cited 2024 Jun 7]. Available from: https://www.cell.com/the-innovation/abstract/S2666-6758(22)00055-8
109. Yan Y yan, Guo Q ru, Wang F hua, Adhikari R, Zhu Z yan, Zhang H yan, et al. Cell-free DNA: hope and potential application in cancer. *Front Cell Dev Biol.* 2021 Feb 22;9:639233.
110. Kim SY, Jeong S, Lee W, Jeon Y, Kim YJ, Park S, et al. Cancer signature ensemble integrating cfDNA methylation, copy number, and fragmentation facilitates multi-cancer early detection. *Exp Mol Med.* 2023 Nov;55(11):2445–60.
111. Bohers E, Viailly PJ, Jardin F. cfDNA sequencing: technological approaches and bioinformatic issues. *Pharmaceuticals.* 2021 Jun 21;14(6):596.
112. Bronkhorst AJ, Ungerer V, Holdenrieder S. The emerging role of cell-free DNA as a molecular marker for cancer management. *Biomol Detect Quantif.* 2019 Mar 18;17:100087.
113. Adashek JJ, Janku F, Kurzrock R. Signed in blood: circulating tumor DNA in cancer diagnosis, treatment and screening. *Cancers.* 2021 Jul 18;13(14):3600.
114. Campos-Carrillo A, Weitzel JN, Sahoo P, Rockne R, Mokhnatkin JV, Murtaza M, et al. Circulating tumor DNA as an early cancer detection tool. *Pharmacol Ther.* 2019 Dec 18;107458.
115. Arisi MF, Dotan E, Fernandez SV. Circulating tumor DNA in precision oncology and its applications in colorectal cancer. *Int J Mol Sci.* 2022 Apr 18;23(8):4441.
116. Lin D, Shen L, Luo M, Zhang K, Li J, Yang Q, et al. Circulating tumor cells: biology and clinical significance. *Signal Transduct Target Ther.* 2021 Nov 22;6(1):404.
117. Agashe R, Kurzrock R. Circulating tumor cells: from the laboratory to the cancer clinic. *Cancers.* 2020 Sep;12(9):2361.

118. Prasoppokakorn T, Buntho A, Ingrungruanglert P, Tiyarattanachai T, Jaihan T, Kulkraisri K, et al. Circulating tumor cells as a prognostic biomarker in patients with hepatocellular carcinoma. *Sci Rep.* 2022 Nov 4;12(1):18686.
119. Dasgupta A, Lim AR, Ghajar CM. Circulating and disseminated tumor cells: harbingers or initiators of metastasis? *Mol Oncol.* 2017 Jan;11(1):40–61.
120. Kejíík Z, Kaplánek R, Dytrych P, Masařík M, Veselá K, Abramenko N, et al. Circulating tumour cells (CTCs) in NSCLC: from prognosis to therapy design. *Pharmaceutics.* 2021 Nov 5;13(11):1879.
121. Ju S, Chen C, Zhang J, Xu L, Zhang X, Li Z, et al. Detection of circulating tumor cells: opportunities and challenges. *Biomark Res.* 2022 Aug 13;10:58.
122. Descamps L, Le Roy D, Deman AL. Microfluidic-based technologies for CTC isolation: a review of 10 years of intense efforts towards liquid biopsy. *Int J Mol Sci.* 2022 Feb 10;23(4):1981.
123. Turner SA, Abou Shaar R, Yang Z. The basics of commonly used molecular techniques for diagnosis, and application of molecular testing in cytology. *Diagn Cytopathol.* 2023 Jan;51(1):83–94.
124. Saliminejad K, Khorram Khorshid HR, Soleymani Fard S, Ghaffari SH. An overview of microRNAs: Biology, functions, therapeutics, and analysis methods. *J Cell Physiol.* 2019 May;234(5):5451–65.
125. Condrat CE, Thompson DC, Barbu MG, Bugnar OL, Boboc A, Cretoiu D, et al. miRNAs as biomarkers in disease: latest findings regarding their role in diagnosis and prognosis. *Cells.* 2020 Jan 23;9(2):276.
126. Ouyang T, Liu Z, Han Z, Ge Q. MicroRNA detection specificity: recent advances and future perspective. *Anal Chem.* 2019 Mar 5;91(5):3179–86.
127. Gayosso-Gómez LV, Ortiz-Quintero B. Circulating MicroRNAs in blood and other body fluids as biomarkers for diagnosis, prognosis, and therapy response in lung cancer. *Diagnostics.* 2021 Mar 2;11(3):421.
128. Galvão-Lima LJ, Morais AHF, Valentim RAM, Barreto EJSS. miRNAs as biomarkers for early cancer detection and their application in the development of new diagnostic tools. *Biomed Eng OnLine.* 2021 Feb 16;20:21.
129. Singh AK, Kumar K, Singh LB, Ahuja A, Choudhury S, Manoj ML, et al. Omics technology: role and future in providing biotic and abiotic stress tolerance to plants. In: Sharma A, editor. *Microbes and signaling biomolecules against plant stress: strategies of plant-microbe relationships for better survival* [Internet]. Singapore: Springer; 2021. p. 151–68. [cited 2024 Jun 7]. Available from: https://doi.org/10.1007/978-981-15-7094-0_8
130. Williams GA, Liede S, Fahy N, Aittomaki K, Perola M, Helander T, et al. Annex A: what is genomics? Definitions and applications. In: *Regulating the unknown: a guide to regulating genomics for health policy-makers* [Internet]. European Observatory on Health Systems and Policies; 2020 [cited 2024 Jun 28]. Available from: https://www.ncbi.nlm.nih.gov/books/NBK569502/
131. Satam H, Joshi K, Mangrolia U, Waghoo S, Zaidi G, Rawool S, et al. Next-generation sequencing technology: current trends and advancements. *Biology.* 2023 Jul 13;12(7):997.
132. Tefferi A. Genomics basics: DNA structure, gene expression, cloning, genetic mapping, and molecular tests. *Semin Cardiothorac Vasc Anesth.* 2006 Dec;10(4):282–90.
133. Dong Z, Chen Y. Transcriptomics: advances and approaches. *Sci China Life Sci.* 2013 Oct;56(10):960–7.
134. Al-Amrani S, Al-Jabri Z, Al-Zaabi A, Alshekaili J, Al-Khabori M. Proteomics: concepts and applications in human medicine. *World J Biol Chem.* 2021 Sep 27;12(5):57–69.
135. Qiu S, Cai Y, Yao H, Lin C, Xie Y, Tang S, et al. Small molecule metabolites: discovery of biomarkers and therapeutic targets. *Signal Transduct Target Ther.* 2023 Mar 20;8(1):1–37.
136. Qiu S, Cai Y, Yao H, Lin C, Xie Y, Tang S, et al. Small molecule metabolites: discovery of biomarkers and therapeutic targets. *Signal Transduct Target Ther.* 2023 Mar 20;8(1):1–37.
137. Subramanian I, Verma S, Kumar S, Jere A, Anamika K. Multi-omics data integration, interpretation, and its application. *Bioinforma Biol Insights.* 2020 Jan 31;14:1177932219899051.
138. Dai X, Shen L. Advances and trends in omics technology development. *Front Med.* 2022 Jul 1;9:911861.
139. Kim D, Kim Y, Son N, Kang C, Kim A. Recent omics technologies and their emerging applications for personalised medicine. *IET Syst Biol.* 2017 Apr 19;11(3):87–98.
140. Plebani M. Chapter 3 - "Omics" translation: a challenge for laboratory medicine. In: Wehling M, editor. *Principles of translational science in medicine.* 3rd ed. [Internet]. Boston: Academic Press; 2021. p. 21–32. [cited 2024 Jun 11]. Available from: https://www.sciencedirect.com/science/article/pii/B9780128204931000210

141. Krishnan G, Singh S, Pathania M, Gosavi S, Abhishek S, Parchani A, et al. Artificial intelligence in clinical medicine: catalyzing a sustainable global healthcare paradigm. *Front Artif Intell.* 2023 Aug 29;6:1227091.
142. Pinto-Coelho L. How artificial intelligence is shaping medical imaging technology: a survey of innovations and applications. *Bioengineering.* 2023 Dec 18;10(12):1435.
143. McGenity C, Clarke EL, Jennings C, Matthews G, Cartlidge C, Freduah-Agyemang H, et al. Artificial intelligence in digital pathology: a systematic review and meta-analysis of diagnostic test accuracy. *NPJ Digit Med.* 2024 May 4;7(1):1–19.
144. Sebastian AM, Peter D. Artificial intelligence in cancer research: trends, challenges and future directions. *Life.* 2022 Nov 28;12(12):1991.
145. Askin S, Burkhalter D, Calado G, El Dakrouni S. Artificial intelligence applied to clinical trials: opportunities and challenges. *Health Technol.* 2023;13(2):203–13.
146. Zhang B, Shi H, Wang H. Machine Learning and AI in cancer prognosis, prediction, and treatment selection: a critical approach. *J Multidiscip Healthc.* 2023 Jun 26;16:1779–91.
147. Hesse BW, Kwasnicka D, Ahern DK. Emerging digital technologies in cancer treatment, prevention, and control. *Transl Behav Med.* 2021 Nov 30;11(11):2009–17.
148. Fitzgerald RC, Antoniou AC, Fruk L, Rosenfeld N. The future of early cancer detection. *Nat Med.* 2022 Apr;28(4):666–77.
149. Watters KE, Kirkpatrick J, Palmer MJ, Koblentz GD. The CRISPR revolution and its potential impact on global health security. *Pathog Glob Health.* 2021;115(2):80–92.
150. Khalifa M, Albadawy M. AI in diagnostic imaging: revolutionising accuracy and efficiency. *Comput Methods Programs Biomed Update.* 2024 Jan 1;5:100146.
151. Jørgensen SH, Bøgh N, Hansen ESS, Væggemose M, Wiggers H, Laustsen C. Hyperpolarized MRI – an update and future perspectives. *Semin Nucl Med.* 2022 May 1;52(3):374–81.
152. Kandalai S, Li H, Zhang N, Peng H, Zheng Q. The human microbiome and cancer: a diagnostic and therapeutic perspective. *Cancer Biol Ther.* 2023;24(1):2240084.

14

Emerging Technologies in Neurological Disease Diagnosis

Benjamin Tagoe, Louisa Quainoo, Emmanuel Kwaku Ofori, Seth Kwabena Amponsah, and Yashwant V. Pathak

14.1 Introduction

The nervous system can be affected by over 600 disorders, including dementia, multiple sclerosis (MS), Parkinson's disease (PD), brain tumors, epilepsy, stroke, and traumatic brain injuries. Typical symptoms of neurological disorders include pain, seizures, muscle weakness, difficulty with coordination, and loss of consciousness [1]. Additionally, several infections can also affect the nervous system: bacterial infections like *Mycobacterium tuberculosis* and *Neisseria meningitidis*, fungal infections like *Aspergillus* and *Cryptococcus*, parasitic infections like Chagas disease and malaria, and viral infections like West Nile Virus, Zika, and Enteroviruses [2–6]. These atypical neurological disorders can affect a large proportion of the population and are not always associated with specific neurological disorders [7].

Dementia is a progressive neurological disorder that affects cognitive functions such as memory, orientation, reasoning, calculation, language, comprehension, judgment, and the ability to learn. Alzheimer's disease (AD) is the leading cause of dementia, responsible for about 75% of cases due to neurofibrillary tangles and cortical amyloids [8–10]. While dementia mainly affects people over the age of 65, around 2% of cases occur in those younger than 65. The prevalence of dementia doubles every five years with advancing age, and genetic variation increases the risk for about 25% of the population [11, 12].

MS, marked by inflammatory demyelination of the nervous system, is the most prevalent neurological disorder. It primarily affects young individuals and affects around 2.5 million people globally. Magnetic resonance imaging (MRI) is frequently used in diagnosing MS, but there are currently no treatment options for this condition [13].

PD is a chronic neurodegenerative disorder that can manifest with non-motor symptoms such as hyposmia, paresthesia, depression, and pain [14, 15]. PD is a condition with an incidence rate of 4.5–19 per 100,000 people [16] annually. PD can affect individuals of all genders and ages. Treatment approaches vary based on the patient's severity, mental health, and age. Gálvez and colleagues assessed the impact of Binaural Beats on gait, cognition, electroencephalography (EEG) power, anxiety, and functional connectivity in patients with Parkinson's disease on a short-term basis [17].

A stroke is a brain injury that lasts more than 24 hours and has no known cause other than vascular disorder [18]. In developed countries, approximately 75–80% of strokes result from brain ischemia, while intracerebral hemorrhage accounts for 10–15% of cases. Stroke diagnosis is reliable and is based entirely on a physician's clinical assessment [7].

In the past decade, there have been significant technological advancements in the examination of the neurological system. Developments in MRI, particularly high-resolution imaging and functional MRI (fMRI), have substantially improved the ability to identify diseases of the central nervous system. Furthermore, real-time diagnostic data is now available from new digital sensors and wearable

DOI: 10.1201/9781003486909-14

technology, which help with the diagnosis of neurodegenerative diseases [19]. Moreover, whole-exome sequencing has become a common tool in the clinical diagnosis of a number of diseases, including complex neurological disorders [20]. Computer-aided diagnosis (CAD) systems can also assist primary healthcare providers such as neurosurgeons, neurologists, and radiologists in making improved clinical decisions by utilizing artificial (AI) and machine learning (ML) techniques [7].

14.2 Current Methods and Technology for Diagnosis of Neurological Diseases

The landscape of diagnosing neurological diseases is evolving rapidly with the advent of advanced methods and technologies. Traditional diagnostic approaches, often reliant on clinical evaluations and imaging techniques, are now complemented by innovative tools that offer deeper insights and greater precision. Current methods include the use of MRI, single-photon emission computed tomography (SPECT), and genetic testing, which enable real-time monitoring of neurological activity and disease progression.

14.2.1 Magnetic Resonance Imaging

MRI generates comprehensive three-dimensional anatomical images by utilizing a combination of computer-generated radio waves and a strong magnetic field. During an MRI scan, the machine's magnet creates a powerful magnetic field that aligns hydrogen ions within the patient's body. When exposed to radiofrequency waves, these aligned hydrogen ions are temporarily displaced and then return to their original state, emitting a radiofrequency signal. A series of smaller magnetic pulses are used to encode the locations of these echoes, which are then processed by a computer system to generate images [21].

MRI is used to diagnose various conditions, including brain and spinal cord tumors, traumatic brain injury, and stroke. Furthermore, MRI can be employed in diagnosing abnormal brain development, inflammation, vascular irregularities, brain damage related to epilepsy, and infection. MRI is also employed in diagnosing and monitoring conditions such as multiple sclerosis [22]. Over the last 30 years, substantial advances in MRI techniques, as well as the integration of MRI with other diagnostic procedures have greatly aided the creation of novel diagnostic methods. Table 14.1 gives an overview of the current applications of MRI in diagnosing neurological diseases.

14.2.1.1 MRI in Diagnosing MS

MRI has become a cornerstone in the diagnosis of MS, significantly enhancing the accuracy and reliability of detecting this complex neurological disorder. The integration of MRI with medical history and clinical examination has transformed the diagnostic approach, particularly for cases of clinically isolated syndrome, which can present initial symptoms that are ambiguous and overlap with other conditions [21].

MRI is instrumental in diagnosing MS by revealing lesions in the brain indicative of demyelination. These lesions help differentiate MS from other neurological disorders that might present with similar symptoms. Before the advent of MRI, diagnosing MS often relied on less definitive or more invasive techniques, such as lumbar punctures. The introduction of MRI has markedly improved diagnostic precision, providing a clearer picture of brain pathology and leading to more accurate diagnoses across diverse racial, ethnic, and gender groups [21].

The technology behind MRI allows for highly accurate detection of demyelination in the brain. This demyelination disrupts neural transmission and results in a range of physical effects, underscoring the importance of MRI in understanding the extent and impact of the disease. MRI's ability to detect and monitor MS lesions has advanced considerably, offering unparalleled insights into the disease's progression and its effects on brain networks [21].

In terms of accessibility, MRI machines are widely available across medical centers, hospitals, and clinics worldwide. However, disparities in access to MRI reflect broader inequalities in medical care. While MRI provides a high degree of diagnostic accuracy, previous methods could not match its precision in identifying demyelination, often leading to missed or delayed diagnoses [21].

TABLE 14.1

Applications of magnetic resonance imaging in neurological diagnosis [21]

Technique	Applications	References
Susceptibility-weighted MRI	Diagnosis of traumatic brain damage, neurodegenerative disorders, arterial stroke, cerebral amyloid angiopathy, and brain malignancies	[23]
Functional MRI	Assessment of how neurodegenerative diseases like Alzheimer's and Huntington's, trauma, and stroke affect brain function	[24]
Diffusion-tensor imaging MRI	Assessment of Huntington's disease, brain tumors, epilepsy, multiple sclerosis, Parkinson's disease, Williams syndrome, Alzheimer's disease, and fragile X syndrome	[25]
FLAIR MRI	Used in situations of metastasis, multiple sclerosis, subarachnoid hemorrhage, and tuberous sclerosis	[26]
Diffusion-weighted MRI	Diagnosis of stroke caused by acute brain ischemia, white matter diseases, spinal cord injury, peripheral nerve imaging, and brain tumors	[27]
MR spectroscopy	Used for identifying demyelinating disorders, brain neoplasms, infective focal lesions, and inherited metabolic disorders	[28]
Brain volumetric analysis	Applied in the evaluation of dementia, multiple sclerosis, epilepsy, and traumatic brain injury	[29]

MRI scans are capable of identifying varying degrees of lesion presence in the brain. While a single lesion may be difficult to interpret, multiple lesions typically confirm an MS diagnosis. The presence of numerous lesions usually correlates with a more advanced stage of MS, indicating widespread involvement of brain networks. Accurate interpretation of MRI results depends on the expertise of trained technologists and radiologists. Misinterpretation or oversight by inadequately trained personnel can significantly impact the validity of test results [30].

Despite its widespread adoption as a best practice in medical diagnostics, MRI is not infallible. In rare cases, MRI images may appear normal or inconclusive for MS. When this occurs, additional diagnostic methods, like evoked potentials, spinal fluid analysis, or alternative imaging techniques, are employed to provide a definitive diagnosis [30]. The combination of MRI with these supplementary techniques ensures a comprehensive approach to diagnosing and managing MS.

14.2.1.2 Diffusion-Weighted MRI in Diagnosing Acute Stroke

Diffusion-weighted MRI (dwMRI) has emerged as a valuable tool in the early detection and diagnosis of acute ischemic stroke. Recent studies highlight the technique's potential not only in detecting ischemic stroke but also in distinguishing brain tumors, mapping brain fibers, and assessing conditions such as epilepsy and neurotoxicity [31]. The primary advantage of dwMRI lies in its ability to detect changes in brain tissue much earlier than traditional MRI methods. One of the most significant benefits of dwMRI is its ability to identify ischemic stroke-related changes 30 minutes after onset, compared to the eight hours required for conventional MRI [31]. This early detection is crucial because it allows for timely intervention, potentially improving patient outcomes by addressing pathological changes before they become pronounced.

In the context of ischemic stroke, dwMRI offers superior identification of the stroke onset area compared to conventional MRI. The technique enhances accuracy in localizing affected regions within the first 48 hours of the stroke. Moreover, dwMRI has shown promise in prognosis assessments for patients who have undergone thrombectomy following an ischemic stroke. Research utilizing dwMRI-based predictive algorithms has demonstrated its ability to accurately forecast the risk of disability, achieving a high level of precision for all patients studied [32].

Despite its widespread availability, the expertise required to perform and interpret dwMRI is less common, leading to disparities in access. Factors such as geographic location and insurance coverage can influence availability, and while disparities in stroke assessment and diagnosis have not been extensively studied, they remain a concern. Timeliness is critical in the diagnosis and treatment of ischemic stroke. Traditional MRI methods typically require at least eight hours to detect significant changes in brain tissue, whereas dwMRI can reveal alterations much sooner. This rapid detection ability is essential for initiating appropriate treatments and improving patient outcomes [31]. Furthermore, dwMRI measures water displacement over distances of 1–20 micrometers [33]. The identification of lesions through dwMRI provides valuable insights into patient outcomes, with more extensive lesion presence linked to poorer functional outcomes at three months post-hospital discharge. Patients with lesions identified by dwMRI are nearly six times more likely to experience worse functional outcomes and have a lower chance of recovering in a 2–3-month time frame [34].

For accurate results, dwMRI should be requested by primary healthcare providers knowledgeable about ischemic stroke and dwMRI, administered by trained technologists, and interpreted by experienced radiologists. Inaccurate results can arise if these criteria are not met. A key challenge in the broader adoption of dwMRI is the high cost of hardware upgrades necessary for enhanced image quality and strength. Additionally, translating technological advances into clinical practice must consider patient safety, post-processing methods, and contrast agents [31].

While dwMRI offers significant advantages, it is not without limitations. The technique can produce images of lower quality, with increased noise and artifacts compared to conventional MRI sequences. The effectiveness of dwMRI is also constrained by power and hardware limitations. Nonetheless, ongoing improvements in acquisition times and technology are enhancing image resolution and reducing artifacts, gradually addressing these challenges [31].

14.2.1.3 Functional MRI and Its Application

Functional MRI (fMRI) is a noninvasive imaging technique that measures slight changes in blood flow while a patient performs activities like moving and speaking within an MRI scanner. By tracking blood flow and oxygen levels, fMRI provides insights into neuronal activity in the brain. This allows for precise identification of brain regions responsible for essential functions such as thinking, speaking, seeing, moving, and sensing. Furthermore, because fMRI can detect abnormal neural activity, it is also used to assess the impact of conditions like stroke, trauma, AD, and other disorders in the brain [35].

14.2.2 Genetic Testing in Diagnosing Neurological Disorders

Genetic testing has become an integral tool in neurology, especially for diagnosing a wide range of neurological disorders when clinical examinations and other diagnostic methods fail to provide a definitive diagnosis. Disorders such as PD, Kennedy's disease, AD, Huntington's disease, Duchenne muscular dystrophy, and amyotrophic lateral sclerosis, among others, are commonly diagnosed through genetic testing. Additionally, genetic testing plays a crucial role in guiding treatment plans for various conditions, including autism [36].

This technique marks a significant advancement in neurological diagnostic capabilities by pinpointing the specific gene or genes responsible for a patient's condition. This ability to provide a clear diagnosis is consistent across different ethnic, racial, and gender sub-populations across the globe, offering equitable benefits in identifying the genetic basis of neurological disorders. Unlike traditional diagnostic methods that often focus on identifying the symptoms or impairments themselves, genetic testing reveals the underlying genetic causes of these conditions. Moreover, genetic testing can offer predictive insights into how a disorder may progress, even before symptoms fully manifest [21].

Genetic sequencing has been available as a practical tool since the mid-2000s, following the development of next-generation sequencing and the commercialization of related tools. Despite its widespread use, there are disparities in access due to the relatively high cost of genetic testing. Although the costs are gradually decreasing, the technique remains expensive, and insurance coverage is not always guaranteed. Consequently, individuals unable to afford out-of-pocket expenses may face limited access to this diagnostic option [21].

The limitations of previous diagnostic techniques primarily revolved around their inability to identify the specific gene responsible for a condition. In some cases, these older methods could not conclusively diagnose a particular disorder. Conversely, genetic testing can detect specific genetic variants in a patient's genome that are associated with a particular condition. This identification not only clarifies the physiological pathways involved in the disorder but also suggests potential treatment options [36].

Before ordering genetic testing, a thorough clinical examination is essential to guide the process. A multidisciplinary team, including a physician familiar with genetic disorders, a genetic counselor, a geneticist, and a pathologist should be involved. The genetic counselor, in particular, plays a vital role in helping patients understand their diagnosis and make informed decisions based on the test results. Testing should be conducted in an accredited laboratory to ensure the accuracy and reliability of the results [21].

Despite its potential, the widespread adoption of genetic testing as a standard medical practice faces challenges. The high cost of genetic testing remains a significant barrier, as does the availability of trained personnel to administer and interpret the tests. It is important to note that while genetic testing can identify the genetic basis of a condition, it does not offer insight into the severity of the physical deficits or impairments that may arise from the condition. Therefore, while genetic testing is a powerful tool for diagnosis, it must be used in conjunction with other clinical assessments to fully understand a patient's condition and plan appropriate treatments [21].

14.2.3 Single-Photon Emission Computed Tomography

SPECT is a sophisticated nuclear imaging method used to evaluate specific brain activities. It can be used in the diagnosis of neurological and psychiatric disorders. SPECT enables healthcare providers to investigate and monitor the underlying pathophysiology of complex brain disorders. For instance, SPECT scans are instrumental in diagnosing stroke, AD, epilepsy, and dementia [37]. The technique produces an accurate three-dimensional map of how blood flows through the brain, which can reveal altered blood flow and blocked blood vessels, aiding in the diagnosis and assessment of vascular brain diseases [21].

14.2.3.1 SPECT with DaTscan™ for Diagnosing Parkinsonian Syndromes

The Food and Drug Administration (FDA) authorized the use of ioflupane i-123, also marketed as DaTscan™, a radiopharmaceutical agent in 2011 with the goal of helping with the identification of different Parkinsonian disorders. When injected into the bloodstream, DaTscan™ can help in the management of depression. Upon reaching the brain, DaTscan™ binds to dopamine transporters located in dopaminergic neurons. The SPECT imaging system, which detects the radioactive signals emitted by DaTscan™, then generates a detailed map showing the locations and quantities of these neurons in the brain. By highlighting the areas where dopaminergic neurons are damaged, this imaging technique can reveal the presence and severity of PD [38].

Although DaTscan™ can accurately diagnose PD, it may not provide further information beyond what a comprehensive clinical exam can reveal. However, there are certain cases where DaTscan™ can enhance the diagnostic process. Research suggests that DaTscan™ can be particularly useful in distinguishing between PD and other forms of Parkinsonism, such as drug-induced or vascular Parkinsonism. DaTscan™ is primarily FDA-approved for distinguishing between PD and essential tremor. Although clinicians can often differentiate between these two conditions by closely observing the characteristics of a patient's tremors, there are instances where making a definitive diagnosis through clinical examination alone may not be sufficient. In such cases, DaTscan™ can provide the additional diagnostic clarity needed [39].

14.2.4 Electromyography and Its Clinical Applications

Electromyography (EMG) is a diagnostic tool that records the electrical activity in skeletal muscles, providing essential insights into muscle and nerve function. When muscles are damaged or nerves are impaired, they produce abnormal electrical signals, which can be detected through EMG. This ability makes EMG particularly useful in diagnosing a range of conditions, including nerve and muscle disorders, amyotrophic lateral sclerosis (ALS), and spinal nerve root compression. A specific variation of EMG, known as surface electromyography (sEMG), involves the placement of multiple electrodes on the skin to capture muscle activity just beneath the surface. Although sEMG cannot detect electrical signals from muscles located as deep within the body as those measured by traditional needle-based EMG, it offers the advantage of obtaining information over a broader area of muscle tissue [21]. Additionally, sEMG's effectiveness and utility have greatly improved over time, largely due to significant advancements in analytical tools used to interpret sEMG signals [40]. Today, sEMG is widely employed in neurophysiological research [41] and in rehabilitation practices [42]. Despite its potential, the clinical adoption of sEMG has been limited, though a number of neurophysiologists advocate for its broader use in clinical settings [40, 41].

Currently, sEMG is applied clinically in several key areas. It is used to assess muscle coordination, particularly during clinical gait analysis. It also aids in the functional diagnosis and monitoring of therapy outcomes for neurological disorders such as cerebral palsy and stroke. sEMG is also useful for examining orthopedic disorders, such as back pain and degenerative joint disease [41]. However, widespread clinical use of sEMG is hampered by the lack of standardized protocols and consensus on its application. For example, while sEMG shows promise in assessing muscle co-contraction during gait in individuals with neurological impairments, the absence of agreed-upon standards prevents it from being routinely recommended for this purpose [43].

14.3 Emerging Technologies for Diagnosing Neurological Disorders

Emerging technologies are revolutionizing the diagnosis of neurological disorders, offering new avenues for early detection and more accurate assessments. Among these advancements, machine-learning-based computer-aided diagnosis (ML-CAD) systems stand out for their ability to analyze complex data and identify patterns indicative of neurological disorders [7]. ML-CAD tools leverage AI to enhance the interpretation of imaging and clinical data, improving diagnostic accuracy and efficiency [7]. In parallel, the development of advanced biomarkers is providing critical insights into neurological diseases. These biomarkers, whether derived from blood, cerebrospinal fluid, or digital sources, offer valuable information about disease presence, progression, and response to treatment [44]. By integrating ML-CAD with emerging biomarkers, healthcare providers can achieve a more comprehensive understanding of neurological disorders, leading to more precise diagnoses and personalized treatment strategies.

14.3.1 Machine-Learning-Based Computer-Aided Diagnosis

A computer-aided diagnosis system enhances clinical decision-making for neurologists, neurosurgeons, radiologists, and other medical professionals by employing AI, advanced signal processing, and ML techniques in an automated system. In recent years, research in this area has significantly accelerated. Figure 14.1 illustrates a standard ML-based CAD system comprising five stages: a) signal transformation, b) feature extraction, c) feature dimensionality reduction, d) optimal feature selection or ranking, and e) classification [7].

14.3.1.1 Input Data

Input data for CAD systems often comprise signals and/or images. In the case of PD, many CAD systems rely on speech analysis and EEG for diagnosis. Image-based methods typically employ SPECT and MRI scans [7]. For epilepsy, a frequently used resource is the EEG dataset from Bonn University. In

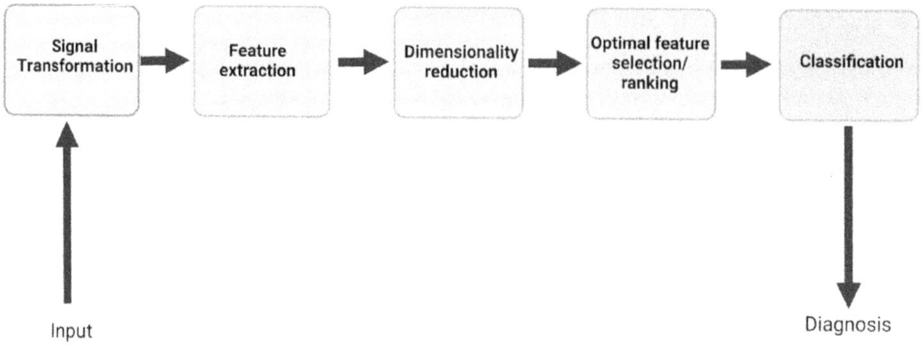

FIGURE 14.1 A typical machine-learning-based computer-aided diagnosis system [7].

diagnosing MS, T1- and T2-weighted MRI scans are commonly used, where T1 and T2 refer to the intervals between magnetic pulses and the timing of image capture. Systems designed for AD predominantly use T2-weighted MRI scans from the Open Access Series of Imaging Studies (OASIS) and Alzheimer's Disease Neuroimaging Initiative (ADNI) databases [7].

14.3.1.2 Image Transformation

In image processing, the initial step usually involves eliminating redundant information, which is followed by feature extraction. This process involves collecting pertinent details necessary for extracting relevant features [7].

14.3.1.3 Feature Extraction

The signal-based approach often uses the Discrete Wavelet Transform (DWT) to decompose signals into high and low-frequency components [7]. The curvelet transform, which is a more advanced form of DWT, represents images from various angles and scales. Additionally, higher-order spectra (HOS) features are employed for representing and extracting these features. The extracted features are designed to uncover subtle patterns within the input data [45, 46].

Image preprocessing techniques involve intensity normalization, adaptive histogram equalization [47], and background subtraction to highlight regions of interest [48]. For image analysis, gray-level co-occurrence matrix features are commonly used, with entropy and energy metrics frequently discussed in the literature [49, 50]. Additionally, wavelet-based energy and entropy features are applied. Statistical measures such as Zernike moments, Hu's moments, statistical moments, and central moments are also employed in developing CAD systems for neurological disorders, incorporating both signal- and image-based approaches [7].

14.3.1.4 Dimensionality Reduction

Feature extraction algorithms can sometimes produce redundant landscapes, which increases processing demands and can make real-time applications impractical. To address this, various dimensionality reduction techniques are commonly employed. Independent component analysis (ICA), linear discriminant analysis (LDA), and principal component analysis (PCA) are among the most frequently used methods. Additionally, advanced variants of PCA, such as kernel PCA, have also been explored in the literature [7].

14.3.1.5 Optimal Feature Selection and Ranking

To achieve optimal classification performance, it is essential to eliminate redundant information from features. For problems involving multiple classes, analysis of variance (ANOVA) is typically the method of choice. Effective feature selection techniques include the Student's *t*-test, entropy measures, Wilcoxon rank tests, Bhattacharyya distance, receiver operating characteristic (ROC) analysis, as well as optimization methods such as particle swarm optimization, genetic algorithms, and ant colony optimization [7]. Researchers often combine different selection strategies to identify the most relevant features [51]. Max-relevance feature and Fuzzy logic-based min-redundancy selection methods have been employed for diagnosing PD [52].

14.3.1.6 Feature Classification

Classification methods generally consist of two stages: training and testing. These models are first trained using historical data before being applied to classify new cases. Different classifiers employed for diagnosing neurological disorders include probabilistic neural networks, support vector machines (SVM) with polynomial kernel functions, Naive Bayes, linear discriminant analysis, *k*-nearest neighbors, random forests, and Gaussian mixture models. Support vector machines are among the most commonly used classifiers. Recently, an enhanced probabilistic neural network has been employed to effectively diagnose PD [53–56].

14.3.2 Deep Learning-Based Techniques

Deep learning methods have been created to overcome the limitations of traditional ML approaches. Convolutional neural networks (CNNs) represent a key advancement in this field. They provide several advantages over conventional ML-based CAD systems. CNNs are designed with a multilayer architecture that efficiently processes large datasets, handles imbalanced data, and produces unbiased results. Typically, CNNs include convolutional, pooling, and fully connected layers in their architecture [57].

Additional layers can be incorporated into CNNs to address particular needs. CNN-based methods have proven effective in diagnosing neurological disorders [7]. For early detection of issues, a more intricate network design may be required. Deeper architectures enhance the ability to extract detailed features from signals by applying kernels defined at each layer [57]. Deep neural network techniques have been utilized to tackle complex challenges across various domains, such as pavement crack detection, image recognition, vehicle type identification, structural damage assessment, transportation systems, big data time series forecasting, computer-brain interfaces, and concrete strength estimation [7]. Several researchers have developed CAD systems using deep learning techniques, which excel at identifying patterns in biological signals and images. Recent studies have demonstrated the effectiveness of these techniques in both signal-based and image-based CAD systems [58–60].

Deep learning methods are categorized into two types: supervised learning and unsupervised learning. CNNs fall under supervised learning, while autoencoders are part of unsupervised learning. For instance, Antoniades et al. [61] used deep learning to analyze epileptic intracranial EEG data, while Johansen et al. [62] applied CNNs to various fields including epileptiform spike detection [63], vehicle type identification [64], transportation systems [65], big data time series forecasting [57], concrete strength estimation[66], and computer-brain interfaces [67].

Ullah et al. [68] applied deep learning methods for diagnosing epilepsy, while Martinez-Murcia et al. utilized CNNs to analyze neuroimaging data for PD [69]. Figure 14.2 shows a common CNN architecture featuring convolutional layers, fully connected layers, max-pooling, and a softmax layer. More recent advancements include 3D CNNs and CNN-Recurrent Neural Network (RNN) models, which are being used for diagnosing PD, epilepsy, and AD [70]. Different variations of CNNs are being tested for detecting PD and ischemic stroke. While CNN-based methods generally outperform traditional handcrafted techniques, they often require a larger number of training examples to achieve optimal performance.

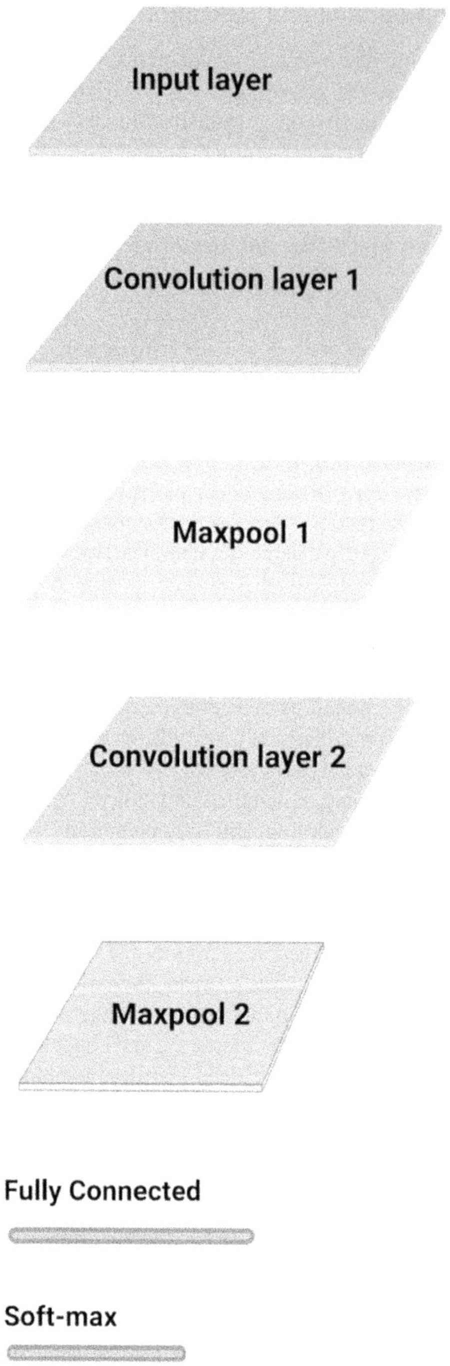

FIGURE 14.2 Conventional framework of convolutional neural networks [7].

14.3.3 Electrical Impedance Myography

A low-intensity, high-frequency electrical current is delivered to a specific muscle or muscle group during electrical impedance myography (EIM), and the voltages that arise are recorded [69]. This noninvasive technique has been proposed as a possible main diagnostic tool and is helpful in assessing a variety of neuromuscular disorders [71–74].

While EIM shows promise in neurological disease diagnosis, its primary use among clinicians and researchers has been to evaluate disease severity, monitor progression over time, and assess therapeutic responses. Notably, EIM has been utilized in clinical trials for several neuromuscular conditions, such as ALS, spinal muscular atrophy, Duchenne muscular dystrophy, sarcopenia, and facioscapulohumeral muscular dystrophy [71, 73]. This technique allows for easier or more sensitive muscle evaluation compared to traditional methods.

There is a growing number of researchers who use EIM in assessing neuromuscular disorders and total muscle health. These studies are focused on direct therapeutic applications or technology developments. It is expected that bioimpedance theory will progressively become part of the conventional toolsets for neuromuscular assessments as the medical community learns more about it and becomes acquainted with the uses of EIM [71].

14.3.4 Digital Biomarkers in Diagnosing Neurological Diseases

Digital biomarkers are an emerging technology that holds promise for diagnosing and managing neurological diseases. By leveraging data collected from digital devices like smartphones, wearables, and other connected tools, digital biomarkers offer a new way to assess and monitor health conditions in a more dynamic and continuous manner. These biomarkers consist of quantifiable physiological and behavioral data points that provide valuable insights into an individual's health status, particularly concerning neurological diseases [75].

One of the most promising applications of digital biomarkers lies in their ability to facilitate early diagnosis. For example, in AD, changes in cognitive functions such as memory, speech patterns, and motor skills can serve as early warning signs. Through smartphone applications that analyze speech patterns, it is possible to detect subtle cognitive shifts that might otherwise go unnoticed until the disease has progressed. Similarly, in PD, wearable devices can monitor key motor functions such as tremors, gait, and balance. These metrics are crucial for both diagnosing the condition and managing its progression [76].

Beyond early diagnosis, digital biomarkers are revolutionizing the continuous monitoring of patients with chronic neurological conditions. Traditionally, such patients would require frequent in-person visits to assess their condition. Digital biomarkers, however, enable the collection of real-time data in everyday environments, offering a more accurate and holistic view of a patient's health over time. This continuous data stream allows for the early detection of any changes, enabling more timely interventions [77].

Standardizing procedures and developing certified reference materials and methodologies are essential for the effective implementation of biomarkers [78, 79]. Recent diagnostic criteria for multiple sclerosis now incorporate the presence of cerebrospinal fluid (CSF) oligoclonal bands [80]. The success of CSF biomarkers in diagnosing AD has encouraged research into other neurodegenerative conditions, such as frontotemporal dementia, PD, and dementia with Lewy bodies. Innovative protein aggregation assays, originally designed for prion diseases, now present new opportunities for diagnosing tau, α-synuclein and TAR DNA binding protein-43 pathologies [81]. These assays hold the potential to be used in diagnosing α-synucleinopathies and other related disorders in the future.

Blood-based biomarkers have greatly advanced neurology research. Despite initial doubts about the viability of peripheral markers due to the constraints of the blood-brain barrier, recent technological progress has enabled the detection of low-concentration analytes in various biofluids. Cutting-edge equipment, such as single molecule molecule arrays (SIMOA) and mass spectrometry, now provide high analytical sensitivity [75]. Neurofilaments in the blood serve as indicators of neuronal damage in a range of neurological conditions, including neurodegenerative diseases, traumatic brain injury, peripheral neuropathies, multiple sclerosis, and neurological damage associated with coronavirus disease 2019 (COVID-19). This represents a major breakthrough in the field [82–84].

The capability to measure central nervous system indicators from a readily accessible source enables the use of blood markers to monitor disease progression in both clinical settings and research studies. Blood levels of neurofilament light protein (NfL) are useful for evaluating disease progression in conditions such as multiple sclerosis, cardiac arrest, and traumatic brain injury, among other applications.

Besides NfL, several other blood analytes show potential for clinical use. Recently, methods for detecting various isoforms of phosphorylated tau have also been reported [85].

All of these assays can detect AD with excellent accuracy and are predicted to become clinically useful. Imaging markers in neurology have improved significantly. Novel MRI modalities are crucial for analyzing small changes in brain structure in various neurological disorders [75]. New Tesla-MRI scanners offer excellent resolution to detect minute changes in neurological disorders. The discovery of radiotracers capable of binding protein aggregates in the brain marked a significant advancement in imaging research. Amyloid positron emission tomography, employing Pittsburgh compound B, was the first to be produced. Other 18F-based radiotracers have since followed suit [86].

Radiotracers have received approval in several countries for diagnosing AD. More recently developed tau tracers are being utilized in the treatment of chronic traumatic encephalopathy, AD, and other tauopathies [87].

14.4 Ethical Considerations, Effective Governance, and Regulation of Neurotechnology

The rapid convergence of neurotechnologies with other emerging fields, particularly AI, has introduced a level of unpredictability and complexity that complicates their regulation. As these technologies increasingly intertwine, their combined effects become more difficult to foresee, making effective regulation and anticipation of long-term impact a significant challenge. While the excitement surrounding the potential of neurotechnologies is understandable and should be encouraged, it is equally important to acknowledge their limitations and address valid concerns related to governance, regulation, patient safety (especially in the context of invasive technologies), and critical considerations of ethics and human rights [88–90].

Many neurotechnologies remain in the research and development stage, and the process of bringing these innovations into clinical practice is often protracted and fraught with challenges. Successfully navigating the technological, clinical, ethical, legal, and commercial obstacles requires a collaborative effort. The United Nations Educational, Scientific and Cultural Organization (UNESCO) has highlighted the profound ethical implications of neurotechnologies, which have the capacity to decode and alter perception, behavior, emotion, cognition, and memory. These capabilities raise significant concerns about mental privacy and the potential modification of identity, beliefs, and desires, ultimately challenging the essence of our "humanness". Consequently, there is a growing call for the establishment of specialized "neuro-rights" that would encompass concepts such as mental privacy (the right to control access to one's neural data) and cognitive liberty, which refers to the freedom to govern one's mental processes, cognition, and consciousness [88, 90, 91].

To protect personal data privacy, especially as private companies may seek to collect and commercialize this data for marketing and consumer engagement, robust governance frameworks are essential. As neurotechnologies evolve, enabling not only the reading of brain data but also the potential to influence it, the risk of "brain hacking" becomes a genuine concern. This term describes the potential manipulation or weaponization of individuals' behaviors, thoughts, and feelings. While this scenario has not yet materialized, it represents a significant future risk that demands proactive discussions, agreements, and the implementation of ethical and regulatory frameworks to prevent misuse when the technology becomes feasible [92].

Another critical issue is the increasingly blurred line between medical and consumer neurotechnology [93]. Neurotechnology has been used for decades in managing neurological disorders, but there is now rapid growth in its application within the consumer sector, including areas such as personal well-being, sports, marketing, and even workforce monitoring. This crossover raises concerns about safety and underscores the need for stringent regulations in the development and testing phases to prevent the generation of inaccurate data and potential biases, which could lead to discrimination and other harm [94].

The Organization for Economic Co-operation and Development (OECD) has created the first global standard in the field of neurotechnology in response to the demand for ethical innovation in this field. This standard seeks to support innovation while guiding policymakers and entrepreneurs in tackling the moral, legal, and societal issues raised by cutting-edge neurotechnologies. In order to tackle urgent health challenges and social requirements, the OECD has highlighted a number of structural improvements that could speed up the development of neurotechnologies, provided that these advancements are made responsibly and with the required safeguards in place. These include fostering responsible research by considering ethical, legal, and social issues and encouraging collaboration among all stakeholders throughout the development process. Additionally, anticipatory governance, proactively addressing these issues to implement regulatory frameworks in a timely manner, will be crucial [92].

Promoting open innovation, where public and private stakeholders collaborate, invest, and share assets, can help mitigate the investment risks and high failure rates associated with clinical trials in neurotechnology. It is also important to avoid "neuro-hype" by controlling unproven claims and myths about neurotechnology, promoting realistic expectations through evidence-based policies and guidelines. Last, addressing socioeconomic disparities is vital to ensuring access to neurotechnological innovations, particularly in resource-limited countries. As we move forward with advancements in neurotechnology, it is essential to consider these factors carefully to maximize the significant benefits of these technologies while minimizing any potential risks.

14.5 Conclusion and Future Directions

Neurotechnology is rapidly advancing, with current and future developments poised to significantly alter brain chemistry and create new neural connections within the nervous system [95]. These advancements hold immense therapeutic potential for a wide range of neurological conditions, such as stroke, chronic pain, paralysis, and psychological disorders like anxiety and post-traumatic stress disorder. Already, brain stimulation technologies are being used to help restore damaged brain tissue, demonstrating the profound impact neurotechnology can have on the brain function [96, 97].

Within the next decade, commercial implants designed for memory stimulation are likely to become available. Looking further ahead, within the next 20 years, it is plausible that neurotechnological innovations will enable the manipulation of memories, including the potential to delete negative or traumatic ones. The fields of brain-computer interfaces (BCI) and robotics are also expected to see transformative advancements. For example, these technologies could dramatically improve the lives of individuals who have lost limbs by allowing them to control robotic prosthetics intuitively [92].

Over the coming decades, provided that appropriate regulations are in place, the rapid progress in neurotechnology is likely to yield positive outcomes. These benefits will extend beyond neurology, impacting the diagnosis and management of neurological disorders and contributing to the well-being of individuals and society as a whole. Neurotechnology can help individuals live longer, healthier, and more comfortable lives by improving our understanding of the pathophysiology of diseases and facilitating the adoption of focused treatments and preventive policies. Furthermore, the arrival of revolutionary assistive technology in the home and workplace is imminent, presenting fresh opportunities to improve the lives of many.

To realize these ambitious goals, it is crucial that multiple stakeholders: researchers, clinicians, policymakers, and others, collaborate in the responsible development and implementation of neurotechnologies. Ensuring that the benefits of these technologies are fully realized will require careful consideration of several challenges. One of the most critical challenges is the need for "ground truth", or information that is definitively known to be real or true, which is essential for training and validating neurotechnologies. In the field of neurology, generating such data can be particularly complex due to unclear pathologies, varying diagnostic criteria, and the reliance on observational or subjective data of inconsistent quality. Overcoming these challenges will be key to the successful development and application of neurotechnological innovations.

REFERENCES

1. Thakur KT, Albanese E, Giannakopoulos P, Jette N, Linde M, Prince MJ, Steiner TJ, Dua T. Neurological Disorders. In: Patel V, Chisholm D, Dua T, Laxminarayan R, Medina-Mora ME, editors. Mental, Neurological, and Substance Use Disorders: Disease Control Priorities, Third Edition (Volume 4). Washington (DC): The International Bank for Reconstruction and Development / The World Bank; 2016 Mar 14.
2. Acharya UR, Hagiwara Y, Adeli H. Automated seizure prediction. *Epilepsy & Behav.* 2018;88:251–61. http://dx.doi.org/10.1016/j.yebeh.2018.09.030
3. Bairy GM, Lih OS, Hagiwara Y, Puthankattil SD, Faust O, Niranjan UC, et al. Automated diagnosis of depression electroencephalograph signals using linear prediction coding and higher order spectra features. *J Med Imaging Heal Informatics.* 2017;7:1857–62. http://dx.doi.org/10.1166/jmihi.2017.2204
4. Bhat S, Acharya UR, Adeli H, Bairy GM, Adeli A. Automated diagnosis of autism: in search of a mathematical marker. *Rev Neurosci.* 2014;25. http://dx.doi.org/10.1515/revneuro-2014-0036
5. Sridhar C, Bhat S, Acharya UR, Adeli H, Bairy GM. Diagnosis of attention deficit hyperactivity disorder using imaging and signal processing techniques. *Comput Biol Med.* 2017;88:93–9. http://dx.doi.org/10.1016/j.compbiomed.2017.07.009
6. Amponsah S, Tagoe B. *Drug resistance in antiviral therapy.* In: Shegokar R, Pathak, Y (eds); Viral Drug Delivery Systems. Springer, Cham. 2023. p. 17–26.
7. Raghavendra U, Acharya UR, Adeli H. Artificial intelligence techniques for automated diagnosis of neurological disorders. *Eur Neurol.* 2019;82:41–64. Available from: https://api.semanticscholar.org/CorpusID:208185620
8. Mammone N, Ieracitano C, Adeli H, Bramanti A, Morabito FC. Permutation jaccard distance-based hierarchical clustering to estimate EEG network density modifications in MCI subjects. *IEEE Trans Neural Networks Learn Syst.* 2018;29:5122–35. http://dx.doi.org/10.1109/tnnls.2018.2791644
9. Acharya UR, Fernandes SL, WeiKoh JE, Ciaccio EJ, Fabell MKM, Tanik UJ, et al. Automated detection of Alzheimer's disease using brain MRI images– a study with various feature extraction techniques. *J Med Syst.* 2019;43. http://dx.doi.org/10.1007/s10916-019-1428-9
10. Muolokwu CE, Chaulagain B, Gothwal A, Mahanta AK, Tagoe B, Lamsal B, et al. Functionalized nanoparticles to deliver nucleic acids to the brain for the treatment of Alzheimer's disease. *Front Pharmacol.* 2024;15:1405423. Available from: https://pubmed.ncbi.nlm.nih.gov/38855744
11. Saunders AM, Strittmatter WJ, Schmechel D, St. George-Hyslop PH, Pericak-Vance MA, Joo SH, et al. Association of apolipoprotein E allele ϵ4 with late-onset familial and sporadic Alzheimer's disease. *Neurology.* 1993;43:1467. http://dx.doi.org/10.1212/wnl.43.8.1467
12. Nalbantoglu J, Gilfix BM, Bertrand P, Robitaille Y, Gauthier S, Rosenblatt DS, et al. Predictive value of apolipoprotein E genotyping in Alzheimer's disease: results of an autopsy series and an analysis of several combined studies. *Ann Neurol.* 1994;36:889–95. http://dx.doi.org/10.1002/ana.410360614
13. Kobelt G, Pugliatti M. Cost of multiple sclerosis in Europe. *Eur J Neurol.* 2005;12:63–7. http://dx.doi.org/10.1111/j.1468-1331.2005.01193.x
14. Nutt JG, Wooten GF. Diagnosis and initial management of Parkinson's disease. *N Engl J Med.* 2005;353:1021–7. http://dx.doi.org/10.1056/nejmcp043908
15. Bhat S, Acharya UR, Hagiwara Y, Dadmehr N, Adeli H. Parkinson's disease: cause factors, measurable indicators, and early diagnosis. *Comput Biol Med.* 2018;102:234–41. http://dx.doi.org/10.1016/j.compbiomed.2018.09.008
16. Shinde S, Prasad S, Saboo Y, Kaushick R, Saini J, Pal PK, et al. Predictive markers for Parkinson's disease using deep neural nets on neuromelanin sensitive MRI. *NeuroImage Clin.* 2019;22:101748. Available from: https://pubmed.ncbi.nlm.nih.gov/30870733
17. Gálvez G, Recuero M, Canuet L, Del-Pozo F. Short-term effects of binaural beats on EEG power, functional connectivity, cognition, gait and anxiety in Parkinson's disease. *Int J Neural Syst.* 2018;28:1750055. http://dx.doi.org/10.1142/s0129065717500551
18. Hatano S. Experience from a multicentre stroke register: a preliminary report. *Bull World Health Organ.* 1976;54:541–53.
19. Granziera C, Woelfle T, Kappos L. Development and implementation of new diagnostic technologies in neurology. *Nat Rev Neurol.* 2022;18:445–6. http://dx.doi.org/10.1038/s41582-022-00692-z

20. Retterer K, Juusola J, Cho MT, Vitazka P, Millan F, Gibellini F, et al. Clinical application of whole-exome sequencing across clinical indications. *Genet Med.* 2016;18:696–704. http://dx.doi.org/10.1038/gim.2015.148
21. National Academies of Sciences, Engineering and MH and MDB on HCSC on IN or ID or ET. *Advances in the diagnosis and evaluation of disabling physical health conditions.* [Internet]. Washington (DC): National Academies Press; 2023. Available from: https://www.ncbi.nlm.nih.gov/books/NBK593686/
22. NINDS (National Institute of Neurological Disorders and Stroke). *Neurological diagnostics tests and procedures fact sheet.* 2022 [Internet]. 2022 [cited 2024 Aug 11]. Available from: https://www.ninds.nih.gov/neurological-diagnostic-tests-and-procedures-fact-sheet
23. Halefoglu AM, Yousem DM. Susceptibility weighted imaging: clinical applications and future directions. *World J Radiol.* 2018;10:30–45. Available from: https://pubmed.ncbi.nlm.nih.gov/29849962
24. Baggio HC, Junqué C. Functional MRI in Parkinson's disease cognitive impairment [Internet]. In: *International Review of Neurobiology.* Elsevier; 2019. p. 29–58. http://dx.doi.org/10.1016/bs.irn.2018.09.010
25. Soares JM, Marques P, Alves V, Sousa N. A hitchhiker's guide to diffusion tensor imaging. *Front Neurosci.* 2013;7:31. Available from: https://pubmed.ncbi.nlm.nih.gov/23486659
26. Kates R, Atkinson D, Brant-Zawadzki M. Fluid-attenuated inversion recovery (FLAIR). *Top Magn Reson Imaging.* 1996;8:389–96. http://dx.doi.org/10.1097/00002142-199612000-00005
27. Baliyan V, Das CJ, Sharma R, Gupta AK. Diffusion weighted imaging: technique and applications. *World J Radiol.* 2016;8:785–98. Available from: https://pubmed.ncbi.nlm.nih.gov/27721941
28. Oz G, Alger JR, Barker PB, Bartha R, Bizzi A, Boesch C, et al. Clinical proton MR spectroscopy in central nervous system disorders. *Radiology.* 2014;270:658–79. Available from: https://pubmed.ncbi.nlm.nih.gov/24568703
29. Bash S, Tanenbaum L. Quantitative volumetry is revolutionizing neuroimaging. *Appl Radiol.* 2021;38–42. http://dx.doi.org/10.37549/ar2728
30. Dobson R, Giovannoni G. Multiple sclerosis - a review. *Eur J Neurol.* 2019;26(1):27–40.
31. Chilla G, Tan CH, Xu C, Poh CL. Diffusion weighted magnetic resonance imaging and its recent trend-a survey. *Quant Imaging Med Surg.* 2015;5:407–22.
32. Raoult H, Lassalle MV, Parat B, Rousseau C, Eugène F, Vannier S, et al. DWI-based algorithm to predict disability in patients treated with thrombectomy for acute stroke. *AJNR Am J Neuroradiol.* 2020;41:274–9. Available from: https://pubmed.ncbi.nlm.nih.gov/32001446
33. Charles-Edwards EM, deSouza NM. Diffusion-weighted magnetic resonance imaging and its application to cancer. *Cancer Imaging.* 2006;6:135–43. Available from: https://pubmed.ncbi.nlm.nih.gov/17015238
34. Garg RK, Khan J, Dawe RJ, Conners J, John S, Prabhakaran S, et al. The influence of diffusion weighted imaging lesions on outcomes in patients with acute spontaneous intracerebral hemorrhage. *Neurocrit Care.* 2020;33:552–64. Available from: https://pubmed.ncbi.nlm.nih.gov/32072457
35. MC L. Magnetic resonance imaging (MRI) in neurologic disorders. [Internet]. *Merck Manual.* 2022 [cited 2024 Aug 11]. Available from: https://www.merckmanuals.com/en-ca/professional/neurologic-disorders/neurologic-tests-and-procedures/magnetic-resonance-imaging-mri-in-neurologic-disorders
36. K F. Genetic testing for neurological diseases. [Internet]. *Natl. Institutes Heal.* 2014 [cited 2024 Aug 11]. Available from: https://www.genome.gov/Multimedia/Slides/GenomicsinMedicine2014-2015/Fischbeck_4_4_14.pdf
37. Sinai C. Brain spect scan [Internet]. 2023 [cited 2024 Aug 11]. Available from: https://www.cedars-sinai.org/programs/imaging-center/exams/nuclear-medicine/brain-spect-scan.html
38. APDA. What role does DaTscan have in the diagnosis of Parkinson's disease. [Internet]. 2022 [cited 2024 Aug 11]. Available from: https://www.apdaparkinson.org/article/what-is-a-datscan-and-should-i-get-one/
39. Roussakis A-A, Piccini P, Politis M. Clinical utility of DaTscanTM (123I-Ioflupane Injection) in the diagnosis of Parkinsonian Syndromes. *Degener Neurol Neuromuscul Dis.* 2013;3:33–9. Available from: https://pubmed.ncbi.nlm.nih.gov/30890892
40. Felici F, Del Vecchio A. Surface electromyography: what limits its use in exercise and sport physiology? *Front Neurol.* 2020;11:578504. Available from: https://pubmed.ncbi.nlm.nih.gov/33240204

41. Campanini I, Disselhorst-Klug C, Rymer WZ, Merletti R. Surface EMG in Clinical assessment and neurorehabilitation: barriers limiting its use. *Front Neurol.* 2020;11:934. Available from: https://pubmed.ncbi.nlm.nih.gov/32982942
42. Kotov-Smolenskiy AM, Khizhnikova AE, Klochkov AS, Suponeva NA, Piradov MA. Surface EMG: applicability in the motion analysis and opportunities for practical rehabilitation. *Hum Physiol.* 2021;47:237–47. http://dx.doi.org/10.1134/s0362119721020043
43. Rosa MCN, Marques A, Demain S, Metcalf CD, Rodrigues J. Methodologies to assess muscle co-contraction during gait in people with neurological impairment – A systematic literature review. *J Electromyogr Kinesiol.* 2014;24:179–91. http://dx.doi.org/10.1016/j.jelekin.2013.11.003
44. Lleó A. Biomarkers in neurological disorders: a fast-growing market. *Brain Commun.* 2021;3:fcab086–fcab086. Available from: https://pubmed.ncbi.nlm.nih.gov/33977270
45. Shao Y, Celenk M. Higher-order spectra (HOS) invariants for shape recognition. *Pattern Recognit.* 2001;34:2097–113. http://dx.doi.org/10.1016/s0031-3203(00)00148-5
46. Chua KC, Chandran V, Acharya UR, Lim CM. Application of higher order statistics/spectra in biomedical signals—A review. *Med Eng Phys* [Internet]. 2010;32:679–89. http://dx.doi.org/10.1016/j.medengphy.2010.04.009
47. Pizer SM, Amburn EP, Austin JD, Cromartie R, Geselowitz A, Greer T, et al. Adaptive histogram equalization and its variations. *Comput Vision, Graph Image Process* [Internet]. 1987;39:355–68. http://dx.doi.org/10.1016/s0734-189x(87)80186-x
48. Malladi R, Sethian JA, Vemuri BC. Shape modeling with front propagation: a level set approach. *IEEE Trans Pattern Anal Mach Intell* [Internet]. 1995;17:158–75. http://dx.doi.org/10.1109/34.368173
49. Kapur JN. Information of order α and type β. *Proc Indian Acad Sci - Sect A* [Internet]. 1968;68:65–75. http://dx.doi.org/10.1007/bf03047688
50. Shannon CE. A mathematical theory of communication. *Bell Syst Tech J* [Internet]. 1948;27:379–423. http://dx.doi.org/10.1002/j.1538-7305.1948.tb01338.x
51. Nemati S, Basiri ME, Ghasem-Aghaee N, Aghdam MH. A novel ACO–GA hybrid algorithm for feature selection in protein function prediction. *Expert Syst Appl* [Internet]. 2009;36:12086–94. http://dx.doi.org/10.1016/j.eswa.2009.04.023
52. Peng H, Long F, Ding C. Feature selection based on mutual information criteria of max-dependency, max-relevance, and min-redundancy. *IEEE Trans Pattern Anal Mach Intell* [Internet]. 2005;27:1226–38. http://dx.doi.org/10.1109/tpami.2005.159
53. Larose DT. *Discovering knowledge in data* [Internet]. Wiley; 2004. http://dx.doi.org/10.1002/0471687545
54. Amit Y, Geman D. Shape quantization and recognition with randomized trees. *Neural Comput* [Internet]. 1997;9:1545–88. http://dx.doi.org/10.1162/neco.1997.9.7.1545
55. Berge A, Schistad Solberg AH. Structured gaussian components for hyperspectral image classification. *IEEE Trans Geosci Remote Sens* [Internet]. 2006;44:3386–96. http://dx.doi.org/10.1109/tgrs.2006.880626
56. Hirschauer TJ, Adeli H, Buford JA. Computer-aided diagnosis of Parkinson's disease using enhanced probabilistic neural network. *J Med Syst* [Internet]. 2015;39. http://dx.doi.org/10.1007/s10916-015-0353-9
57. Tan JH, Hagiwara Y, Pang W, Lim I, Oh SL, Adam M, et al. Application of stacked convolutional and long short-term memory network for accurate identification of CAD ECG signals. *Comput Biol Med* [Internet]. 2018;94:19–26. http://dx.doi.org/10.1016/j.compbiomed.2017.12.023
58. Koziarski M, Cyganek B. Image recognition with deep neural networks in presence of noise – Dealing with and taking advantage of distortions. *Integr Comput Aided Eng* [Internet]. 2017;24:337–49. http://dx.doi.org/10.3233/ica-170551
59. Torres JF, Galicia A, Troncoso A, Martínez-Álvarez F. A scalable approach based on deep learning for big data time series forecasting. *Integr Comput Aided Eng* [Internet]. 2018;25:335–48. http://dx.doi.org/10.3233/ica-180580
60. Cheng D, Liu M. *Classification of Alzheimer's disease by cascaded convolutional neural networks using PET images* [Internet]. Lecture Notes in Computer Science Springer International Publishing; 2017. p. 106–13. http://dx.doi.org/10.1007/978-3-319-67389-9_13

61. Antoniades A, Spyrou L, Took CC, Sanei S. Deep learning for epileptic intracranial EEG data [Internet]. 2016 IEEE 26th International Workshop on Machine Learning Signal Process. IEEE; 2016. http://dx.doi.org/10.1109/mlsp.2016.7738824
62. Johansen AR, Jin J, Maszczyk T, Dauwels J, Cash SS, Westover MB. Epileptiform spike detection via convolutional neural networks. *Proc IEEE Int Conf Acoust Speech Signal Process ICASSP* [Internet]. 2016;2016:754–8. [cited 2016 May 19]. Available from: https://pubmed.ncbi.nlm.nih.gov/29527131
63. Lin Y, Nie Z, Ma H. Structural damage detection with automatic feature-extraction through deep learning. *Comput Civ Infrastruct Eng* [Internet]. 2017;32:1025–46. http://dx.doi.org/10.1111/mice.12313
64. Molina-Cabello MA, Luque-Baena RM, López-Rubio E, Thurnhofer-Hemsi K. Vehicle type detection by ensembles of convolutional neural networks operating on super-resolved images. *Integr Comput Aided Eng* [Internet]. 2018;25:321–33. http://dx.doi.org/10.3233/ica-180577
65. Hashemi H, Abdelghany K. End-to-end deep learning methodology for real-time traffic network management. *Comput Civ Infrastruct Eng* [Internet]. 2018;33:849–63. http://dx.doi.org/10.1111/mice.12376
66. Rafiei MH, Khushefati WH, Demirboga R, Adeli H. Supervised deep restricted Boltzmann machine for estimation of concrete. *ACI Mater J* [Internet]. 2017;114. http://dx.doi.org/10.14359/51689560
67. Li W, Li M, Zhou H, Chen G, Jin J, Duan F. A Dual stimuli approach combined with convolutional neural network to improve information transfer rate of event-related potential-based brain-computer interface. *Int J Neural Syst* [Internet]. 2018;28:1850034. http://dx.doi.org/10.1142/s012906571850034x
68. Ullah I, Hussain M, Qazi E-H, Aboalsamh H. An automated system for epilepsy detection using EEG brain signals based on deep learning approach. *Expert Syst Appl* [Internet]. 2018;107:61–71. http://dx.doi.org/10.1016/j.eswa.2018.04.021
69. Martinez-Murcia FJ, Górriz JM, Ramírez J, Ortiz A. Convolutional neural networks for neuroimaging in Parkinson's disease: is preprocessing needed? *Int J Neural Syst* [Internet]. 2018;28:1850035. http://dx.doi.org/10.1142/s0129065718500351
70. Tjepkema-Cloostermans MC, de Carvalho RC V, van Putten MJAM. Deep learning for detection of focal epileptiform discharges from scalp EEG recordings. *Clin Neurophysiol* [Internet]. 2018;129:2191–6. http://dx.doi.org/10.1016/j.clinph.2018.06.024
71. Sanchez B, Rutkove SB. Electrical impedance myography and its applications in neuromuscular disorders. *Neurotherapeutics* [Internet]. 2017;14:107–18. Available from: https://pubmed.ncbi.nlm.nih.gov/27812921
72. Cebrián-Ponce Á, Irurtia A, Carrasco-Marginet M, Saco-Ledo G, Girabent-Farrés M, Castizo-Olier J. Electrical impedance myography in health and physical exercise: a systematic review and future perspectives. *Front Physiol* [Internet]. 2021;12:740877. Available from: https://pubmed.ncbi.nlm.nih.gov/34594243
73. Spieker AJ, Narayanaswami P, Fleming L, Keel JC, Muzin SC, Rutkove SB. Electrical impedance myography in the diagnosis of radiculopathy. *Muscle Nerve* [Internet]. 2013/09/11. 2013;48:800–5. Available from: https://pubmed.ncbi.nlm.nih.gov/23483460
74. Tarulli A, Esper GJ, Lee KS, Aaron R, Shiffman CA, Rutkove SB. Electrical impedance myography in the bedside assessment of inflammatory myopathy. *Neurology* [Internet]. 2005;65:451–2. http://dx.doi.org/10.1212/01.wnl.0000172338.95064.cb
75. Youn B-Y, Ko Y, Moon S, Lee J, Ko S-G, Kim J-Y. Digital biomarkers for neuromuscular disorders: a systematic scoping review. *Diagnostics (Basel, Switzerland)* [Internet]. 2021;11:1275. Available from: https://pubmed.ncbi.nlm.nih.gov/34359358
76. Dorsey ER, Papapetropoulos S, Xiong M, Kieburtz K. The first frontier: digital biomarkers for neurodegenerative disorders. *Digit biomarkers* [Internet]. 2017;1:6–13. Available from: https://pubmed.ncbi.nlm.nih.gov/32095743
77. Kourtis LC, Regele OB, Wright JM, Jones GB. Digital biomarkers for Alzheimer's disease: the mobile/wearable devices opportunity. *NPJ Digit Med* [Internet]. 2019/02/21. 2019;2:9. Available from: https://pubmed.ncbi.nlm.nih.gov/31119198
78. Lleó A, Cavedo E, Parnetti L, Vanderstichele H, Herukka SK, Andreasen N, et al. Cerebrospinal fluid biomarkers in trials for Alzheimer and Parkinson diseases. *Nat Rev Neurol* [Internet]. 2014;11:41–55. http://dx.doi.org/10.1038/nrneurol.2014.232
79. Blennow K, Hampel H, Weiner M, Zetterberg H. Cerebrospinal fluid and plasma biomarkers in Alzheimer disease. *Nat Rev Neurol* [Internet]. 2010;6:131–44. http://dx.doi.org/10.1038/nrneurol.2010.4

80. Thompson AJ, Banwell BL, Barkhof F, Carroll WM, Coetzee T, Comi G, et al. Diagnosis of multiple sclerosis: 2017 revisions of the McDonald criteria. *Lancet Neurol* [Internet]. 2018;17:162–73. http://dx.doi.org/10.1016/s1474-4422(17)30470-2
81. Green AJE, Zanusso G. Prion protein amplification techniques [Internet]. *Handb. Clin. Neurol.* Elsevier; 2018. p. 357–70. http://dx.doi.org/10.1016/b978-0-444-63945-5.00019-2
82. Khalil M, Teunissen CE, Otto M, Piehl F, Sormani MP, Gattringer T, et al. Neurofilaments as biomarkers in neurological disorders. *Nat Rev Neurol* [Internet]. 2018;14:577–89. http://dx.doi.org/10.1038/s41582-018-0058-z
83. Aamodt AH, Høgestøl EA, Popperud TH, Holter JC, Dyrhol-Riise AM, Tonby K, et al. Blood neurofilament light concentration at admittance: a potential prognostic marker in COVID-19. *J Neurol* [Internet]. 2021;268:3574–83. [cited 2021 Mar 20]. Available from: https://pubmed.ncbi.nlm.nih.gov/33743046
84. Amponsah SK, Tagoe B, Adams I, Bugyei KA. Efficacy and safety profile of corticosteroids and non-steroidal anti-inflammatory drugs in COVID-19 management: a narrative review. *Front Pharmacol* [Internet]. 2022;13:1063246. Available from: https://pubmed.ncbi.nlm.nih.gov/36532785
85. Moscoso A, Grothe MJ, Ashton NJ, Karikari TK, Rodriguez JL, Snellman A, et al. Time course of phosphorylated-tau181 in blood across the Alzheimer's disease spectrum. *Brain* [Internet]. 2021;144:325–39. Available from: https://pubmed.ncbi.nlm.nih.gov/33257949
86. Klunk WE, Engler H, Nordberg A, Wang Y, Blomqvist G, Holt DP, et al. Imaging brain amyloid in Alzheimer's disease with Pittsburgh compound-B. *Ann Neurol* [Internet]. 2004;55:306–19. http://dx.doi.org/10.1002/ana.20009
87. Stern RA, Adler CH, Chen K, Navitsky M, Luo J, Dodick DW, et al. Tau positron-emission tomography in former national football league players. *N Engl J Med* [Internet]. 2019/04/10. 2019;380:1716–25. Available from: https://pubmed.ncbi.nlm.nih.gov/30969506
88. UNESCO. *The risks and challenges of neurotechnologies for human rights* [Internet]. UNESCO; 2023. http://dx.doi.org/10.54678/pogs7778
89. Müller O, Rotter S. Neurotechnology: current developments and ethical issues. *Front Syst Neurosci* [Internet]. 2017;11:93. Available from: https://pubmed.ncbi.nlm.nih.gov/29326561
90. M I. Common human rights challenges raised by different applications of neurotechnologies in the biomedical field. Rep Comm by Comm Bioeth Counc Eur. Cedex: Strasbourg.
91. Wajnerman Paz A. Is mental privacy a component of personal identity? *Front Hum Neurosci* [Internet]. 2021;15:773441. Available from: https://pubmed.ncbi.nlm.nih.gov/34720912
92. Bhidayasiri R. The grand challenge at the frontiers of neurotechnology and its emerging clinical applications. *Front Neurol* [Internet]. 2024;15:1314477. Available from: https://pubmed.ncbi.nlm.nih.gov/38299015
93. Paek AY, Brantley JA, Evans BJ, Contreras-Vidal JL. Concerns in the blurred divisions between medical and consumer neurotechnology. *IEEE Syst J* [Internet]. 2020/12/18. 2021;15:3069–80. Available from: https://pubmed.ncbi.nlm.nih.gov/35126800
94. Yuste R. Advocating for neurodata privacy and neurotechnology regulation. *Nat Protoc* [Internet]. 2023;18:2869–75. http://dx.doi.org/10.1038/s41596-023-00873-0
95. Alosaimi F, Boonstra JT, Tan S, Temel Y, Jahanshahi A. The role of neurotransmitter systems in mediating deep brain stimulation effects in Parkinson's disease. *Front Neurosci* [Internet]. 2022;16:998932. Available from: https://pubmed.ncbi.nlm.nih.gov/36278000
96. Bava JM, Wang Z, Bick SK, Englot DJ, Constantinidis C. Improving visual working memory with cholinergic deep brain stimulation. *Brain Sci* [Internet]. 2023;13:917. Available from: https://pubmed.ncbi.nlm.nih.gov/37371395
97. Xu M, Li Y, Zhang C, Ma Y, Zhang L, Yang Y, et al. Efficacy of scalp stimulation for multidomain cognitive impairment in patients with post-stroke cognitive impairment and dementia: a network meta-analysis and meta-regression of moderators. *J Evid Based Med* [Internet]. 2023;16:505–19. http://dx.doi.org/10.1111/jebm.12568

15

Electrophoresis: A Current Tool in the Diagnosis of Protein and Lipid Disorders

Richmond Owusu Ateko

15.1 Introduction

Electrophoresis has emerged as a fundamental tool in clinical diagnostics due to its ability to separate and analyze molecules based on their size, charge, and mobility in an electric field [1]. Electrophoresis is crucial in diagnosing various disorders, particularly those involving proteins and lipids [2]. Proteins and lipids are essential components of biological systems, performing diverse functions vital for cellular structure, signaling, and metabolism. Dysregulation or abnormalities in protein and lipid profiles can indicate underlying health conditions, ranging from inherited genetic disorders to metabolic diseases.

This chapter explores the application of electrophoresis techniques in diagnosing protein and lipid disorders, highlighting their significance in modern healthcare. By leveraging electrophoresis principles, clinicians can obtain valuable insights into the composition and distribution of proteins and lipids in biological samples, aiding in identifying and characterizing pathological conditions. Electrophoresis offers a versatile platform for diagnostic evaluation, from detecting aberrant protein patterns indicative of hemoglobinopathies to assessing lipid profiles associated with hyperlipidemia.

This chapter will explore the principles of electrophoresis, the techniques available, and their utility in diagnosing a spectrum of protein and lipid disorders. Additionally, the chapter will discuss clinical applications, challenges, and future perspectives surrounding electrophoresis use in clinical practice. By elucidating the role of electrophoresis in diagnosing protein and lipid disorders, this chapter aims to underscore its significance as a valuable tool in modern healthcare diagnostics.

15.2 Brief History of Electrophoresis Techniques

The history of electrophoresis began around 1807 when Russian Chemists Peter Ivanovich Strakhov and Ferdinand Frederic Reuss first observed the electrokinetic phenomenon. They noticed that clay particles dispersed in water moved when a constant electric current was applied [3]. Michaelis officially coined the word "electrophoresis", derived from the Greek words "elektron" (amber), historically associated with electricity, and "phorein" (to carry) [4]. However, Arne Tiselius significantly advanced the technique in the 1930s. He developed the first electrophoretic apparatus in 1937, known as the "Tiselius apparatus", for moving-boundary electrophoresis [5]. This apparatus opened up new possibilities for using electrophoresis to analyze chemical mixtures.

A significant limitation of the Tiselius apparatus was its ineffectiveness in separating compounds with similar electrophoretic properties. In response to this challenge, new electrophoresis techniques were developed in the late 1940s, employing solid or gel matrices to achieve better separation. These techniques allowed compounds to be separated into discrete, stable bands, improving both the clarity and

DOI: 10.1201/9781003486909-15

stability of the results. In 1950, Tiselius recognized the significance of these advancements and coined the term "zone electrophoresis" to describe these methods [6]. In 1955, Oliver Smithies introduced starch gel as a medium in electrophoresis, leading to the widespread adoption of zone electrophoresis gained widespread use [7]. This innovation and the subsequent use of polyacrylamide and other gel types significantly enhanced protein separation efficiency. Throughout the 20th century, controlling factors such as pore size and polyacrylamide gel stability remained a major challenge, even with significant advances in high-resolution electrophoresis techniques. A significant breakthrough occurred in the early 2000s with standardized polymerization times for polyacrylamide gels. As a result, researchers could conduct detailed structural analyses with greater accuracy and reliability, greatly enhancing biochemical studies of complex protein mixtures. [4]

Since the 1950s, electrophoresis methods have significantly diversified, with continuous development in new techniques and applications. Innovations such as capillary electrophoresis, affinity electrophoresis, free flow electrophoresis, electroblotting, isotachophoresis, preparative native polyacrylamide gel electrophoresis (PAGE), and pulsed-field gel electrophoresis have emerged. These advancements have expanded electrophoresis's capabilities in scientific research, allowing for more precise and varied analysis of molecular components [4].

15.3 Principle of Electrophoresis

Electrophoresis is a laboratory technique that separates molecules based on size, charge, and shape. The principle underlying electrophoresis is that charged molecules will move through a conductive medium, such as a gel, when subjected to an electric field [1]. Molecules like proteins, deoxyribonucleic acid (DNA), and ribonucleic acid (RNA) carry a charge. When placed in an electric field, these molecules will move toward the electrode with an opposite charge. Positively charged molecules migrate to the cathode (negative electrode), and negatively charged molecules travel to the anode (positive electrode) [8].

The charged molecules move through various mediums, including compact materials such as paper, films, or gels (like agarose or polyacrylamide). The choice of medium affects the resolution and the separation quality; gels provide a porous matrix that sieves molecules based on size and shape [9]. A buffer system maintains a stable pH and ionic strength, which is crucial for consistent electrophoretic movement. Although the movement of the charged molecules is constant under specified conditions, it is influenced by their shape, size, charge, and temperature. Electrophoretic conditions are defined by both the electrical parameters (current, voltage, and power) and various medium-specific factors, such as ionic strength, pH value, viscosity, and pore size, which influence the movement of molecules [10]. The electrophoresis unit generally consists of a chamber where a supporting medium, such as gel, is placed. It includes electrodes to create an electric field and buffer reservoirs to maintain pH and conductivity. The medium can be supported horizontally or vertically, and a lid or cover is used to maintain a stable environment. The power supply controls the voltage and current applied to the gel [11].

15.4 Types of Electrophoresis

Electrophoresis can be classified into various types, as shown in Figure 15.1. This classification depends on the medium used, the specific application, and the type of analysis required. This chapter will not cover all types of electrophoresis but will instead focus on the protein and lipid analysis techniques.

15.4.1 Electrophoresis Methods for Protein Analysis

This section explores some of the electrophoretic techniques utilized in protein analysis. Electrophoresis methods are indispensable tools in molecular biology, biochemistry, and proteomics. They have proven effective in studying clinically significant proteins and aiding in elucidating their characteristics.

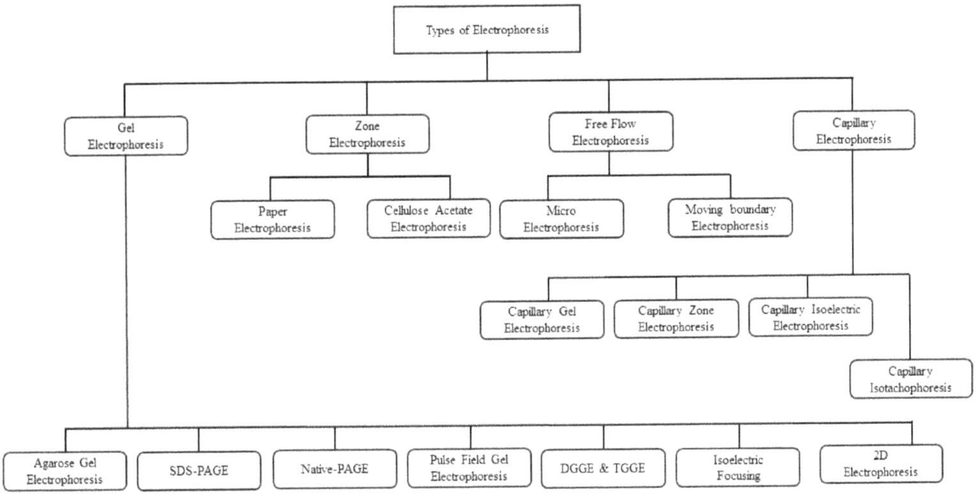

FIGURE 15.1 Types of electrophoresis.

15.4.1.1 Free Flow Electrophoresis

Free flow electrophoresis (FFE) is a highly adaptable method that employs a continuous-flow system to separate proteins based on their charge and size. This method operates in a liquid medium, allowing for the separation of proteins in their native state [12]. This method is particularly advantageous for separating large quantities of proteins and for preparative applications, as it can process samples continuously without the need for gel matrices [1]. The FFE apparatus comprises a separation chamber where the sample is injected into a flowing buffer. An electric field is applied perpendicular to the flow direction, causing proteins to migrate based on their charge [13]. One key benefit of FFE is its ability to maintain protein functionality, making it suitable for studies involving enzyme activity, protein-protein interactions, and protein-ligand binding.

15.4.1.2 Paper Electrophoresis

Paper electrophoresis is a simple and cost-effective method used to separate and analyze amino acids, peptides, and proteins [14]. This approach uses high-quality filter paper or electrophoresis paper. The paper strip is placed between two buffer reservoirs, arranged either horizontally or vertically, and connected to the ends of the strip directly or using wicks or gauze [15]. After the electrophoretic process, direct densitometric analysis can detect the separated molecules on the paper strip [16]. Interestingly, the combination of paper electrophoresis and chromatography was instrumental in determining the cause of sickle cell anemia [17]. Despite its simplicity and historical use, paper electrophoresis presents several challenges. These include limited resolution, variability in paper quality and consistency, the need for large sample amounts, and low sensitivity.

15.4.1.3 Cellulose Acetate Electrophoresis

Cellulose acetate was introduced as an alternative to paper in electrophoresis due to the challenges of using paper. It is preferred because it does not adsorb substances and does not have impurities like nitrogen, hemicellulose, and lignin compounds. Additionally, cellulose acetate exhibits greater homogeneity and a more uniform pore size compared to paper [1]. The procedures for using cellulose acetate in electrophoresis are identical to those for paper. This method is beneficial for the clinical analysis of serum and the separation of hemoglobin from blood samples [16].

15.4.1.4 Capillary Isoelectric Focusing Electrophoresis

Capillary isoelectric focusing separates protein molecules based on their isoelectric points. A pH gradient is made in a capillary tube by filling it with an ampholyte solution. As the analytes migrate through the tube, they stop moving and become electrically neutral at their specific isoelectric points. This method effectively separates proteins and peptides with discrete isoelectric points. However, it is time-consuming as it requires isoelectric point calibration, and resolving complex samples can be challenging [18, 19].

15.4.1.5 Capillary Gel Electrophoresis

Capillary gel electrophoresis is a powerful analytical technique that employs a sieving matrix, typically a cross-linked polymer, within a capillary tube to achieve high-resolution separation of molecules. During the electrophoretic process, larger molecules move more slowly through the matrix than smaller ones, enabling effective separation. This method helps separate proteins and allows for the accurate determination of differences in molecular weights. Capillary gel electrophoresis has been successfully employed in analyzing complex protein samples such as bovine immunoglobulin G and human erythrocyte membrane proteins, achieving high reproducibility and quantification accuracy [20]. However, a significant drawback is that the reliance on the gel matrix for separation makes capillary gel electrophoresis time-consuming [21–23].

15.4.1.6 Agarose Gel Electrophoresis

Agarose gel electrophoresis (AGE) is typically used to separate DNA fragments but can also effectively separate high molecular weight proteins. Agarose, a natural polysaccharide derived from seaweed, has large pore sizes that make it suitable for separating large plasma proteins. [24]. Native agarose gels can be used to electrophorese proteins and protein-protein complexes in a horizontal gel system. This method offers advantages such as simplicity in setup, short runtime, and avoiding toxic components [24, 25]. While agarose gel electrophoresis primarily separates larger proteins, Wu and Kusukawa developed a sodium dodecyl sulfate (SDS) agarose gel method in 1998 that can resolve smaller proteins [26]. The findings demonstrate that AGE, traditionally used for nucleic acid separation, has been successfully adapted for protein analysis, yielding promising results.

15.4.1.7 Polyacrylamide Gel Electrophoresis

Polyacrylamide gel electrophoresis is the preferred technique for analyzing protein mixtures, assessing protein purity, and determining molecular weights. The polyacrylamide matrix is formed by polymerizing acrylamide monomers with a cross-linking agent, typically N, N′ -methylene-bisacrylamide (bisacrylamide) [27]. The cross-linking process is catalyzed by ammonium persulfate (APS) and N, N, N′, N′-tetramethylethylenediamine (TEMED) [12] (Figure 15.2). Polyacrylamide gels have smaller pores than agarose gels, making them more suitable for separating proteins. The pore size can be adjusted by varying the acrylamide-to-cross-linker ratios, allowing for the separation of proteins with different molecular weights [28]. Acrylamide concentration and pore size are inversely related, so the acrylamide concentration can be tailored to the specific proteins that need to be separated, providing the required polyacrylamide pore size. Table 15.1 provides a general guideline for selecting the appropriate gel concentration based on the protein size.

Protein PAGE is typically performed using a discontinuous buffer in a vertical gel system (Figure 15.3). The electrophoretic system consists of two chambers: an upper chamber that houses the negative electrode and a lower chamber that contains the positive electrode [29]. The polymerization occurs between two glass plates. Once the gel has polymerized, it is positioned so that the top part is immersed in the upper chamber buffer while the bottom part is placed in the lower chamber buffer. When current is applied, the charged analytes and the buffer ions move through the gel from the upper to the lower chamber. This movement separates the analytes based on their size, with smaller molecules moving

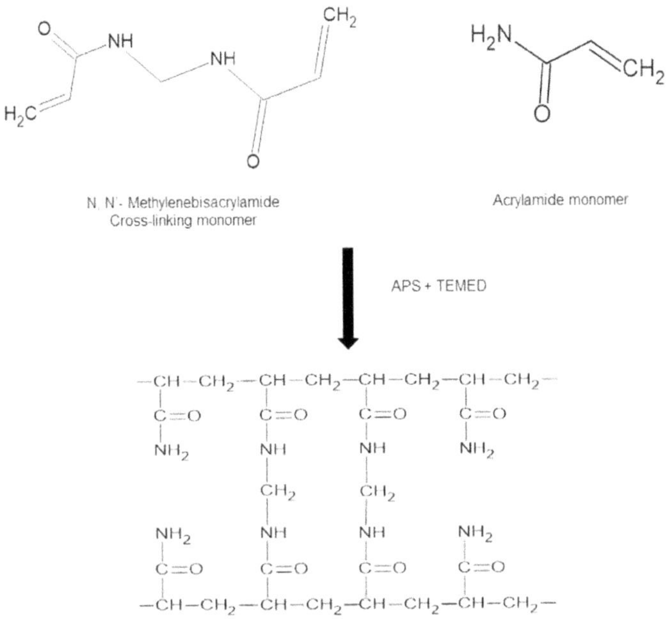

FIGURE 15.2 Polymerization of bis-acylamide with acrylamide monomer.

TABLE 15.1

Acrylamide concentration and protein separation range

Acrylamide concentration (%)	Polypeptide separation range (kDa) (amino acid length)
8	25–200 (225–1800)
10	15–100 (135–900)
12.5	10–70 (90–630)
15	8–60 (55–550)
20	4–40 (36–360)

faster, resulting in fragments of different sizes [1]. Native PAGE and SDS-PAGE are the two main types of polyacrylamide gel electrophoresis [30].

Native PAGE is commonly used to separate proteins in their natural forms based on size, charge, and shape at the pH of the running buffer [12]. This method maintains the native conformation of proteins, making it particularly useful for studying protein-protein interactions, protein folding, and enzyme activity. Native PAGE is performed in a non-denaturing buffer system, allowing proteins to retain their functional structure [1]. However, it may not provide accurate molecular-weight estimates, as the migration rate can be influenced by factors other than molecular weight, such as shape and charge. An advantage of this technique is that native gel proteins can be isolated and used to make antibodies that can be used for proteomic work and structural studies [16, 31].

Sodium dodecyl sulfate-polyacrylamide gel electrophoresis (SDS-PAGE) is widely used to separate proteins based on their molecular weights. This method utilizes sodium dodecyl sulfate, an anionic detergent, which denatures proteins by unfolding them and giving them a negative charge proportional

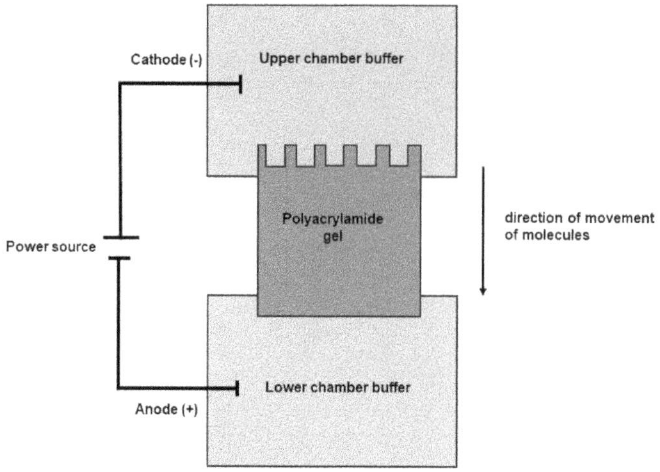

FIGURE 15.3 Polyacrylamide gel electrophoresis.

to their length [28]. The resulting uniform charge-to-mass ratio enables the separation of proteins based solely on size during electrophoresis. The proteins travel through the gel toward the anode, with smaller proteins moving faster and larger proteins moving more slowly. The most popular SDS-PAGE dye is Coomassie Brilliant Blue R-250, which stains the protein bands blue. In contrast, silver stains, which offer better sensitivity, color the protein bands black or brown [32, 33]. SDS-PAGE is commonly used to analyze protein purity, determine subunit composition, and estimate molecular weights. Thus, it is an essential tool for protein research, providing valuable information about protein structure and function.

15.4.2 Electrophoretic Methods for Lipid Analysis

This section explores electrophoretic techniques in lipid and lipoprotein analysis, highlighting their importance and applications. The primary methods include capillary electrophoresis, AGE, and polyacrylamide gradient gel electrophoresis (PGGE). These techniques have significantly contributed to understanding lipid composition, structure, and function and have advanced the study of lipid-related diseases.

15.4.2.1 Capillary Electrophoresis

Capillary electrophoresis has emerged as a practical analytical tool for lipid analysis, offering high selectivity and sensitivity for a diverse range of lipid classes. The method separates lipids based on their charge-to-mass ratio within a capillary tube under an applied electric field. In addition to its high resolution, capillary electrophoresis requires only small sample volumes, making it an efficient and effective tool for lipid analysis [34].

Capillary electrophoresis has been used to identify various lipids, including fatty acids, glycerolipids, sphingolipids, and sterols [35]. In this technique, the lipid components in a mixture are separated by their differential migration, influenced by electrophoretic force and electroosmotic flow. Recently, a method for fractionating plasma for lipid analysis using capillary electrophoresis has been developed and implemented in different species, yielding quantitative results [36]. When coupled with mass spectrometry, capillary electrophoresis enhances lipid profiling capabilities. It is particularly valuable in clinical research and settings where lipids play crucial roles in pathophysiological conditions such as atherosclerosis [34].

15.4.2.2 Agarose Gel Electrophoresis

Agarose gel electrophoresis is a reliable method for separating and analyzing lipids based on their size and charge, especially in lipoprotein profiling. The agarose gel provides a stable medium that supports the migration of lipid-protein complexes under electrophoretic conditions [37]. One of the primary applications of this technique in lipid analysis is the characterization of lipoproteins, which are complexes of lipids and proteins essential for lipid transport in the bloodstream. Researchers or clinicians can visualize and differentiate various lipoprotein fractions, such as high-density lipoproteins (HDL), low-density lipoproteins (LDL), and very low-density lipoproteins (VLDL), using a variety of staining techniques [38, 39]. This capability is crucial for studying lipid metabolism and diagnosing lipid-related disorders, including cardiovascular diseases.

Agarose gel electrophoresis offers several advantages, including simplicity, relatively low cost, and the ability to handle large sample volumes. Additionally, it preserves the native state of lipid-protein complexes, allowing for subsequent functional assays. However, AGE has limitations in resolution compared to other electrophoretic techniques, such as capillary electrophoresis, which may be more suitable for separating complex lipid mixtures or identifying minor lipid components [34]. Despite these limitations, its simplicity and cost-effectiveness make it a popular diagnosis choice in resource-limited clinical settings. For example, a broad β band on AGE suggests dysbetalipoproteinemia (dysβ) [40].

15.4.2.3 Non-denaturing Polyacrylamide Gradient Gel Electrophoresis

Non-denaturing polyacrylamide gradient gel electrophoresis is an effective method for analyzing lipoproteins. This technique employs a gradient gel with varying acrylamide concentrations from top to bottom, enabling the separation of a wide range of lipoprotein sizes. Previous studies have utilized PGGE to analyze LDL and HDL subclasses as a simpler and more cost-effective alternative to ultracentrifugation [41, 42]. In 2003, Blom et al. described a modified version of the non-denaturing PGGE specifically for separating apoB-containing lipoproteins. The method used a 2–8% acrylamide gradient gel and effectively separated LDL particles, triglyceride-rich lipoproteins (TGRL), and their remnants [43]. Polyacrylamide gradient gel electrophoresis is a valuable tool for detecting subtle changes in lipoprotein particle size and diagnosing lipid disorders.

15.5 Protein Disorders

Protein disorders or proteinopathies arise from several factors, including genetic mutations, environmental stressors, and post-translational modifications. These factors can cause proteins to misfold, aggregate, or become dysfunctional, leading to cellular damage and disease [44]. Protein disorders can affect various organ systems and are associated with multiple diseases, from neurodegenerative conditions to metabolic syndromes, as shown in Table 15.2.

TABLE 15.2

Some protein disorders and associated defective proteins

Protein disorder	Defective protein (s)
Alzheimer's disease	Amyloid β peptide; Tau protein
Cerebral β-amyloid angiopathy	Amyloid β peptide
Parkinson's disease	α-Synuclein
Amyotrophic lateral sclerosis	Superoxide dismutase, ubiquilin-2
Huntington's disease	Huntington
Type II diabetes	Islet amyloid polypeptide, amylin
Cystic fibrosis	Cystic fibrosis transmembrane conductance regulator (CFTR) protein
Sickle cell anemia	Hemoglobin
Nephrogenic diabetes insipidus	Aquaporin-2/vasopressin
Multiple myeloma	Antibody light chain
α1 antitrypsin deficiency	$\alpha 1$ antitrypsin

Neurodegenerative diseases like Alzheimer's, Parkinson's, and Huntington's are among the most studied protein disorders. They are marked by the buildup of misfolded proteins, forming aggregates and plaques that disrupt normal cellular functions and eventually result in neuronal death [45].

Protein disorders play a significant role in neurodegenerative diseases and metabolic diseases. Enzyme deficiencies due to protein misfolding or degradation can lead to metabolic imbalances, as seen in conditions like cystic fibrosis and Gaucher's disease. Cystic fibrosis, for example, is caused by mutations in the CFTR protein, leading to its misfolding and improper function, resulting in thick mucus accumulation and respiratory complications [46].

15.5.1 Role of Electrophoresis in Diagnosing Protein Disorders

Serum protein electrophoresis (SPE) is a popular laboratory method that analyzes and separates serum proteins based on size and charge. It is an essential diagnostic tool for diagnosing protein disorders by identifying abnormalities in protein structure and function [47]. Various support mediums, such as agarose, cellulose acetate, and capillary mediums, are used for separating serum proteins, as discussed in Section 15.4.1. Serum protein electrophoresis is extensively used to diagnose various conditions, including acute and chronic inflammations, monoclonal gammopathies, nephropathy, liver diseases, and malnutrition [48]. Furthermore, SPE serves as a screening tool for detecting unexplained physiological changes, including pathological fractures, peripheral neuropathy, infections, kidney failure, anemia, hypercalcemia, proteins in urine, and renal dysfunction [49].

Serum protein fractions are typically categorized into five fractions based on their electrophoretic mobilities: albumin, $\alpha 1$, $\alpha 2$, β , and γ globulin [50] (Figure 15.4). Albumin, the most abundant fraction, is crucial in maintaining osmotic balance and transporting substances such as hormones and fatty acids. The globulin fraction includes $\alpha 1$, $\alpha 2$, β , and γ globulins, each serving specific functions such as lipid transport and immune defense [49]. Analyzing these serum proteins using techniques like electrophoresis helps diagnose proteinopathies and detect abnormalities in protein levels.

15.5.2 Protein Disorders Diagnosed Using Electrophoresis

Some common protein disorders diagnosed using electrophoresis include monoclonal gammopathies, hemoglobinopathies, nephrotic syndrome, $\alpha 1$ antitrypsin deficiency, and amyloidosis.

15.5.2.1 Monoclonal Gammopathies

Monoclonal gammopathies are a group of disorders that involve the abnormal growth of a single clone of plasma cells in the bone marrow, leading to the production of large amounts of monoclonal immunoglobulins, also known as M-proteins. The spectrum of monoclonal gammopathies includes benign conditions, such as monoclonal gammopathy of undetermined significance (MGUS), and more severe diseases like multiple myeloma and related plasma cell neoplasms [47]. M-proteins are typically detected

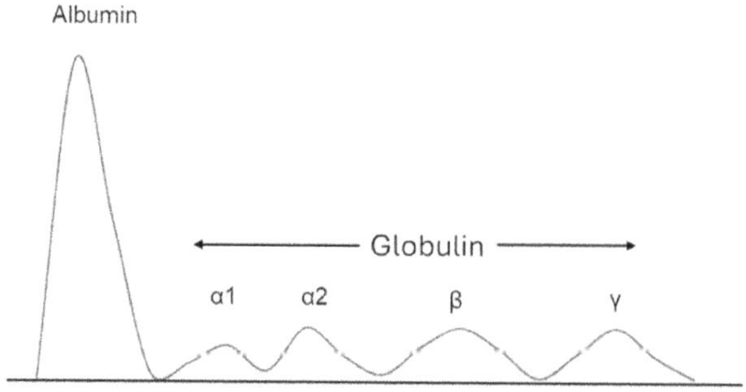

FIGURE 15.4 Normal pattern of serum protein electrophoresis.

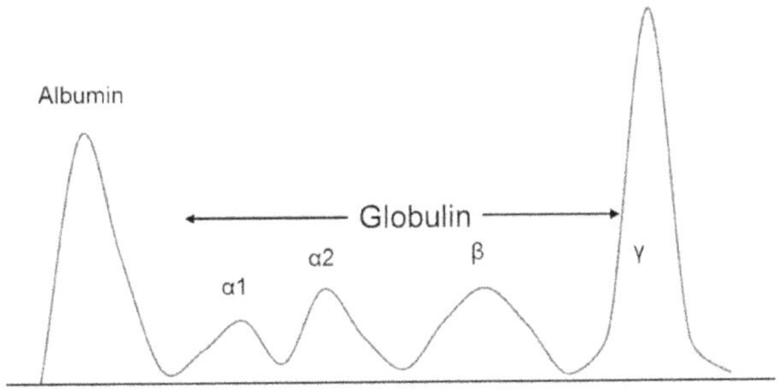

FIGURE 15.5 Abnormal pattern of serum protein electrophoresis.

using electrophoresis in the serum or urine, employing methods like agarose gel electrophoresis or capillary zone electrophoresis [51].

Multiple myeloma represents the most severe form of monoclonal gammopathy, where malignant plasma cells accumulate in the bone marrow and interfere with the production of normal blood cells. M-proteins are a hallmark feature of multiple myeloma and can be detected using serum protein electrophoresis [52] (Figure 15.5).

MGUS, conversely, is a common benign condition where abnormal plasma cells produce M-proteins without causing significant health problems initially. However, MGUS carries a risk of progressing to multiple myeloma or related disorders in a small percentage of cases. Regular monitoring through electrophoresis helps clinicians assess the risk of progression and decide on appropriate management strategies [53]. Waldenström macroglobulinemia is another rare monoclonal gammopathy characterized by abnormal plasma cells' excessive production of IgM monoclonal immunoglobulins. Electrophoresis techniques are essential for diagnosing and monitoring Waldenström macroglobulinemia, distinguishing it from other types of gammopathies based on the specific characteristics of the immunoglobulin involved [47].

Protein electrophoresis offers a simpler and cost-effective method for diagnosing and classifying monoclonal gammopathies by identifying and quantifying M-proteins in serum or urine samples [54]. This technique helps differentiate between various gammopathies and provides valuable information for disease management and prognosis. Early detection through electrophoresis allows for timely initiation of treatment in symptomatic patients and close monitoring of individuals at risk for disease progression.

15.5.2.2 Hemoglobinopathies

Hemoglobin electrophoresis separates the different hemoglobin types according to their charge and size to identify abnormal hemoglobin variants. This technique is beneficial for diagnosing conditions such as sickle cell disease, thalassemia, and other hemoglobin variants like hemoglobin C (HbC), hemoglobin D (HbD), and hemoglobin E (HbE) [55].

In hemoglobin electrophoresis, a blood sample is applied to a gel or capillary system in either acidic or alkaline buffers. When an electric current is applied, normal adult hemoglobin (HbA) and other variants migrate at different rates, forming distinct bands. These bands can be visualized and compared to known standards. The resulting pattern shows the types and proportions of hemoglobin present in the sample, enabling accurate diagnosis of hemoglobinopathies [56]. By analyzing these patterns, clinicians can diagnose various hemoglobinopathies, determine carrier status, and guide treatment decisions. For instance, identifying a predominant HbS band confirms a diagnosis of sickle cell disease, while an elevated HbA2 level suggests beta-thalassemia. Hemoglobin electrophoresis is also essential in newborn screening programs, enabling early detection and management of hemoglobin disorders.

15.5.2.3 Nephrotic Syndrome

Nephrotic syndrome typically presents with significant proteinuria, hypoalbuminemia, hyperlipidemia, and edema [50]. Electrophoresis plays a crucial role in diagnosing and managing this condition by analyzing the protein content in blood and urine samples [57]. This technique helps identify abnormalities in protein levels and types, providing essential information for accurate diagnosis and effective management of nephrotic syndrome.

In nephrotic syndrome, serum protein electrophoresis typically shows a reduction in the albumin and γ globulin fractions but an increase in the $\alpha 2$ fraction. In cases of severe nephrotic syndrome, all fractions except the $\alpha 2$ fraction are reduced [49, 58]. Urine protein electrophoresis complements SPE by detecting and characterizing the types of proteins excreted in the urine, which is particularly useful for diagnosing nephrotic syndrome due to the significant proteinuria associated with the condition [59]. A study by Mehta et al. [2022] found similar results when comparing urine and serum protein electrophoresis using polyacrylamide gel in patients with nephrotic syndrome. These patients exhibited proteins, such as β globulins and albumin, in their urine. The study emphasized the importance of using both urine and serum protein electrophoresis to diagnose and differentiate the various stages of nephrotic syndrome [57].

15.5.2.4 $\alpha 1$ antitrypsin deficiency

$\alpha 1$ antitrypsin (AAT) deficiency is a genetic disorder that affects the production of the AAT protein, crucial for protecting the lungs from inflammation. When deficient, there are lower levels or dysfunctional forms of AAT, leading to uncontrolled activity of neutrophil elastase, which can cause damage to the lungs and liver disease. The clinical manifestations of AAT deficiency can vary widely, ranging from asymptomatic individuals to those with severe lung and liver disease. Symptoms can include shortness of breath, wheezing, chronic cough with sputum production, recurrent respiratory infections, fatigue, jaundice, and other signs of liver disease in infants and adults [60, 61].

Diagnosing AAT deficiency typically involves genetic testing to identify mutant variants, combined with electrophoresis techniques such as serum protein electrophoresis and isoelectric focusing. Serum protein electrophoresis enables the visualization of the $\alpha 1$ globulin band, where AAT protein is typically detected. In individuals with AAT deficiency, this band may show reduced or absent presence, indicating lower levels of AAT protein. Both capillary and agarose gel electrophoresis can be used for serum protein electrophoresis [62]. A recent study by Fernández-Gomez in Spain using capillary serum electrophoresis in free solution demonstrated the effectiveness of using SPE in screening for AAT with 91% sensitivity [61]. In resource-limiting settings, SPE can serve as a useful screening test for AAT before more detailed tests, like genetic tests, are conducted for confirmation.

15.5.2.5 Amyloidosis

Amyloidosis is a group of rare but serious diseases that involve the unusual buildup of amyloid proteins in various tissues and organs. These amyloid deposits can disrupt normal organ function, leading to a range of clinical symptoms depending on the organs affected [63]. The most prevalent form of systemic amyloidosis is amyloid-light-chain (AL) amyloidosis. This condition arises when plasma cells in the bone marrow produce abnormal light chains, which then aggregate to form amyloid deposits [64]. Electrophoresis can aid clinicians in effectively diagnosing amyloidosis by identifying the type of amyloid protein involved and monitoring the progression of the disease.

Serum protein electrophoresis coupled with immunofixation electrophoresis (IFE) is a routine screening tool for diagnosing amyloidosis. Serum protein electrophoresis can reveal the presence of monoclonal immunoglobulin light chains, either kappa or lambda, often associated with the disease. Meanwhile, IFE can detect and characterize these monoclonal immunoglobulins or light chains in the serum or urine, which indicate AL amyloidosis. Combining SPE, IFE, and urine protein electrophoresis can detect 90% of affected patients [63]. Additionally, capillary electrophoresis offers high resolution and sensitivity, aiding in the detection of monoclonal proteins and differentiation between types of amyloidosis [65].

15.6 Lipid Disorders

Lipid disorders, often called dyslipidemias, encompass abnormalities in blood lipid levels, including cholesterol, triglycerides, and associated lipoproteins [66]. Hyperlipidemia is the most prevalent type of dyslipidemia and is characterized by elevated cholesterol levels, triglycerides, LDL cholesterol (LDL-c), and reduced HDL cholesterol (HDL-c) levels. Hyperlipidemia poses a significant risk factor for developing cardiovascular diseases (CVDs) such as coronary artery disease (CAD), stroke, and peripheral artery disease (PAD) [67].

The traditional classification of dyslipidemia, developed by Frederickson in the 1960s, categorized the disorder into five types based on distinct lipoprotein patterns and phenotypes identified through electrophoresis and ultracentrifugation [68] (Table 15.3). However, dyslipidemia is now more commonly classified as either primary or secondary, depending on the underlying cause.

Primary hyperlipidemias are genetic disorders that disrupt lipid metabolism, leading to abnormal lipid levels in the blood. These inherited conditions often result in elevated cholesterol and triglyceride levels, increasing the risk of cardiovascular diseases. There are several types of primary hyperlipidemias, each characterized by specific genetic mutations and lipid abnormalities. Familial hypercholesterolemia (FH) is the most common form caused by variants in the LDL receptor gene [69]. This leads to elevated LDL-c levels, significantly raising the risk of premature coronary artery disease due to LDL-c accumulation in the blood. Another highly atherogenic primary hyperlipidemia is dysbetalipoproteinemia, which results from variants in the apolipoprotein (apo) E gene. The disorder is marked by the accumulation of lipoprotein remnants in the blood, resulting in elevated cholesterol and triglyceride levels. Dysbetalipoproteinemia is associated with an increased risk of atherosclerosis and cardiovascular diseases such as CAD and PAD [70].

Secondary hyperlipidemias are lipid disorders that result from underlying conditions, lifestyle factors, or medications rather than genetic mutations [71, 72]. Unlike primary hyperlipidemias, which are inherited, secondary hyperlipidemias arise from external factors that affect lipid metabolism. Common diseases that result in hyperlipidemia include diabetes mellitus, hypothyroidism, obesity, chronic kidney disease, and liver disorders [73, 74]. Additionally, lifestyle factors such as a diet high in saturated fats and trans fats, excessive alcohol consumption, and lack of physical activity can trigger hyperlipidemia. Certain medications, including corticosteroids, beta-blockers, and diuretics, can also induce or exacerbate lipid abnormalities [75].

TABLE 15.3

Dyslipidemia classification according to Fredrickson

Hyperlipoproteinemia type	Name	Lipoproteins affected	Lipids affected
I	Familial hyperchlomicronemia	Elevated CM	Elevated TG
IIa	Familial hypercholesterolemia	Elevated LDL	Elevated TC
IIb		Elevated LDL, VLDL	Elevated TG, TC
III	Familial dysbetalipoproteinemia	Elevated VLDL, IDL	Elevated TG, TC
IV	Familial hypertriglyceridemia	Elevated VLDL	Elevated TG
V	Familial combined hyperlipidemia	Elevated CM, VLDL	Elevated TG, TC

CM = Chylomicron; TG = Triglyceride; TC = Total cholesterol; LDL = Low-density lipoprotein; VLDL = Very-low-density lipoprotein; IDL = Intermediate-density lipoprotein

15.6.1 Role of Electrophoresis in Diagnosing Lipid Disorders

Electrophoresis is essential for diagnosing lipid disorders by separating and analyzing lipoprotein fractions in blood samples. This technique can identify and quantify the various lipoproteins based on their electrophoretic mobility, which is influenced by their size, shape, and charge. Electrophoresis is particularly valuable in diagnosing lipid disorders for several reasons. First, it characterizes lipoproteins, allowing the identification of abnormal patterns indicative of specific lipid disorders. Additionally, electrophoresis differentiates between various lipoproteins, aiding in diagnosing mixed hyperlipidemia, where multiple lipoprotein fractions are elevated [43]. This differentiation is essential for accurate diagnosis and the development of tailored treatment plans.

Inherited conditions like FH and dysβ can be effectively diagnosed using electrophoresis. Significantly elevated LDL levels identify familial hypercholesterolemia, whereas dysβ shows increased IDL. Electrophoresis plays a crucial role in detecting these distinct patterns, aiding in accurate diagnosis. Moreover, electrophoresis can detect secondary lipid disorders resulting from medical conditions, medications, or lifestyle factors. Abnormal lipoprotein patterns identified through electrophoresis may indicate underlying conditions such as diabetes, hypothyroidism, or the impact of specific medications.

15.6.2 Lipid Disorders Diagnosed Using Electrophoresis

15.6.2.1 Familial Hypercholesterolemia

Familial hypercholesterolemia is primarily caused by variants in the LDL receptor (LDLR) gene, *APOB* gene or proprotein convertase subtilisin/kexin type 9 (PCSK9) gene [76, 77]. These genetic alterations impair the body's ability to clear LDL-c from the blood, leading to elevated LDL-c levels. The high level of LDL-c in individuals with FH significantly increases their risk of CVDs. Early detection and management of FH are critical to prevent severe cardiovascular events. Despite its importance, FH remains undiagnosed in many regions due to insufficient screening practices [78].

Diagnosing FH involves identifying these genetic mutations and analyzing lipid profiles to determine elevated LDL-c levels and abnormal lipoprotein patterns. Researchers and clinicians can use electrophoretic techniques such as AGE and PAGE to identify abnormal lipoprotein patterns indicative of FH. Agarose gel electrophoresis is a simple yet affordable method that can effectively identify and quantify LDL particles. It helps assess LDL-c levels and detect abnormal lipoprotein patterns indicative of FH by providing a visual representation of the various lipoprotein bands [79, 80]. Non-denaturing polyacrylamide gel electrophoresis can separate LDL particles into different subclasses, providing information about particle size distribution [81]. In 2014, Pathak and colleagues introduced a cost-effective native PAGE method for lipoprotein sub-fractionation. This method could particularly be advantageous in diagnosing FH in regions with limited access to expensive techniques [82].

15.6.2.2 Dysbetalipoproteinemia

Dysbetalipoproteinemia, or familial type III hyperlipoproteinemia, is a rare hereditary disorder characterized by abnormal lipoprotein metabolism resulting in elevated plasma cholesterol and triglyceride levels, cutaneous and subcutaneous lesions, and an increased risk of premature vascular disease [83]. This autosomal disorder has delayed penetrance and requires additional genetic defects or environmental factors ("second hit") to precipitate hyperlipidemia [84]. Diagnosis of this highly atherogenic disorder often relies on ultracentrifugation, which is expensive and not widely available in most clinical settings [85]. Thus, alternative methods have been sought to screen for this order, particularly in patients with mixed hyperlipidemia.

Electrophoresis has been instrumental in diagnosing dysβ. Fredrickson and colleagues initially used paper electrophoresis to identify *β*-lipoproteins in whole plasma, marking the first diagnosis of this condition [86]. However, this technique was insufficient for identifying a significant proportion of dysβ patients [87]. Consequently, various electrophoretic methods, including immunoelectrophoresis, PAGE, and agarose gel with magnesium chloride/heparin, were developed over the years to improve the diagnosis of dysβ in serum or whole plasma [43]. While these techniques were relatively simple and inexpensive, they lacked the specificity and sensitivity needed for definitive diagnosis.

Non-denaturing polyacrylamide gradient gel electrophoresis for apoB-containing lipoproteins has significantly improved the screening for dysβ in patients with mixed hyperlipidemia. This technique allows multiple samples to be analyzed simultaneously on a single gel, enabling easy comparisons between samples and standards for LDL particle size. Furthermore, it requires only small sample volumes (about 100 μl), making it both practical and efficient for identifying apoB-containing lipoproteins and their subtypes [43].

The non-denaturing PGGE method involves preparing a 2–8% acrylamide gradient to separate apoB-containing lipoproteins. After the electrophoretic process, the gels are visually examined, and LDL particle sizes are categorized into five groups based on size, ranging from A (largest) to B (smallest). The presence of VLDL-IDL-sized lipoproteins without LDL is indicative of the dysβ phenotype. This method provides a detailed assessment of lipoprotein subtypes and offers greater diagnostic sensitivity compared to traditional agarose gel electrophoresis. Consequently, PGGE is a valuable tool for screening and diagnosing dysβ, especially in resource-limited settings where advanced diagnostic equipment may be scarce.

15.7 Challenges and Limitations

Despite the widespread use of electrophoresis methods for separating and analyzing biomolecules like proteins and lipids, these techniques face several challenges and limitations that can impact their effectiveness and reliability. This section discusses some challenges and proposes strategies for overcoming them.

15.7.1 Limited Sensitivity and Specificity

One of the primary challenges is the limited sensitivity and specificity of some electrophoresis methods, which can result in incomplete or inaccurate identification of biomolecules. Traditional methods like paper and agarose gel electrophoresis often fail to distinguish closely related molecular species [88]. More refined techniques, such as PAGE and CE, can be employed to enhance sensitivity and specificity. Additionally, incorporating fluorescence labeling and immunoblotting can improve the detection and identification of specific proteins.

15.7.2 Large Sample Volumes

Another challenge is that some electrophoresis techniques require relatively large sample volumes, which can be problematic when dealing with scarce or precious samples [89]. This limitation can hinder the analysis of valuable or limited biological materials, such as rare proteins from endangered species. To overcome this, using miniaturized electrophoresis systems, such as microfluidic devices, can significantly reduce the required sample volume. These devices minimize sample usage and offer faster separation times and the potential for high-throughput analysis [90]. Additionally, optimizing sample preparation protocols and improving the sensitivity of detection methods can further mitigate the issue of limited sample availability, making electrophoresis more practical and efficient for a broader range of applications.

15.7.3 Resolving Complex Mixtures

Some electrophoretic techniques also struggle to resolve complex mixtures of biomolecules, particularly when the components have similar physical properties. This challenge can result in overlapping bands and unclear separation, making identifying and quantifying individual molecules problematic [91]. Such limitations can lead to complications in analyzing complex biological samples, where precise separation is crucial for accurate results.

Multidimensional electrophoresis techniques, such as 2D gel electrophoresis, can enhance resolution by separating molecules based on multiple properties, such as isoelectric point and molecular weight [1]. Additionally, combining electrophoresis with advanced techniques like mass spectrometry (MS) can provide detailed analysis and identification of complex mixtures [92].

15.7.4 Gel Preparation and Handling

Gel preparation and handling, especially when using PAGE, can be labor intensive and prone to inconsistencies leading to variability in results. These challenges arise from the meticulous process required to cast and handle the gels, which can affect the quality and reproducibility of the results [93]. However, using pre-cast gels or automating the gel preparation process can help mitigate this limitation, enhance consistency, and reduce human error. Furthermore, optimizing gel composition and running conditions can improve reproducibility, ensuring more reliable and accurate separation of biomolecules.

15.7.5 Technical Expertise and Cost

While electrophoresis is an essential tool for analyzing biomolecules, operating advanced equipment often requires significant expertise. The effective application of some current electrophoretic techniques necessitates a specific skill level and understanding of the underlying principles. This expertise is crucial for optimizing separation conditions and interpreting results accurately. Additionally, the need for specialized equipment and consumables can lead to high costs. For instance, capillary gel electrophoresis, although robust and reliable for protein analysis, incurs substantial expenses due to the cost of capillaries, matrices, and detection systems [21]. Furthermore, techniques like 2D gel electrophoresis provide high resolution and reproducibility, but the need for pre-labeling of proteins and sophisticated imaging equipment adds to the expense [94]. Consequently, the high costs associated with some electrophoretic techniques can be prohibitive for some laboratories, particularly those with limited funding, and may influence their choice of methods used for diagnostic purposes.

Investing in training programs for laboratory staff can help build the necessary expertise for effective electrophoresis. Developing and promoting cost-effective electrophoresis systems can also make these technologies more accessible. Collaborating with well-equipped institutions and resource sharing can also alleviate financial constraints, ensuring broader access to advanced diagnostic tools.

15.8 Future Perspectives

Since its introduction in the 19th century, electrophoresis has evolved significantly and continues to hold great promise for advancing clinical diagnostics and research. One key area of ongoing improvement is the sensitivity and specificity of electrophoretic techniques in detecting biomarkers associated with various diseases. Improvements in gel compositions, detection methods (such as immunoblotting and fluorescent labeling) and integration with other technologies like MS are expected to enhance the precision of biomolecule analysis [92].

Second, moving toward miniaturization and automation of electrophoretic systems, like microfluidic devices, promises to transform how clinicians diagnose diseases [95]. These techniques require small sample volumes, have short run times, and facilitate point-of-care testing, thereby enhancing accessibility and efficiency in healthcare settings.

Future electrophoresis systems may also be able to handle high-throughput analysis and multiplexing capabilities. This technology will enable the simultaneous detection and quantification of multiple biomarkers from a single sample, offering comprehensive diagnostic insights and personalized treatment strategies. For instance, a study by Hu et al. in 2022 demonstrated the use of a capillary electrophoresis-based multiplex PCR assay for carrier screening in a Chinese population, highlighting the potential for multiplexing in electrophoresis [96].

Last, the future of electrophoresis techniques in personalized medicine is promising due to their ability to precisely profile biomarkers and therapeutic targets. Electrophoresis will be instrumental in analyzing therapeutic proteins and drug targets, aiding in developing drugs tailored to individual patient characteristics [97]. This personalized approach is expected to enhance therapeutic efficacy and patient outcomes.

15.9 Conclusion

This chapter explored the utility of electrophoresis as a current tool in diagnosing protein and lipid disorders. Electrophoresis has been used extensively by researchers and clinicians to separate and analyze biomolecules. Different electrophoretic techniques provide effective means to screen for and diagnose common protein and lipid disorders, offering significant benefits, particularly in resource-limiting settings.

Moreover, the advancements in electrophoresis, including developing more sensitive and specific techniques, have enhanced its diagnostic accuracy and reliability. The coupling of electrophoresis to other analytical methods and automation of processes promise to improve diagnostic efficiency further. In the future, electrophoresis is expected to remain an essential tool in clinical diagnostics, contributing to better patient care and management by enabling precise and comprehensive analysis of protein and lipid disorders.

REFERENCES

1. Rana B, Joshi GK. Chapter 11 - Electrophoresis: basic principle, types, and applications. In: Bhatt AK, Bhatia RK, Bhalla TC, editors. *Basic biotechniques for bioprocess and bioentrepreneurship.* Academic Press, New York; 2023. p. 183–93.
2. Yamauchi K. Electrophoretic analysis of serum lipoproteins: its usefulness and problems. *Rinsho Byori.* 2014;62(11):1079–87.
3. Reuss FF. Sur un nouvel effet de l'électricité galvanique. *Mem Soc Imp Natur Moscou.* 1809;2:327–37.
4. Michov B. *Electrophoresis fundamentals: essential theory and practice.* Walter De Gruyter, GmbH & Co KG, Berlin; 2022.
5. Tiselius A. A new apparatus for electrophoretic analysis of colloidal mixtures. *Trans Faraday Soc.* 1937;33(0):524–31.
6. Vesterberg O. A short history of electrophoretic methods. *Electrophoresis.* 1993;14(12):1243–9.
7. Smithies O. Zone electrophoresis in starch gels: group variations in the serum proteins of normal human adults. *Biochem J.* 1955;61(4):629–41.
8. Principles of Electrophoresis. *A guide to protein isolation.* Dordrecht: Springer Netherlands; 2002. p. 115–49.
9. Westermeier R. *Electrophoresis in practice: a guide to methods and applications of dna and protein separations.* John Wiley & Sons, New Jersey; 2016.
10. Fritsch RJ, Krause I. Electrophoresis. In: Caballero B, editor. *Encyclopedia of food sciences and nutrition.* 2nd ed. Oxford: Academic Press; 2003. p. 2055–62.
11. Karki P. Gel electrophoresis system- Apparatus, parts, types and examples. 2022. Available from: https://microbenotes.com/gel-electrophoresis-system-apparatus-parts-types-examples/.
12. Santos-Hernández M, Recio I, Amigo L. Electrophoresis. In: McSweeney PLH, McNamara JP, editors. *Encyclopedia of dairy sciences.* 3rd ed. Oxford: Academic Press; 2022. p. 370–81.
13. Staubach S, Tertel T, Walkenfort B, Buschmann D, Pfaffl MW, Weber G, et al. Free flow electrophoresis allows quick and reproducible preparation of extracellular vesicles from conditioned cell culture media. *Extracell Vesicles Circ Nucl Acids.* 2022;16;3(1):31-48.

14. Owen JA. Paper electrophoresis of proteins and protein-bound substances in clinical investigations. In: Sobotka H, Stewart CP, editors. *Advances in Clinical Chemistry*. Elsevier, Amsterdam; 1958. Vol. 1. p. 237–300.
15. Smith I. *Zone electrophoresis*. Elsevier, Amsterdam; 2013.
16. Walker J. Electrophoretic techniques. In: Wilson K, Walker J, editors. *Principles and techniques of biochemistry and molecular biology*. 7th ed. Cambridge: Cambridge University Press; 2010. p. 399–432.
17. Ingram VM. Abnormal human haemoglobins. I. The comparison of normal human and sickle-cell haemoglobins by fingerprinting. *Biochim Biophys Acta*. 1958;28(3):539–45.
18. Kilár F. Recent applications of capillary isoelectric focusing. *Electrophoresis*. 2003;24(22–23):3908–16.
19. Silvertand LHH, Toraño JS, van Bennekom WP, de Jong GJ. Recent developments in capillary isoelectric focusing. *J Chromatogr A*. 2008;1204(2):157–70.
20. Lin C, Cotton F, Boutique C, Dhermy D, Vertongen F, Gulbis B. Capillary gel electrophoresis: separation of major erythrocyte membrane proteins. *J Chromatogr B Biomed Sci Appl*. 2000;742(2):411–9.
21. Zhu Z, Lu JJ, Liu S. Protein separation by capillary gel electrophoresis: a review. *Anal Chim Acta*. 2012;709:21–31.
22. Bhimwal R, Rustandi RR, Payne A, Dawod M. Recent advances in capillary gel electrophoresis for the analysis of proteins. *J Chromatogr A*. 2022;1682:463453.
23. Hajba L, Jeong S, Chung DS, Guttman A. Capillary gel electrophoresis of proteins: historical overview and recent advances. *Trends Analyt Chem*. 2023;162:117024.
24. Krizek DM, Rick ME. Agarose gel electrophoresis of proteins. *Curr Protoc Cell Biol*. 2002;Chapter 6:Unit 6.7.
25. Kim R. Native agarose gel electrophoresis of multiprotein complexes. *Cold Spring Harb Protoc*. 2011;2011(7):884–7.
26. Wu M, Kusukawa N. SDS agarose gels for analysis of proteins. *BioTechniques*. 1998;24(4):676–8.
27. Gelfi C, Righetti PG. Polymerization kinetics of polyacrylamide gels I. Effect of different cross-linkers. *Electrophoresis*. 1981;2(4):213–9.
28. Srinivas PR. Introduction to protein electrophoresis. *Methods Mol Biol*. 2019;1855:23–9.
29. Stellwagen NC. Electrophoresis of DNA in agarose gels, polyacrylamide gels and in free solution. *Electrophoresis*. 2009;30(S1):S188–S95.
30. Isbir T, Kirac D, Demircan B, Dalan B. Gel electrophoresis. In: Maloy S, Hughes K, editors. *Brenner's encyclopedia of genetics*. 2nd ed. San Diego: Academic Press; 2013. p. 165–7.
31. Nowakowski AB, Wobig WJ, Petering DH. Native SDS-PAGE: high resolution electrophoretic separation of proteins with retention of native properties including bound metal ions. *Metallomics*. 2014;6(5):1068–78.
32. Al-Tubuly AA. SDS-PAGE and Western blotting. In: George AJT, Urch CE, editors. *Diagnostic and therapeutic antibodies*. Totowa, NJ: Humana Press; 2000. p. 391–405.
33. Manns JM. SDS-polyacrylamide gel electrophoresis (SDS-PAGE) of proteins. *Curr Protoc Microbiol*. 2011;22(1):A.3M.1–A.3M.13.
34. Otieno AC, Mwongela SM. Capillary electrophoresis-based methods for the determination of lipids—A review. *Anal Chim Acta*. 2008;624(2):163–74.
35. Poinsot V, Ta HY, Meang VO, Perquis L, Gavard P, Pipy B, et al. A digest of capillary electrophoretic methods applied to lipid analyzes. *Electrophoresis*. 2019;40(1):190–211.
36. Valdivia AO, Cray C, Bhattacharya SK. Capillary electrophoresis plasma fractionation for lipids analysis. *Methods Mol Biol*. 2023;2625:175–81.
37. Noble RP. Electrophoretic separation of plasma lipoproteins in agarose gel. *J Lipid Res*. 1968;9(6):693–700.
38. Greenspan P, Mao FW, Ryu BH, Gutman RL. Advances in agarose gel electrophoresis of serum lipoproteins. *J Chromatogr A*. 1995;698(1–2):333–9.
39. Kido T, Kurata H, Matsumoto A, Tobiyama R, Musha T, Hayashi K, et al. Lipoprotein analysis using agarose gel electrophoresis and differential staining of lipids. *J Atheroscler Thromb*. 2001;8(1):7–13.
40. Marshall WJ, Ballantyne FC. Current clinical laboratory practice: investigation of plasma lipids--which tests and when? *Br Med J (Clin Res Ed)*. 1986;292(6536):1652–4.
41. Dormans TP, Swinkels DW, de Graaf J, Hendriks JC, Stalenhoef AF, Demacker PN. Single-spin density-gradient ultracentrifugation vs gradient gel electrophoresis: two methods for detecting low-density-lipoprotein heterogeneity compared. *Clin Chem*. 1991;37(6):853–8.

42. Gambert P, Bouzerand-Gambert C, Athias A, Farnier M, Lallemant C. Human low density lipoprotein subfractions separated by gradient gel electrophoresis: composition, distribution, and alterations induced by cholesteryl ester transfer protein. *J Lipid Res.* 1990;31(7):1199–210.
43. Blom DJ, Byrnes P, Jones S, Marais AD. Non-denaturing polyacrylamide gradient gel electrophoresis for the diagnosis of dysbetalipoproteinemia. *J Lipid Res.* 2003;44(1):212–7.
44. Luheshi LM, Crowther DC, Dobson CM. Protein misfolding and disease: from the test tube to the organism. *Curr Opin Chem.* 2008;12(1):25–31.
45. Chaudhuri TK, Paul S. Protein-misfolding diseases and chaperone-based therapeutic approaches. *FEBS J.* 2006;273(7):1331–49.
46. Yadav K, Yadav A, Priyanka P, Pandey V, Dwivedi U. Protein misfolding diseases and therapeutic approaches. *Curr Protein Pept Sc.* 2019;20(12):1226–45..
47. Ramanathan S, Narasimhachar Srinivas C. *Serum protein electrophoresis and its clinical applications.* IntechOpen, London; 2020.
48. Mondal S, Pradhan R, Chakraborty A, Chatterjee S. Diagnostic role of serum protein electrophoresis. *Indian J Public Health Res Dev.* 2023;14(2):273–78.
49. Kraševac MG, Tašner T. Clinical significance of serum protein electrophoresis. *Zdrav Vestn.* 2019;88(11–12):593.
50. Lee S, Lin I, Yen T, Chu F. The role of protein electrophoresis in differential diagnosis of renal disorders. *J Urol Ren Dis.* 2018;2018:1101.
51. Genzen JR, Murray DL, Abel G, Meng QH, Baltaro RJ, Rhoads DD, et al. Screening and diagnosis of monoclonal gammopathies: an international survey of laboratory practice. *Arch Pathol Lab Med.* 2018;142(4):507–15.
52. Tripathy S. The role of serum protein electrophoresis in the detection of multiple myeloma: an experience of a corporate hospital. *J Clin Diagn Res.* 2012;6(9):1458–61.
53. Mouhieddine TH, Weeks LD, Ghobrial IM. Monoclonal gammopathy of undetermined significance. *Blood.* 2019;133(23):2484–94.
54. Abdalla IA, Tabbara IA. Nonsecretory multiple myeloma. *South Med J.* 2002;95(7):761–4.
55. Sabath DE. The role of molecular diagnostic testing for hemoglobinopathies and thalassemias. *Int J Lab Hematol.* 2023;45(S2):71–8.
56. Mario N, Baudin B, Bruneel A, Janssens J, Vaubourdolle M. Capillary zone electrophoresis for the diagnosis of congenital hemoglobinopathies. *Clin Chem.* 1999;45(2):285–8.
57. Mehta AM, Shenoy RP, Varashree B, Mundkur SC, Biswas M. Electrophoretic pattern of serum and urinary proteins in nephrotic syndrome. *Biomedicine.* 2022;42(3):478–83.
58. Park EM, Kim JS, Kim JM. Electrophoretic patterns of protein in nephrotic syndrome. *Ann Lab Med.* 1985;5(1):35–44.
59. Chew ST, Fitzwilliam J, Indridason OS, Kovalik EC. Role of urine and serum protein electrophoresis in evaluation of nephrotic-range proteinuria. *Am J Kidney Dis.* 1999;34(1):135–9.
60. Greene CM, Marciniak SJ, Teckman J, Ferrarotti I, Brantly ML, Lomas DA, et al. α1-Antitrypsin deficiency. *Nat Rev Dis Prim.* 2016;2(1):16051.
61. Fernández-Gomez B, Menao-Guillén S, Fernandez Gonzalez A, Arruebo Muñio M, Ramos Alvarez M, Inda Landaluce M, et al. Utility of the serum protein electrophoresis in the opportunistic screening for the deficiency of alpha-1 antitrypsin. *Diagnostics.* 2023;13(17):2778.
62. Kherouf H, De Faverges G, Dumont P, Bourgerette E, N'Guyen T, Moquet O. Alpha-1 antitrypsin deficiency in a French General Hospital: fortuitous detection rather than efficient screening. *Adv Respir Med.* 2018;86(4):179–82.
63. Baker KR, Rice L. The Amyloidoses: clinical features, diagnosis and treatment. *Methodist DeBakey Cardio Vasc J.* 2012;8(3):3.
64. Palladini G, Merlini G. What is new in diagnosis and management of light chain amyloidosis? *Blood.* 2016;128(2):159–68.
65. Goldsmith SR, Stockerl-Goldstein K. What do the elevated protein levels mean in my patients with myeloma, amyloidosis, and related disorders? *Am J Med.* 2022;135:S24–S9.
66. Berberich AJ, Hegele RA. A modern approach to dyslipidemia. *Endocr Rev.* 2022;43(4):611–53.
67. Verma N. Introduction to hyperlipidemia and its treatment: a review. *Int J Curr Pharm.* 2016;9(1):6.
68. Fredrickson DS, Lees RS. A system for phenotyping hyperlipoproteinemia. *Circulation.* 1965;31(3):321–7.

69. Marks D, Thorogood M, Neil HAW, Humphries SE. A review on the diagnosis, natural history, and treatment of familial hypercholesterolaemia. *Atherosclerosis.* 2003;168(1):1–14.
70. Koopal C, Retterstol K, Sjouke B, Hovingh GK, Ros E, de Graaf J, et al. Vascular risk factors, vascular disease, lipids and lipid targets in patients with familial dysbetalipoproteinemia: a European cross-sectional study. *Atherosclerosis.* 2015;240(1):90–7.
71. Yanai H, Yoshida H. Secondary dyslipidemia: its treatments and association with atherosclerosis. *Glob Health Med.* 2021;3(1):15–23.
72. Vodnala D, Rubenfire M, Brook RD. Secondary causes of dyslipidemia. *Am J Cardiol.* 2012;110(6):823–5.
73. Agrawal S, Zaritsky JJ, Fornoni A, Smoyer WE. Dyslipidaemia in nephrotic syndrome: mechanisms and treatment. *Nat Rev Nephrol.* 2018;14(1):57–70.
74. Pearce EN. Hypothyroidism and dyslipidemia: modern concepts and approaches. *Curr Cardiol Rep.* 2004;6:451–6.
75. Majanović S, Cvijanović Peloza O, Detel D, Kenđel Jovanović G, Bakula M, Rahelic D, et al. *Dyslipidemia: current perspectives and implications for clinical practice.* IntechOpen, London. 2021.
76. Berberich AJ, Hegele RA. The complex molecular genetics of familial hypercholesterolemia. *Nat Rev Cardiol.* 2019;16(1):9–20.
77. Vrablik M, Tichý L, Freiberger T, Blaha V, Satny M, Hubacek JA. Genetics of familial hypercholesterolemia: new insights. *Front Genet.* 2020;11:574474.
78. Goldberg AC, Hopkins PN, Toth PP, Ballantyne CM, Rader DJ, Robinson JG, et al. Familial hypercholesterolemia: screening, diagnosis and management of pediatric and adult patients: clinical guidance from the national lipid association expert panel on familial hypercholesterolemia. *J Clin Lipidol.* 2011;5(3 Suppl):S1–8.
79. Nauck M, Winkler K, März W, Wieland H. Quantitative determination of high-, low-, and very-low-density lipoproteins and lipoprotein(a) by agarose gel electrophoresis and enzymatic cholesterol staining. *Clin Chem.* 1995;41(12):1761–7.
80. Chary A, Hedayati M. Review of laboratory methods to determine HDL and LDL subclasses and their clinical importance. *Rev Cardiovasc Med.* 2022;23(4):147.
81. Nakano T, Inoue I, Seo M, Takahashi S, Awata T, Komoda T, et al. Rapid and simple profiling of lipoproteins by polyacrylamide-gel disc electrophoresis to determine the heterogeneity of low-density lipoproteins (LDLs) including small, dense LDL. *Recent Pat Cardiovasc Drug Discov.* 2009;4(1):31–6.
82. Pathak M, Chaudhary N, Rathore AS. Development of a low-cost, high-throughput native polyacrylamide gel electrophoresis (N-PAGE) protocol for lipoprotein sub-fractionation using Quality by Design approach. *J Phar Biomed Anal.* 2014;92:119–26.
83. Koopal C, Marais AD, Visseren FL. Familial dysbetalipoproteinemia: an underdiagnosed lipid disorder. *Curr Opin Endocrinol Diabetes Obes.* 2017;24(2):133–9.
84. Mahley RW, Huang Y, Rall SC, Jr. Pathogenesis of type III hyperlipoproteinemia (dysbetalipoproteinemia). Questions, quandaries, and paradoxes. *J Lipid Res.* 1999;40(11):1933–49.
85. Hopkins PN, Brinton EA, Nanjee MN. Hyperlipoproteinemia type 3: the forgotten phenotype. *Curr Atheroscler Rep.* 2014;16(9):440.
86. Fredrickson DS, Levy RI, Lees RS. Fat transport in lipoproteins--an integrated approach to mechanisms and disorders. *N Engl J Med.* 1967;276(4):215–25 contd.
87. Masket BH, Levy RI, Fredrickson DS. Use of polyacrylamide-gel electrophoresis in differentiating type III hyperlipoproteinemia. *J Lab Clin Med.* 1973;81(5):794–802.
88. Nanthasurasak P, Cabot JM, See HH, Guijt RM, Breadmore MC. Electrophoretic separations on paper: past, present, and future-A review. *Anal Chim Acta.* 2017;985:7–23.
89. Duncombe TA, Herr AE. Use of polyacrylamide gel moving boundary electrophoresis to enable low-power protein analysis in a compact microdevice. *Anal Chem.* 2012;84(20):8740–7.
90. Ou X, Chen P, Huang X, Li S, Liu BF. Microfluidic chip electrophoresis for biochemical analysis. *J Sep Sci.* 2020;43(1):258–70.
91. Zhang Z, Zhang F, Liu Y. Recent advances in enhancing the sensitivity and resolution of capillary electrophoresis. *J Chromatogr Sci.* 2013;51(7):666–83.
92. Schiffer E, Mischak H, Novak J. High resolution proteome/peptidome analysis of body fluids by capillary electrophoresis coupled with MS. *Proteomics.* 2006;6(20):5615–27.

93. Boot CS, Luvai A, Neely RDG. The clinical and laboratory investigation of dysbetalipoproteinemia. *Crit Rev Clin Lab Sci.* 2020.
94. Gao W. Analysis of protein changes using two-dimensional difference gel electrophoresis. *Methods Mol Biol.* 2014;1105:17–30.
95. Theodoridis K, Stergiopoulos F, Bechtsis D, Nikolaidis N, Triantafyllidis D, Tsagaris A, et al. An innovative and fully automated system for gel electrophoresis. In: Pierucci S, Manenti F, Bozzano GL, Manca D, editors. *Computer aided chemical engineering.* Elsevier; 2020. Vol. 48. p. 847–52.
96. Hu P, Tan J, Yu F, Shao B, Zhang F, Zhang J, et al. A capillary electrophoresis-based multiplex PCR assay for expanded carrier screening in the eastern Han Chinese population. *NPJ Genom Med.* 2022;7(1):15.
97. Su J, Yang L, Sun Z, Zhan X. Personalized drug therapy: innovative concept guided with proteoformics. *Mol Cell Proteomics.* 2024;23(3):100737.

16

Chemiluminescent Assay: Current Mainstream in Immunological and Serological Testing

Nathaniel Ebo Aidoo and Emmanuel Kwaku Ofori

16.1 Introduction

Chemiluminescent assay (CLA) is a technique that uses the emission of light resulting from a chemical reaction between labeled molecules to detect and quantify specific substances in samples [1]. In general, luminescence is the emission of visible or near-visible (λ = 300–800 nm) radiation generated when an electron transitions from an excited state to a ground state. The resultant potential energy in the atom is released in the form of light [2]. There are different types of luminescence, each differing in how they achieve the excited state. In chemiluminescence, light is produced by a chemical reaction. This chemiluminescent substance is excited through an oxidation reaction, forming an intermediate [3]. When this intermediate returns to a stable ground state, a photon is released, which the luminescent signal instrument detects. The emitted luminescence indicates the presence of the antigen. The intensity of the luminescence corresponds to the amount of the specific biological molecule present in the sample. Various substrates are used for chemiluminescence, with luminol and its derivatives being the most widely used [4].

Compared to absorbance and fluorescence assays, chemiluminescent (CL) assays offer higher sensitivity due to their lower background signals. However, many CL-based reactions have low quantum efficiency, resulting in weak luminescence, which can limit their application in analytical assays [5]. Recently, the use of nanomaterials has significantly improved CL assays. These nanomaterials, with their exceptional optical, electronic, and catalytic properties, enhance the performance of CL assays by serving as catalysts and fluorescence acceptors [5].

16.2 Advantages of Chemiluminescence Assay

Chemiluminescence (CL) assays offer several significant advantages over traditional detection techniques, making them a powerful tool in analytical and diagnostic applications. One of the primary benefits of CL assays is their high sensitivity [6]. Unlike absorbance and fluorescence assays, CL does not require an external light source, which minimizes light scattering and enhances the signal-to-noise ratio (SNR). This intrinsic feature allows for a broader linear dynamic range and improved detection sensitivity [6]. Since the discovery that horseradish peroxidase (HRP) can catalyze the oxidation of luminol by hydrogen peroxide, resulting in amplified CL signals, a variety of CL substrates have been developed, including acridinium ester, peroxyoxalate, and 1,2-dioxetane and their derivatives. These advancements have significantly enhanced the sensitivity and versatility of CL assays.

Chemiluminescent assays can be automated, significantly reducing the time and labor required for testing [2]. Automation enhances efficiency by enabling consistent and accurate handling of numerous

DOI: 10.1201/9781003486909-16

samples simultaneously. This capability is particularly essential in high-throughput settings like clinical laboratories, where large volumes of tests need to be processed swiftly and accurately. Rapid turnaround times are crucial in these environments to ensure timely diagnosis and treatment, allowing healthcare providers to make prompt and informed decisions regarding patient care. Additionally, automation minimizes human error, ensures standardization, and optimizes resource utilization, further improving laboratory operations' overall workflow and reliability.

Chemiluminescent assays provide both qualitative and quantitative data, enabling the detection of specific antibodies and precisely measuring their concentrations [7, 8]. This dual capability is essential for comprehensively understanding the immune response to various diseases, including COVID-19. By identifying the presence of specific antibodies, these assays can confirm exposure to the virus or the success of vaccination. Furthermore, by quantifying antibody levels, they can monitor the progression of the immune response and the effectiveness of treatments over time. This information is crucial for tailoring individual patient care, developing public health strategies, and guiding decisions on booster vaccinations and other interventions.

Other advantages of chemiluminescence assays include rapid acquisition of the analytical signal, high signal intensity, high stability of reagents and their conjugates, absence of interfering emissions (i.e., high specificity), low consumption of reagents, random access, reduced incubation time, and full compatibility with immunology assay protocols (homogenous or non-homogenous).

16.3 Types of Chemiluminescence Assay

16.3.1 Direct Chemiluminescence Assay

Direct chemiluminescence (CL) involves the direct emission of light from a chemical reaction in which the target analyte is labeled directly with a chemiluminescent compound. When the labeled analyte binds to its specific antibody or receptor, the chemiluminescent label produces light upon the addition of the appropriate substrate [3]. One of the earliest examples of direct CL dates back to 1928 and involves the oxidation of luminol by hydrogen peroxide (H_2O_2) [9]. This reaction produces a strong blue light emission with a peak wavelength of 425 nm, observable through a reverse intersystem crossing (rISC). The emission duration can range from a second to several hours, influenced by factors such as the amount of reacting species, the presence of specific additives, and the method of "feeding" the reaction.

16.3.1.1 Direct Chemiluminescence (CL) by Luminol and Its Derivatives

Luminol is commonly used in aqueous solutions where H_2O_2 acts as the oxidant. However, it can also be oxidized by other agents like ozone, singlet oxygen ($1O_2$), and hypochlorites in the presence of transition metal ions [10]. In aprotic solvents, such as dimethyl sulfoxide (DMSO), luminol's chemiluminescence depends on the pH (requiring basic conditions) and the presence of oxygen (O2) [11, 12]. The decomposition of the dianionic cyclic peroxide intermediate ($CP2^-$), formed during the reaction, leads to chemiexcitation and subsequent light emission [13].

Catalysts, such as horseradish peroxidase (HRP), can enhance the chemiluminescence of luminol. HRP, for example, produces a luminol free radical from luminol anions, thereby amplifying the light emission [3]. Additionally, cobalt-doped hydroxyapatite nanoparticles (CoHA-NPs) have been shown to enhance luminol CL intensity significantly, due to the formation of metal-hydroperoxide intermediates on their surface.

16.3.1.2 Direct Chemiluminescence by Chemiluminescence from Other Probes

Beyond luminol, various other compounds have been developed for direct CL applications. Cypridina luciferin, for instance, emits blue light upon oxidation by molecular oxygen, catalyzed by cypridina luciferase [14–16]. Other notable chemiluminescent compounds include peroxyoxalates, dioxetane, acridinium, and chromone derivatives.

16.3.1.3 Direct Chemiluminescence by Peroxyoxalate

Peroxyoxalate chemiluminescence (PO-CL) is a base-catalyzed reaction where an aromatic oxalic ester reacts with H_2O_2 in the presence of a fluorophore, generating light [17]. This reaction produces high-energy intermediates, such as 1,2-dioxetanedione, which decompose to emit light [18]. Imidazole is commonly used as a catalyst in this reaction, enhancing the chemiluminescence efficiency [19].

16.3.1.4 Direct Chemiluminescence by Acridinium Esters

Acridinium ester derivatives are another significant class of CL molecules. These compounds become luminescent upon activation, producing light through a dioxetane intermediate [20–24]. Acridinium derivatives are valued for their high quantum yields and simplicity of synthesis, making them suitable for various sensing and analytical applications [24–26].

16.3.2 Indirect Chemiluminescence

Indirect chemiluminescence (CL) involves a process where the energy from a chemiexcited molecule (energy donor, D) is transferred to another molecule (energy acceptor, E), which then becomes excited and emits light. This energy transfer can occur through various mechanisms, with Förster Resonance Energy Transfer (FRET) and Dexter Energy Transfer being the primary modes [3].

16.3.2.1 Mechanisms of Energy Transfer

16.3.2.1.1 Förster Resonance Energy Transfer

To achieve a highly efficient CL-initiated cascade FRET, adherence to a three-criteria rule has been reported [27].

- In FRET, the donor and acceptor molecules do not need to be in direct contact but must be within a proximity of about 1–10 nm.
- The efficiency of energy transfer depends on the lifetime of the donor's excited state and the overlap between the emission spectrum of the donor and the absorption spectrum of the acceptor. A higher degree of overlap results in more efficient energy transfer.
- FRET is particularly effective when the donor is a CL reagent and the acceptor is a fluorophore, a process referred to as Chemiluminescence Resonance Energy Transfer (CRET).

16.3.2.1.2 Dexter Energy Transfer

Unlike FRET, Dexter energy transfer requires direct overlap of the wavefunctions of the donor and acceptor, implying close proximity and physical contact between the molecules [27].

16.3.2.2 Modes of Indirect Chemiluminescence Emission

16.3.2.2.1 Intermolecular CL Emission

This occurs when the donor and acceptor molecules are separate entities. The distance between them plays a crucial role in the efficiency of energy transfer [3]. Examples include systems where the energy is transferred from a chemiexcited intermediate to an acceptor molecule, leading to secondary emission. For instance, spiroadamantane 1,2-dioxetanes have been used in vivo to visualize enzymatic activity through CL emission.

16.3.2.2.2 Intramolecular CL Emission

This occurs when the donor and acceptor are part of the same molecule, often linked covalently. This setup generally leads to a more efficient energy transfer due to the fixed proximity. For example, a CL probe for imaging pH in live animals was developed using a 1,2-dioxetane scaffold linked to a pH-sensitive fluorophore [3].

16.4 Current Applications of Chemiluminescence Assay in Immunology and Serology

16.4.1 Exploring Autoimmune Diseases

Chemiluminescence assays offer valuable insights into the pathophysiology of autoimmune diseases. They provide a means to monitor disease activity, assess immune function, and explore potential therapeutic interventions. The intricate interplay between antibodies, immune complexes, and cellular responses forms the basis of many applications in autoimmune disease research. In autoimmune diseases like systemic lupus erythematosus (SLE), rheumatoid arthritis (RA), and vasculitis, immune complexes contribute to tissue damage by activating neutrophils [28]. Chemiluminescence assays have demonstrated the presence of immune complexes on the surface of polymorphonuclear leukocytes (PMNs) and their role in inducing reactive oxygen species (ROS) production [29]. Conversely, fluid-phase IgG can modulate ROS generation by PMNs, highlighting the complex regulatory mechanisms involved in immune responses and tissue damage [30].

Familial studies of autoimmunity have utilized chemiluminescence assays to investigate genetic predispositions and immune system dysregulation [31]. Researchers have identified potential genetic markers associated with disease susceptibility by studying monocyte phagocytic activity in families with autoimmune diseases. These findings contribute to our understanding of the genetic factors influencing autoimmune disorders and aid in developing personalized treatment approaches. Alterations in nitric oxide (NO) metabolism have been implicated in neuroimmunologic disorders, impacting disease prognosis and treatment outcomes. Chemiluminescence assays have been employed to evaluate the effects of NO-modulating compounds on leukocyte and erythrocyte adhesion properties in multiple sclerosis patients [32]. Such studies elucidate the role of NO-dependent pathways in disease pathogenesis and suggest novel therapeutic targets for intervention. Regulation of ROS emissions is central to autoimmune disease pathogenesis, influencing various cellular processes such as growth, apoptosis, and immune responses. Chemiluminescence assays, in conjunction with molecular techniques like PCR/RT-PCR, enable the assessment of redox signaling pathways and the expression of components of the NADPH oxidase system in autoimmune tissues [33]. This study provided insights into the molecular mechanisms underlying tissue damage and immune dysregulation in autoimmune disorders.

Moreover, chemiluminescence assays facilitate the evaluation of immune function and infection risk in autoimmune patients. For example, in primary Sjogren's syndrome, activation of neutrophils may contribute to increased susceptibility to bacterial infections [28]. Chemiluminescence assays have been utilized to assess neutrophil function and metabolic changes, guiding therapeutic decisions and disease management strategies.

In summary, chemiluminescence assays serve as indispensable tools in autoimmune disease research, offering valuable insights into disease mechanisms, genetic predispositions, immune dysregulation, and therapeutic interventions. By elucidating the complex interplay between antibodies, immune complexes, and cellular responses, these assays contribute to our understanding of autoimmune pathophysiology and aid in the development of targeted therapies for improved patient outcomes.

16.4.2 To Study Immunodeficiency Disorders

Chemiluminescence assays offer valuable insights into the pathophysiology of immunodeficiency disorders, providing a means to assess immune function, evaluate treatment efficacy, and explore underlying mechanisms.

Chemiluminescence assays have been instrumental in investigating the effects of highly active antiretroviral treatment on neutrophil and monocyte function in patients with moderately advanced HIV-1 infection. These assays measure the functional activity of granulocytes by assessing chemotaxis and oxidative burst, crucial aspects of an immune response [34]. By comparing chemiluminescence levels in patients and healthy controls, researchers can evaluate the efficacy of specific therapies and identify individuals who may not respond adequately to antimicrobial treatments.

Furthermore, chemiluminescence assays offer a valuable tool for evaluating genotoxic effects in infants born to HIV-positive women receiving antiretroviral nucleoside analog drugs [35]. By employing a PCR-based chemiluminescence detection method, researchers can assess mitochondrial DNA copy numbers, providing insights into the potential adverse effects of antiretroviral therapy on mitochondrial function in newborns. In primary immunodeficiencies, where many etiologies remain elusive, chemiluminescence assays have been instrumental in uncovering new alterations in cellular responses [36]. These findings contribute to our understanding of disease pathogenesis and may guide the development of improved treatment strategies for patients with immunodeficiency disorders.

Moreover, chemiluminescence assays offer promise for addressing clinical challenges associated with measuring chemotaxis, a critical aspect of immune function [37]. By quantifying cell migration through ATP content determination using chemiluminescence, researchers can overcome the limitations of conventional methods and explore abnormalities in chemotactic responses more accurately and efficiently. In summary, chemiluminescence assays serve as valuable tools in the study of immunodeficiency disorders, providing insights into immune function, treatment efficacy, and underlying pathogenic mechanisms. By leveraging the sensitivity and versatility of chemiluminescence techniques, researchers can advance our understanding of these complex disorders and develop more effective diagnostic and therapeutic strategies for patients affected by immunodeficiency.

16.4.3 To Study Infectious Diseases

Chemiluminescence (CL) assays have emerged as powerful tools in the study of infectious diseases, providing insights into immune function, pathogen interactions, and the efficacy of therapeutic interventions. The utility of CL in this context is evident across various aspects of infectious disease research, from immune response assessment to pathogen detection and monitoring treatment outcomes.

One notable application of CL assays is in understanding changes in immune function associated with aging. Elderly populations are particularly susceptible to infections and tumors due to alterations in their immune responses [38]. Braga et al. demonstrated that elderly individuals exhibit reduced luminol-amplified CL compared to younger controls. This reduction in CL signals a weakened immune response, suggesting the potential use of CL assays to determine the necessity for vaccines and immunomodulators in elderly populations to bolster their defenses against infectious diseases. CL assays are also instrumental in studying the interaction between pathogens and host immune cells. For instance, Aldinil et al. utilized CL to analyze the interaction between Treponema pallidum and isolated rat Kupffer cells, measuring the production of ROS to assess phagocytic activity [39]. Similarly, Carlyon et al. used CL to evaluate the effects of *Anaplasma phagocytophilum* on neutrophils' NADPH oxidase assembly and ROS production, highlighting alterations in phagocytic responses due to infection [40].

Opsonization significantly enhances neutrophils' phagocytic efficiency, which is crucial for pathogen destruction. The oxidative burst of neutrophils, a key component of this process, can be measured using luminol-enhanced CL [41–43]. This technique assesses oxidative bursts in both opsonized and non-opsonized states, providing valuable information on the immune system's readiness to combat various pathogens. Additionally, CL assays can investigate the opsonic requirements for phagocytosis of different bacterial serotypes [44].

The inflammatory response involves recruiting neutrophils to infection sites. Hofman et al. studied this process by evaluating transepithelial migration and phagocytosis using luminol-mediated CL, demonstrating the role of neutrophils in controlling inflammation during infections [45]. Furthermore, CL assays facilitate the rapid and quantitative detection of pathogens. The Digene Hybrid Capture System, for instance, uses CL to detect and quantify cytomegalovirus DNA in leukocytes, offering a fast and objective measure of viral activity even when clinical symptoms are not present [46].

Monitoring infection progression and treatment efficacy is another critical application of CL assays. Barbour et al. used CL to evaluate the activation state of neutrophils in patients with active bacterial infections, noting that CL production decreases with effective therapy [47]. This correlation underscores the potential of CL assays in assessing patient responses to treatment. CL assays can also highlight defects in immune cell function in various diseases. For example, leukocytes from diabetic patients exhibit a reduced CL response, indicating impaired bacterial killing capacity, which may explain their heightened susceptibility to infections [48]. Moreover, CL assays can measure oxidative stress and inflammation in patients, using markers like C-reactive protein and ferritin to evaluate disease activity and mortality risk.

CL assays have proven invaluable in specific infections and conditions. In the study of postoperative infections, reduced CL responses reflect decreased microbicidal capacity of granulocytes [49]. In sepsis models, CL assays help evaluate the impact of infection on neutrophil function and oxidative stress [50]. Furthermore, CL can assess the capacity of specific antibodies to induce opsonization and enhance phagocytosis of pathogens like *Haemophilus influenzae* [28].

Automated CL immunoassays are also effective for diagnosing infections and monitoring disease progression. For instance, a novel CL immunoassay for human cytomegalovirus showed high sensitivity and specificity for detecting recent infections [51]. Similar methods are used to diagnose infectious mononucleosis and neurocysticercosis [52].

16.4.4 Evaluate Immune Response against Tumors

Chemiluminescence (CL) assays have proven to be powerful tools in evaluating the immune response against tumors, providing critical insights into oxidative stress, the role of ROS, and the effectiveness of various therapeutic interventions. These assays enable the quantification and analysis of superoxide production and other oxidative activities, which are crucial in understanding tumor biology and developing targeted treatments.

One significant application of CL assays in cancer research is the measurement of oxidative stress through superoxide quantification using lucigenin-amplified CL. Tumors often produce higher levels of ROS compared to non-neoplastic tissues, making this a valuable marker for tumor activity and oxidative stress. For instance, the addition of ROS scavengers to the therapy for gastric tumors has been shown to play a role in the prevention of gastric carcinoma [53]. This approach can also be extended to evaluate the efficacy of anti-inflammatory drugs in reducing oxidative stress and tumor progression.

Studies have highlighted the presence of nitric oxide (NO) in the inner mitochondrial membrane and its role in producing superoxide anion and hydrogen peroxide (H_2O_2) [54, 55] These ROS participate in the modulation of cell proliferation and mitochondrial function [56, 57]. In murine tumor models, decreased oxidative phosphorylation and defective tumoral mitochondrial NO-dependent H_2O_2 production have been linked to persistent tumoral growth, mimicking embryonic behavior [58]. This relationship was demonstrated using western blotting analysis with an enhanced CL detection system to monitor changes in oxidative activity. By detecting these oxidative changes, researchers can gain insights into the metabolic state of tumors and the potential mechanisms driving their growth.

Additionally, CL assays have been employed to study the effects of therapeutic agents on tumors. For example, the impact of eniluracil, a drug that inactivates dihydropyrimidine dehydrogenase activity, was assessed on human solid tumors, including colorectal tumors [59]. The use of CL in this context was crucial in demonstrating the reduction of drug resistance in human colorectal cancer. This highlights the utility of CL assays in evaluating the effectiveness of cancer treatments and their impact on tumor metabolism and ROS production.

16.4.5 To Study Endocrine Disorders

Chemiluminescence (CL) assays have emerged as valuable tools in studying endocrine disorders, offering precise and efficient ways to measure hormonal levels and dynamics. These assays are particularly useful in evaluating the pulsatile secretion of hormones and their responses to various physiological changes or disease conditions [28].

One notable application of CL assays in endocrine research is in determining the secretory patterns of growth hormone (GH). N. Shah and colleagues used an ultrasensitive GH CL assay to evaluate the GH secretory responses during a continuous 24-hour intravenous infusion of saline versus the potent hexapeptide, GHRP-2, in estrogen-unreplaced postmenopausal women [60]. This paired, randomized design study provided insights into the kinetics of hormonal responses, showcasing the ability of CL assays to detect subtle changes in hormone levels over time.

CL assays have also been employed to measure the concentrations of human GH and prolactin (PRL) in media and cell extracts. These assays were used to compare the activity of hormone analogs on hormone release by cultures of secreting pituitary adenomas [61]. The nonisotopic, automatic CL assays provided reliable intra- and inter-assay coefficients of variation for GH and PRL, demonstrating their accuracy and reproducibility. This approach enabled researchers to effectively assess the effects of different hormone analogs on pituitary function, facilitating a better understanding of pituitary adenomas and their treatment [61].

In addition to GH and PRL, CL immunoassays have been used to determine the concentrations of adrenocorticotropic hormone (ACTH), luteinizing hormone (LH), and follicle-stimulating hormone (FSH). These assays, conducted using a nonisotopic, automatic CL immunoassay system, yielded consistent intra- and inter-assay coefficients of variation for these hormones [61]. Compared to conventional techniques, the ease of use and shorter time required to obtain results with CL assays make them a superior choice for hormone determination in clinical and research settings. The application of CL assays in endocrine studies extends beyond the measurement of hormone levels. Their high sensitivity and rapid turnaround time are crucial for real-time monitoring of hormonal fluctuations, which is essential in understanding endocrine disorders' pathophysiology and therapeutic interventions' impact. For instance, the ability to accurately measure hormone levels in response to specific stimuli or treatments can help in tailoring individualized therapeutic strategies for patients with endocrine disorders.

16.4.6 Explore the Inflammatory Response of Airways

Chemiluminescence (CL) assays have proven to be instrumental in exploring the inflammatory response of airways, particularly in conditions characterized by oxidative stress and neutrophil (PMN) activity. These assays provide a sensitive and specific method to measure the production of ROS and the activity of immune cells, which are crucial in understanding and managing inflammatory pulmonary diseases.

Oxidative stress during sepsis is a critical factor that contributes to multiorgan injuries. CL techniques have demonstrated that ex vivo treatments with Vitamin E and simvastatin can inhibit the production of superoxide (O2–) radicals by inactivating NADPH oxidase [62]. This finding highlights the potential of CL assays in selecting and evaluating drugs aimed at reducing oxidative stress and its harmful effects during sepsis.

Inflammatory pulmonary diseases, particularly severe asthma, commonly involve increased numbers and activities of PMNs. Lucigenin-amplified CL has emerged as a suitable technique for measuring the activity of alveolar macrophages, especially when PMNs constitute a small proportion of mixed cell populations [63]. This method allows researchers to explore the heightened PMN activity in cells obtained from asthmatic airways, providing insights into the inflammatory processes underlying asthma. Environmental factors, such as inhalation of dust and toxins, are often linked to pulmonary diseases. A luminol-dependent CL assay was developed to study inflammation in phagocytic cells and lung tissue from animals exposed to dust [64]. This assay showed significantly higher CL signals in dust-exposed animals compared to a saline-treated control group, indicating its effectiveness in detecting and quantifying inflammation due to environmental toxins.

Furthermore, CL assays have been used to investigate the effects of treatments on inflammatory responses in pulmonary diseases. For instance, in a rat model of cystic fibrosis, CL assays suggested that ginseng treatment activated PMNs and modulated the IgG response to *Pseudomonas aeruginosa* [65]. This enhanced bacterial clearance and reduced the formation of immune complexes, leading to milder lung pathology. Such findings underscore the therapeutic potential of certain treatments in mitigating inflammatory responses and improving clinical outcomes in cystic fibrosis. Additionally, the role of PMNs in causing pulmonary damage in adult respiratory distress syndrome (ARDS) has been elucidated using CL assays [66]. These assays demonstrated that activated circulating PMNs release high levels of inflammatory mediators, including ROS, contributing significantly to pulmonary damage.

Understanding the functional status of PMNs in ARDS through CL assays can aid in developing strategies to manage and mitigate lung damage in affected patients.

16.4.7 Evaluate Cellular Activation

Chemiluminescence (CL) assays are invaluable in evaluating cellular activation, particularly their ability to measure ROS production and phagocytic cell activity. These assays provide critical insights into the oxidative bactericidal mechanisms of polymorphonuclear leukocytes (PMNs) and mononuclear phagocytes (MNs), identifying intrinsic defects in their function and assessing the effects of various agents, such as drugs and opsonins, on these cells [67].

When various substances stimulate phagocytes, they release highly reactive oxygen species, which can be quantitatively measured using CL [68]. The specificity of these measurements can be enhanced by using superoxide scavengers like superoxide dismutase and selective inhibitors of phagocyte NADPH oxidase. This allows researchers to dissect the contributions of specific ROS to the overall oxidative response. Furthermore, a range of substances, including cytokines, can modulate antigen-induced CL, demonstrating the assay's versatility in studying immune modulation [69]. Luminol, a lipid-soluble substance, is commonly used in CL assays because it can easily penetrate cells and tissues. It enables the measurement of luminescence in single phagocytic cells, groups of cells, and even cells within tissue. The production of ROS such as singlet oxygen, superoxide anion, hydrogen peroxide, hypochlorous acid, and hydroxyl free radicals can be monitored using luminol-dependent CL [70, 71]. This makes it possible to study the dynamic processes of ROS production and their roles in cellular activation and inflammation.

CL techniques are instrumental in examining the initiation and resolution of inflammation. For instance, Towbin et al. developed a CL assay to investigate the balance between interleukin-1 (IL-1) and its receptor antagonist (IL-1ra) during inflammatory reactions [72]. This assay also assessed the impact of anti-inflammatory agents on IL-1 and IL-1ra expression in bodily fluids, highlighting the regulatory mechanisms of inflammation. Luminol-dependent CL is valuable for studying the earliest events in inflammation, as it predominantly reflects the production of hydrogen peroxide (H_2O_2) in conjunction with nitric oxide (NO) and peroxynitrite formation [73–75]. This makes it an effective method for exploring the mechanisms underlying inflammatory responses and evaluating potential therapeutic agents' effects. A novel CL assay has recently been developed to detect the endotoxin activity of lipopolysaccharide (LPS) in whole blood. This assay is based on the in vitro activation of neutrophils and utilizes the priming effects of complement-opsonized immune complexes on the respiratory burst activity of neutrophils. The resulting chemiluminescent emission indicates membrane NADPH oxidase and myeloperoxidase activity disturbances providing a sensitive measure of neutrophil activation [76]. Furthermore, CL assays can analyze NADPH oxidase activity in the presence of inhibitors of the arachidonic acid cascade, aiding in the investigation of phospholipase A2 (PLA2) products and their roles in cellular activation [77]. These assays also allow for the study of the kinetics and magnitude of the oxidative burst capacity of granulocytes from peripheral blood, offering early criteria for cell activation [28]. This has implications for developing immune modulators and future carriers for vaccinal epitopes. Whole blood CL assays offer the advantage of evaluating both oxygen radicals released by phagocytes and serum opsonin activity using minimal blood samples [78]. This makes them particularly useful for the early detection of postoperative infections and for assessing host defenses against infection.

16.4.8 Evaluate Drugs and Chemical Products

Chemiluminescence (CL) assays are highly effective tools for evaluating the effects of drugs and chemical products on cellular and immune responses. These assays utilize the principle of light emission during chemical reactions to measure various biological activities, providing sensitive and quantitative insights into how different substances interact with cells and affect their functions.

One significant application of CL assays is examining antifungal agents' impact on immune responses. For instance, the luminol-enhanced CL assay has been used to study the effects of various antifungal drugs, such as bifonazole, fluconazole, itraconazole, and terbinafine, on the chemiluminescence response of mouse spleen cells [79]. The observed reduction in CL response indicates an inhibition of the cellular immune response, which is critical in understanding the immunomodulatory effects of these drugs. Moreover, the assay can evaluate how antifungal drugs influence the phagocytic activity of polymorphonuclear neutrophils (PMNs). This is particularly important in preventing septic shock, as the drugs can inhibit the PMN-mediated inflammatory cascade without compromising their phagocytic activity [80].

Flavonoids, the primary constituents of many herbal medicines, have been shown to inhibit the growth of *Helicobacter pylori*, a bacterium linked to gastric ulcers and cancer [81]. CL techniques are instrumental in evaluating the anti-*Helicobacter pylori* activity of various flavonoids, including flavanols, flavones, flavonols, and isoflavonoids, by measuring their impact on bacterial growth and survival. In the context of viral infections, neuraminidase inhibitors have been licensed for the prophylaxis and treatment of influenza. CL assays have proven to be rapid and reliable methods for screening large numbers of influenza isolates for susceptibility to these inhibitors, facilitating the development of effective antiviral therapies [82].

The toxicity of chemical products on the vertebrate immune system can also be assessed using CL assays. For example, the effects of permethrin, a new class of insecticides, were evaluated on splenic macrophages using CL techniques. This approach helps determine the immunotoxicity of chemical agents and their potential impact on immune function [83]. Antibiotics that enhance phagocyte functions can be more effective in treating microbial infections. CL assays measure the generation of superoxide anion by neutrophils, providing a quantitative assessment of how certain antibiotics can potentiate phagocyte functions and improve infection outcomes [84].

CL assays are also valuable for exploring the immunogenicity and immune responses against adjuvants. For instance, luminal-dependent CL was used to evaluate the respiratory burst in splenic cells from mice pretreated with various immunostimulants, such as oil-in-water emulsions of muramyl dipeptide and trehalose dimycolate. The enhancement of non-specific resistance to influenza virus infection was found to be related to the chemical structure of these synthetic immunostimulants [85]. Similarly, the antihelminthic agent levamisole, known for non-specifically enhancing immune responses, was examined for its effect on the chemotaxis of human neutrophils and the levels of cellular cyclic nucleotides using CL assays [86].

16.5 Limitations of Chemiluminescence Assay

While CLA offers numerous advantages, they also have notable disadvantages that need careful consideration. Each point below highlights a specific limitation, elaborating on its impact on the effectiveness and feasibility of using CLA in various laboratory settings. One significant disadvantage of CLA is its limited antigen detection capability [2]. While CLA is highly sensitive, it may not detect certain antigens as effectively as other assay methods. This limitation can be particularly problematic when dealing with complex samples or when the target antigen is present at deficient concentrations, potentially leading to false negatives or inaccurate quantification.

Another major drawback is the high costs associated with CLA systems [2]. The initial investment for purchasing CLA analyzers is substantial, often requiring a significant outlay for both the equipment and the necessary reagents. Additionally, ongoing maintenance costs and the need for regular calibration can strain laboratory budgets, especially in smaller or resource-constrained facilities. This high financial barrier may limit the adoption of CLA technology despite its benefits. CLA also suffers from a limited test panel [2]. Unlike other assay methods offering a broader range of detectable analytes, CLA platforms may be restricted in the types and number of tests they can perform. This limitation can be a significant hindrance for laboratories that need to conduct a diverse array of tests, forcing them to rely on multiple assay systems to meet their diagnostic and research needs. Potential interference from sample components or cross-reactivity with other substances is also a concern with CLA [87]. Such interferences can affect the accuracy of the results, leading to false positives or negatives. Laboratories need to be aware of these potential issues and consider them when interpreting test outcomes to avoid erroneous conclusions.

Another issue is the closed analytical systems often associated with CLA platforms [2]. These systems can need more flexibility, limiting the ability to customize or adapt the assay parameters to specific experimental requirements. Laboratories may find this restrictive, particularly when they need to modify protocols or when they aim to integrate CLA with other analytical techniques. In many CL systems, the low background emission level in the absence of the analyte can pose challenges [2]. The CL signals in flow systems, which increase proportionally to the analyte concentration, often appear as sharp peaks on a low, constant blank signal. Because only a small portion of CL emission is measured from this time profile, reactions with complex kinetics may result in non-linear response plots versus analyte concentration. This non-linearity can complicate data interpretation and affect the reliability of the assay results. In summary, while CLA offers high sensitivity and specificity, its disadvantages include high costs, limited antigen detection, and potential interferences. Laboratories must weigh these factors against the benefits of CLA, making informed decisions based on their specific needs, budget constraints, and long-term objectives.

16.6 Future Perspectives and Developments

The future of chemiluminescence immunoassay (CLA) technology is poised for significant advancements, driven by innovative developments aimed at enhancing its analytical performance. Despite its current efficiency, CLA continues to evolve, promising even greater improvements in the years to come. One promising development in CLA technology is the flow-injection chemiluminescent immunoassay (FI-CLA). This method leverages the rapid injection of micro-bubbles into the reaction system, which ensures a more efficient mixing of reagents, reduces incubation times, and improves temperature control. As a result, FI-CLA enhances immunoreaction kinetics and significantly reduces analysis time, making it a valuable innovation for faster and more accurate diagnostics [88, 89].

Currently, CLA technology is limited to discrete tests that measure one autoantibody at a time. However, there is an emerging need for multiparametric tests capable of identifying multiple components of a complex immunological profile in a single analytical step. The use of two-dimensional resolution for CL multiplex immunoassays could meet this need. This technique employs a multichannel sampling strategy combined with various enzyme labels. Following a brief batch incubation, free conjugated enzymes are separated from those bound to immunocomplexes and captured by magnetic microparticles. The subsequent application of a channel-resolved approach allows for the recording of signals from multiple parallel measuring channels, enabling the sequential determination of multiple analytes efficiently and cost-effectively [90, 91]. Additionally, multianalyte assays have been realized using the zone-resolved strategy, which implements arrays where different antigens are immobilized at distinct positions on the solid phase. This setup allows individual immunoreactions to occur simultaneously and be distinctly identified by array detectors [92]. The use of specific charge-coupled device (CCD) equipment has accelerated the development of chemiluminescent imaging techniques, making CLA arrays more convenient compared to those employing alternative labels.

Another significant advancement is applying ultrasensitive chemiluminescence magnetic nanoparticles immunoassay (CL-MBs-nano-immunoassay) technology. This non-competitive and direct-type immunoassay uses magnetic beads as the solid phase and employs gold nanoparticles with double labeling. One label is a monoclonal antibody specific for the analyte, and the other is horseradish peroxidase, which amplifies the luminescent signal from the immunoreaction and the associated enzymatic reaction exponentially. This innovation significantly increases the analytical sensitivity of the CLA method, enhancing its diagnostic capabilities [93, 94].

In conclusion, the evolution of CLA technology is just beginning. Introducing new, more efficient analytical methods based on chemiluminescence principles is expected to continue, reducing costs and improving diagnostic accuracy. This transformation will align antibody diagnostics with established biochemistry and immunoassay methods, providing significant clinical benefits through enhanced diagnostic accuracy and expediency. The future of CLA holds great promise for advancing autoimmune diagnostics and other areas of medical research and clinical practice.

16.7 Conclusion

Chemiluminescent assays (CLA) have emerged as a pivotal technology in immunological and serological testing, offering remarkable sensitivity, specificity, and rapidity. These assays have revolutionized diagnostic capabilities across various applications, including infectious diseases, endocrine disorders, inflammatory responses, cellular activation, and drug evaluation. Despite some limitations, such as high initial costs and technical complexities, the continued innovation and development in CLA technology promise to address these challenges. Advances like flow-injection CLA, multiparametric tests, and ultrasensitive nanoparticle assays are set further to enhance diagnostics' efficiency, flexibility, and accuracy. As CLA technology evolves, it is poised to deliver even greater clinical benefits, solidifying its status as the mainstream method in modern diagnostic testing.

REFERENCES

1. Yang M, Huang J, Fan J, Du J, Pu K, Peng X. Chemiluminescence for bioimaging and therapeutics: recent advances and challenges. *Chem Soc Rev* [Internet]. 2020 Oct 5;49(19):6800–15 [cited 2024 May 30]. Available from: https://pubs.rsc.org/en/content/articlehtml/2020/cs/d0cs00348d
2. Cinquanta L, Fontana DE, Bizzaro N. Chemiluminescent immunoassay technology: what does it change in autoantibody detection? *Autoimmun Highlights* [Internet]. 2017 Dec 1;8(1):1–8 [cited 2024 May 29]. Available from: https://link.springer.com/articles/10.1007/s13317-017-0097-2
3. Tzani MA, Gioftsidou DK, Kallitsakis MG, Pliatsios NV, Kalogiouri NP, Angaridis PA, et al. Direct and indirect chemiluminescence: reactions, mechanisms and challenges. *Molecules* [Internet]. 2021 Dec 1;26(24) [cited 2024 May 26]. Available from: /pmc/articles/PMC8705051/
4. Khan P, Idrees D, Moxley MA, Corbett JA, Ahmad F, Von Figura G, et al. Luminol-based chemiluminescent signals: clinical and non-clinical application and future uses. *Appl Biochem Biotechnol* [Internet]. 2014;173(2):333 [cited 2024 May 30]. Available from: /pmc/articles/PMC4426882/
5. Zhu X, Gao T. Spectrometry. In: Li G. *Nano-inspired biosensors for protein assay with clinical applications.* Elsevier, Amsterdam. 2018 Jan 1. p. 237–64.
6. Yan Y, Shi P, Song W, Bi S. Chemiluminescence and bioluminescence imaging for biosensing and therapy: in vitro and in vivo perspectives. *Theranostics* [Internet]. 2019;9(14):4047 [cited 2024 May 30]. Available from: /pmc/articles/PMC6592176/
7. Alonso R, Roa PL, Suárez M, Bouza E. New automated chemiluminescence immunoassay for simultaneous but separate detection of human immunodeficiency virus antigens and antibodies. *J Clin Microbiol* [Internet]. 2014;52(5):1467–70 [cited 2024 May 30]. Available from: https://journals.asm.org/doi/10.1128/jcm.03486-13
8. Xiang A, Wei F, Lei X, Liu Y, Guo Y. A simple and rapid capillary chemiluminescence immunoassay for quantitatively detecting human serum HBsAg. *Eur J Clin Microbiol Infect Dis* [Internet]. 2013 Dec 1;32(12):1557–64 [cited 2024 May 30]. Available from: https://link.springer.com/article/10.1007/s10096-013-1910-0
9. Albrecht HO. Über die Chemiluminescenz des Aminophthalsäurehydrazids. *Z Phys Chem* [Internet]. 1928 Aug 1;136U(1):321–30 [cited 2024 May 26]. Available from: https://www.degruyter.com/document/doi/10.1515/zpch-1928-13625/html
10. Yue L, Liu YT. Mechanistic insight into pH-dependent luminol chemiluminescence in aqueous solution. *J Phys Chem B* [Internet]. 2020 Sep 3;124(35):7682–93 [cited 2024 May 26]. Available from: https://pubs.acs.org/doi/abs/10.1021/acs.jpcb.0c06301
11. White EH, Roswell DF. The chemiluminescence of organic hydrazides. *Acc Chem Res* [Internet]. 1970 Feb 1;3(2):54–62 [cited 2024 May 26]. Available from: https://pubs.acs.org/doi/pdf/10.1021/ar50026a003
12. White EH, Zafiriou O, Kägi HH, Hill JHM. Chemiluminescence of luminol: the chemical reaction. *J Am Chem Soc* [Internet]. 1964 Mar 1;86(5):940–1 [cited 2024 May 26]. Available from: https://pubs.acs.org/doi/pdf/10.1021/ja01059a050

13. Yue L, Liu YJ. Two conical intersections control luminol chemiluminescence. *J Chem Theory Comput* [Internet]. 2019 Mar 12;15(3):1798–805 [cited 2024 May 26]. Available from: https://pubs.acs.org/doi/abs/10.1021/acs.jctc.8b01114
14. Khakhar A, Starker CG, Chamness JC, Lee N, Stokke S, Wang C, et al. Building customizable auto-luminescent luciferase-based reporters in plants. *Elife*. 2020 Mar 1;9.
15. Johnson FH, Shimomura O. Introduction to the Cypridina system. *Methods Enzymol.* 1978 Jan 1;57(C):331–64.
16. Morin JG. Based on a review of the data, use of the term 'cypridinid' solves the Cypridina/Vargula dilemma for naming the constituents of the luminescent system of ostracods in the family Cypridinidae. *Luminescence* [Internet]. 2011 Jan 1;26(1):1–4 [cited 2024 May 26]. Available from: https://onlinelibrary.wiley.com/doi/full/10.1002/bio.1178
17. Tonkin SA, Bos R, Dyson GA, Lim KF, Russell RA, Watson SP, et al. Studies on the mechanism of the peroxyoxalate chemiluminescence reaction: part 2. Further identification of intermediates using 2D EXSY 13C nuclear magnetic resonance spectroscopy. *Anal Chim Acta*. 2008 May 5;614(2):173–81.
18. Farahani P, Baader WJ. Unimolecular decomposition mechanism of 1,2-dioxetanedione: concerted or biradical? That is the question! *J Phys Chem A* [Internet]. 2017 Feb 16;121(6):1189–94 [cited 2024 May 26]. Available from: https://pubs.acs.org/doi/abs/10.1021/acs.jpca.6b10365
19. Stevani CV, Lima DF, Toscano VG, Baader WJ. Kinetic studies on the peroxyoxalate chemiluminescent reaction: imidazole as a nucleophilic catalyst. *J Chem Soc Perkin Trans 2* [Internet]. 1996 Jan 1;5(5):989–95 [cited 2024 May 26]. Available from: https://pubs.rsc.org/en/content/articlehtml/1996/p2/p29960000989
20. Natrajan A, Wen D. Effect of branching in remote substituents on light emission and stability of chemiluminescent acridinium esters. *RSC Adv* [Internet]. 2014 May 19;4(42):21852–63 [cited 2024 May 26]. Available from: https://pubs.rsc.org/en/content/articlehtml/2014/ra/c4ra02516d
21. Ren L, Cui H. Chemiluminescence accompanied by the reaction of acridinium ester and manganese (II). *Luminescence* [Internet]. 2014 Nov 1;29(7):929–32 [cited 2024 May 26]. Available from: https://onlinelibrary.wiley.com/doi/full/10.1002/bio.2643
22. Nakazono M, Nanbu S, Akita T, Hamase K. Synthesis, chemiluminescence, and application of 2,4-disubstituted phenyl 10-methyl-10λ4-acridine-9-carboxylates. *Dyes Pigments*. 2019 Nov 1;170:107628.
23. Czechowska J, Kawecka A, Romanowska A, Marczak M, Wityk P, Krzymiński K, et al. Chemiluminogenic acridinium salts: a comparison study. Detection of intermediate entities appearing upon light generation. *J Lumin*. 2017 Jul 1;187:102–12.
24. Zadykowicz B, Czechowska J, Ozóg A, Renkevich A, Krzymiński K. Effective chemiluminogenic systems based on acridinium esters bearing substituents of various electronic and steric properties. *Org Biomol Chem* [Internet]. 2015 Dec 23;14(2):652–68 [cited 2024 May 26]. Available from: https://pubs.rsc.org/en/content/articlehtml/2016/ob/c5ob01798j
25. Natrajan A, Sharpe D. Synthesis and properties of differently charged chemiluminescent acridinium ester labels. *Org Biomol Chem* [Internet]. 2013 Jan 17;11(6):1026–39 [cited 2024 May 26]. Available from: https://pubs.rsc.org/en/content/articlehtml/2013/ob/c2ob27190g
26. Weeks I, Beheshti I, McCapra F, Campbell AK, Woodhead JS. Acridinium esters as high-specific-activity labels in immunoassay. *Clin Chem* [Internet]. 1983 Aug 1;29(8):1474–9 [cited 2024 May 26]. Available from: https://dx.doi.org/10.1093/clinchem/29.8.1474
27. Song Q, Yan X, Cui H, Ma M. Efficient cascade resonance energy transfer in dynamic nanoassembly for intensive and long-lasting multicolor chemiluminescence. *ACS Nano* [Internet]. 2020 Mar 24;14(3):3696–702 [cited 2024 May 26]. Available from: https://pubmed.ncbi.nlm.nih.gov/32150394/
28. Rodriguez-Orozco AR, Ruiz-Reyes H, Medina-Serriteno N. Recent applications of chemiluminescence assays in clinical immunology. *Mini Rev Med Chem* [Internet]. 2010 Dec 1;10(14):1393–400 [cited 2024 May 28]. Available from: https://pubmed.ncbi.nlm.nih.gov/20201791/
29. Doll NJ, Wilson MR, Salvaggio JE. Inhibition of polymorphonuclear leukocyte chemiluminescence for detection of immune complexes in human sera. *J Clin Invest* [Internet]. 1980;66(3):457–64 [cited 2024 May 28]. Available from: https://pubmed.ncbi.nlm.nih.gov/6156953/
30. Chedraoui-Silva S, Mantovani B. The role of complement in the modulation by fluid-phase IgG of the production of reactive oxygen species by polymorphonuclear leukocytes stimulated with IgG immune complexes. *Brazil J Med Biol Res* [Internet]. 2003;36(12):1665–72 [cited 2024 May 28]. Available from: https://www.scielo.br/j/bjmbr/a/n96BKKKxGnYxyZhcgwkk8bs/?format=html&lang=en

31. Badr El Din MK. Defective monocyte phagocytic function as a possible genetic marker for rheumatic susceptibility. 1998 [cited 2024 May 28]. Available from: https://iris.who.int/handle/10665/117728
32. Mayer M, Hermanova Z. Effect of nitric oxide metabolism upon peripheral blood chemiluminescence and leukocyte and erythrocyte adherence in multiple sclerosis. *Bratisl Lek Listy* [Internet]. 1999 Jan 1;100(10):531–6 [cited 2024 May 28]. Available from: https://europepmc.org/article/med/10649849
33. Vasantha Rao P, Maddala R, John F, Zigler JS. Expression of nonphagocytic NADPH oxidase system in the ocular lens. *Mol Vis* [Internet]. 2004 Feb 19;10:112–21 [cited 2024 May 28]. Available from: https://europepmc.org/article/med/14978478
34. Mastroianni CM, Lichtner M, Mengoni F, D'Agostino C, Forcina G, D'Ettorre G, et al. Improvement in neutrophil and monocyte function during highly active antiretroviral treatment of HIV-1-infected patients. *AIDS*. 1999;13(8):883–90.
35. Poirier MC, Divi RL, Al-Harthi L, Olivero OA, Nguyen V, Walker B, et al. Long-term mitochondrial toxicity in HIV-uninfected infants born to HIV-infected mothers. *J Acquir Immune Defic Syndr* [Internet]. 2003 Jun 1;33(2):175–83 [cited 2024 May 28]. Available from: https://pubmed.ncbi.nlm.nih.gov/12794551/
36. Di Renzo M, Pasqui AL, Bruni F, Saletti M, Bova G, Chiarion C, et al. Evaluation of some immune functions in a patient affected by common variable immunodeficiency using luminescent techniques. *J Biolumin Chemilumin* [Internet]. 1997 Jul 1;12(4):193–7 [cited 2024 May 28]. Available from: https://europepmc.org/article/med/9481606
37. McCafferty AC, Cree IA. Measurement of cell migration stimulated by interleukin 8: use of ATP chemiluminescence. *Cytokine*. 1994 Jul 1;6(4):450–3.
38. Braga PC, Sala MT, Dal Sasso M, Mancini L, Sandrini MC, Annoni G. Influence of Age on Oxidative Bursts (Chemiluminescence) of Polymorphonuclear Neutrophil Leukocytes. *Gerontology* [Internet]. 1998 Aug 1;44(4):192–7 [cited 2024 May 28]. Available from: https://dx.doi.org/10.1159/000022009
39. Aldini R, Marangoni A, Guardigli M, Sambri V, Giacani L, Montagnani M, et al. Chemiluminescence detection of reactive oxygen species in isolated Kupffer cells during phagocytosis of Treponema pallidum. *Comparative Hepatology*. 2004 Jan 14;3(1):1–2. Available from: https://link.springer.com/articles/10.1186/1476-5926-2-S1-S41
40. Carlyon JA, Latif DA, Pypaert M, Lacy P, Fikrig E. Anaplasma phagocytophilum utilizes multiple host evasion mechanisms to thwart NADPH oxidase-mediated killing during neutrophil infection. *Infect Immun* [Internet]. 2004 Aug;72(8):4772–83 [cited 2024 May 28]. Available from: https://journals.asm.org/doi/10.1128/iai.72.8.4772-4783.2004
41. Teneberg S, Jurstrand M, Karlsson KA, Danielsson D. Inhibition of nonopsonic Helicobacter pylori–induced activation of human neutrophils by sialylated oligosaccharides. *Glycobiology* [Internet]. 2000 Nov 1;10(11):1171–81 [cited 2024 May 28]. Available from: https://dx.doi.org/10.1093/glycob/10.11.1171
42. Danielsson D, Jurstrand M. Nonopsonic activation of neutrophils by Helicobacter pylori is inhibited by rebamipide. *Dig Dis Sci* [Internet]. 1998 Sep 1;43(9 Suppl):167S-173S [cited 2024 May 28]. Available from: https://europepmc.org/article/med/9753245
43. Hansen PS, Go MF, Varming K, Andersen LP, Genta RM, Graham DY, et al. Proinflammatory activation of neutrophils and monocytes by Helicobacter pylori in patients with different clinical presentations. *Infect Immun* [Internet]. 1999;67(6):3171–4 [cited 2024 May 28]. Available from: https://journals.asm.org/doi/10.1128/iai.67.6.3171-3174.1999
44. Matthay KK, Mentzer WC, Wara DW, Preisler HK, Lameris NB, Ammann AJ. Evaluation of the opsonic requirements for phagocytosis of streptococcus pneumoniae serotypes VII, XIV, and XIX by chemiluminescence assay. *Infect Immun* [Internet]. 1981;31(1):228–35 [cited 2024 May 28]. Available from: https://journals.asm.org/doi/10.1128/iai.31.1.228-235.1981
45. Hofman P, Piche M, Far DF, Le Negrate G, Selva E, Landraud L, et al. Increased *Escherichia coli* phagocytosis in neutrophils that have transmigrated across a cultured intestinal epithelium. *Infect Immun* [Internet]. 2000 Feb;68(2):449–55 [cited 2024 May 28]. Available from: https://journals.asm.org/doi/10.1128/iai.68.2.449-455.2000
46. Mazzulli T, Wood S, Chua R, Walmsley S. Evaluation of the digene hybrid capture system for detection and quantitation of human cytomegalovirus viremia in human immunodeficiency virus-infected patients. *J Clin Microbiol* [Internet]. 1996;34(12):2959–62 [cited 2024 May 28]. Available from: https://journals.asm.org/doi/10.1128/jcm.34.12.2959-2962.1996

47. Barbour AG, Allred CD, Solberg CO, Hill HR. Chemiluminescence by polymorphonuclear leukocytes from patients with active bacterial infection. *J Infect Dis* [Internet]. 1980 Jan 1;141(1):14–26 [cited 2024 May 28]. Available from: https://dx.doi.org/10.1093/infdis/141.1.14
48. Shah SV, Wallin JD, Eilenj SD. Chemiluminescence and superoxide anion production by leukocytes from diabetic patients. *J Clin Endocrinol Metab* [Internet]. 1983 Aug 1;57(2):402–9 [cited 2024 May 29]. Available from: https://dx.doi.org/10.1210/jcem-57-2-402
49. Salo M, Perttilä J, Lehtonen OP. Granulocyte chemiluminescence in patients with postoperative infections. *Archives of Surgery* [Internet]. 1988 Jan 1;123(1):17–22 [cited 2024 May 29]. Available from: https://jamanetwork.com/journals/jamasurgery/fullarticle/592865
50. Ahmad H, Ca K. Zymosan-induced luminol-dependent chemiluminescence response of circulating and extravasated leukocytes in experimental sepsis. *Mediators Inflamm* [Internet]. 2004 Apr;13(2):123–5 [cited 2024 May 29]. Available from: https://www.hindawi.com/journals/mi/2004/369438/
51. Revello MG, Gorini G, Gerna G. Clinical evaluation of a chemiluminescence immunoassay for determination of immunoglobulin G avidity to human cytomegalovirus. *Clin Diagn Lab Immunol* [Internet]. 2004 Jul;11(4):801–5 [cited 2024 May 29]. Available from: https://journals.asm.org/doi/10.1128/CDLI.11.4.801-805.2004
52. Feng Z, Li Z, Sui B, Xu G, Xia T. Serological diagnosis of infectious mononucleosis by chemiluminescent immunoassay using capsid antigen p18 of Epstein-Barr virus. *Clinica Chimica Acta.* 2005 Apr 1;354(1–2):77–82.
53. Oliveira CPMS, Kassab P, Lopasso FP, Souza HP, Janiszewski M, Laurindo FRM, et al. Protective effect of ascorbic acid in experimental gastric cancer: reduction of oxidative stress. *World J Gastroenterol* [Internet]. 2003 Mar 1;9(3):446–8 [cited 2024 May 29]. Available from: http://www.wjgnet.com/1007-9327/9/446.asp
54. Boveris A, Valdez LB, Zaobornyj T, Bustamante J. Mitochondrial metabolic states regulate nitric oxide and hydrogen peroxide diffusion to the cytosol. *Biochimica et Biophysica Acta (BBA) - Bioenergetics.* 2006 May 1;1757(5–6):535–42.
55. Radi R, Cassina A, Hodara R. Nitric oxide and peroxynitrite interactions with mitochondria. *Biol Chem* [Internet]. 2002 Apr 12;383(3–4):401–9 [cited 2024 May 29]. Available from: https://www.degruyter.com/document/doi/10.1515/BC.2002.044/html
56. Diebold L, Chandel NS. Mitochondrial ROS regulation of proliferating cells. *Free Radic Biol Med.* 2016 Nov 1;100:86–93.
57. Idelchik M del PS, Begley U, Begley TJ, Melendez JA. Mitochondrial ROS control of cancer. *Semin Cancer Biol.* 2017 Dec 1;47:57–66.
58. Galli S, Labato MI, Bal de Kier Joffé E, Carreras MC, Poderoso JJ. Decreased mitochondrial nitric oxide synthase activity and hydrogen peroxide relate persistent tumoral proliferation to embryonic behavior. *Cancer Res* [Internet]. 2003 Oct 1;63(19):6370–7 [cited 2024 May 29]. Available from: http://cancerres.aacrjournals.org/cgi/content/full/63/19/6370
59. Ahmed FY, Johnston SJ, Cassidy J, O'Kelly T, Binnie N, Murray GI, et al. Eniluracil treatment completely inactivates dihydropyrimidine dehydrogenase in colorectal tumors. *Journal of Clinical Oncology* [Internet]. 1999 Sep 21;17(8):2439–45 [cited 2024 May 29]. Available from: https://ascopubs.org/doi/10.1200/JCO.1999.17.8.2439
60. Shah N, Evans WS, Bowers CY, Veldhuis JD. Tripartite neuroendocrine activation of the human growth hormone (GH) Axis in women by continuous 24-hour GH-releasing peptide infusion: pulsatile, entropic, and nyctohemeral mechanisms. *J Clin Endocrinol Metab* [Internet]. 1999 Jun 1;84(6):2140–50 [cited 2024 May 29]. Available from: https://dx.doi.org/10.1210/jcem.84.6.5687
61. Hofland LJ, Van Der Hoek J, Van Koetsveld PM, De Herder WW, Waaijers M, Sprij-Mooij D, et al. The novel somatostatin analog SOM230 is a potent inhibitor of hormone release by growth hormone- and prolactin-secreting pituitary adenomas in vitro. *J Clin Endocrinol Metab* [Internet]. 2004 Apr 1;89(4):1577–85 [cited 2024 May 29]. Available from: https://dx.doi.org/10.1210/jc.2003-031344
62. Durant R, Klouche K, Delbosc S, Morena M, Amigues L, Beraud JJ, et al. Superoxide anion overproduction in sepsis: effects of vitamin E and simvastatin. *Shock* [Internet]. 2004 Jul;22(1):34–9 [cited 2024 May 29]. Available from: https://journals.lww.com/shockjournal/fulltext/2004/07000/superoxide_anion_overproduction_in_sepsis__effects.6.aspx

63. Ward C, Kelly CA, Stenton SC, Duddridge M, Hendrick DJ, Walters EH. The relative contribution of bronchoalveolar macrophages and neutrophils to lucigenin- and luminol-amplified chemiluminescence. *Eur Respir J* [Internet]. 1990 Oct 1;3(9):1008–14 [cited 2024 May 29]. Available from: https://erj.ersjournals.com/content/3/9/1008
64. Antonini JM, Van Dyke K, Ye Z, DiMatteo M, Reasor MJ. Introduction of luminol-dependent chemiluminescence as a method to study silica inflammation in the tissue and phagocytic cells of rat lung. *Environ Health Perspect* [Internet]. 1994;102(SUPPL. 10):37–42 [cited 2024 May 29]. Available from: https://ehp.niehs.nih.gov/doi/10.1289/ehp.94102s1037
65. Song Z, Kharazmi A, Wu H, Faber V, Moser C, Johansen HK, et al. Effects of ginseng treatment on neutrophil chemiluminescence and immunoglobulin G subclasses in a rat model of chronic *Pseudomonas aeruginosa* pneumonia. *Clin Diagn Lab Immunol* [Internet]. 1998;5(6):882–7 [cited 2024 May 29]. Available from: https://pubmed.ncbi.nlm.nih.gov/9801351/
66. Zimmerman GA, Renzetti AD, Hill HR. Functional and metabolic activity of granulocytes from patients with adult respiratory distress syndrome. Evidence for activated neutrophils in the pulmonary circulation. *Am Rev Respir Dis* [Internet]. 1983;127(3):290–300 [cited 2024 May 29]. Available from: https://pubmed.ncbi.nlm.nih.gov/6830052/
67. Prendergast E, Proctor RA. Simple procedure for measuring neutrophil chemiluminescence. *J Clin Microbiol* [Internet]. 1981;13(2):390–2 [cited 2024 May 29]. Available from: https://pubmed.ncbi.nlm.nih.gov/7204552/
68. Mehrzad J, Duchateau L, Pyörälä S, Burvenich C. Blood and milk neutrophil chemiluminescence and viability in primiparous and pluriparous dairy cows during late pregnancy, around parturition and early lactation. *J Dairy Sci* [Internet]. 2002;85(12):3268–76 [cited 2024 May 29]. Available from: https://pubmed.ncbi.nlm.nih.gov/12512600/
69. Tengler RS, Furukawa K, de Weck AL, Maly FE. Chemiluminescence of mononuclear cells is enhanced during antigen recognition. *J Biolumin Chemilumin* [Internet]. 1993;8(3):159–67 [cited 2024 May 29]. Available from: https://pubmed.ncbi.nlm.nih.gov/8493886/
70. Radi R, Cosgrove TP, Beckman JS, Freeman BA. Peroxynitrite-induced luminol chemiluminescence. *Biochem J* [Internet]. 1993;290 (Pt 1):51–7 [cited 2024 May 29]. Available from: https://pubmed.ncbi.nlm.nih.gov/8382481/
71. Lucisano YM, De-Mello AM, Vasques ER, Mantovani B. Precipitated immune complexes of IgM induce the generation of reactive oxygen species by rabbit polymorphonuclear leucocytes. *Braz J Med Biol Res* [Internet]. 1998;31(6):793–7 [cited 2024 May 29]. Available from: https://pubmed.ncbi.nlm.nih.gov/9698825/
72. Towbin H, Schmitz A, van Oostrum J, Seitz M, Dewald B, Zingel O, et al. Monoclonal antibody based enzyme-linked and chemiluminescent assays for the human interleukin-1 receptor antagonist. Application to measure hIL-1ra levels in monocyte cultures and synovial fluids. *J Immunol Methods* [Internet]. 1994 Mar 29;170(1):125–35 [cited 2024 May 29]. Available from: https://pubmed.ncbi.nlm.nih.gov/8157985/
73. Wang JF, Komarov P, Degroot H. Luminol chemiluminescence in rat macrophages and granulocytes: the role of NO, O_2–/H_2O_2, and HOCl. *Arch Biochem Biophys* [Internet]. 1993 Jul;304(1):189–96 [cited 2024 May 29]. Available from: https://pubmed.ncbi.nlm.nih.gov/8391779/
74. Kikuchi K, Nagano T, Hayakawa H, Hirata Y, Hirobe M. Detection of nitric oxide production from a perfused organ by a luminol-H_2O_2 system. *Anal Chem* [Internet]. 1993 Jul 1;65(13):1794–9 [cited 2024 May 29]. Available from: https://pubmed.ncbi.nlm.nih.gov/8368532/
75. Carreras MC, Pargament GA, Catz SD, Poderoso JJ, Boveris A. Kinetics of nitric oxide and hydrogen peroxide production and formation of peroxynitrite during the respiratory burst of human neutrophils. *FEBS Lett* [Internet]. 1994 Mar 14;341(1):65–8 [cited 2024 May 29]. Available from: https://pubmed.ncbi.nlm.nih.gov/8137924/
76. Romaschin AED, Walker PM. Endotoxin activity in whole blood by neutrophil chemiluminescence—a novel analytical paradigm. *Clin Chem* [Internet]. 2000 Sep 1;46(9):1504–6 [cited 2024 May 29]. Available from: https://dx.doi.org/10.1093/clinchem/46.9.1504
77. Daniels I, Lindsay MA, Keany CIC, Burden RP, Fletcher J, Haynes AP. Role of arachidonic acid and its metabolites in the priming of NADPH oxidase in human polymorphonuclear leukocytes by peritoneal dialysis effluent. *Clin Diagn Lab Immunol* [Internet]. 1998;5(5):683–9 [cited 2024 May 29]. Available from: https://journals.asm.org/doi/10.1128/cdli.5.5.683-689.1998

78. Fujisawa M, Kojima K, Beppu T, Futagawa S, Kuwahara K, Hiramatsu K. Early diagnosis of postoperative infection: assessment of whole blood chemiluminescence. *Surg Today* [Internet]. 2000;30(4):309–18 [cited 2024 May 29]. Available from: https://link.springer.com/article/10.1007/s005950050592
79. Abruzzo GK, Fromtling RA, Turnbull TA, Giltinan DM. Effects of bifonazole, fluconazole, itraconazole, and terbinafine on the chemiluminescence response of immune cells. *J Antimicrob Chemother* [Internet]. 1987 Jul 1;20(1):61–8 [cited 2024 May 29]. Available from: https://dx.doi.org/10.1093/jac/20.1.61
80. Khan HA. Effect of fluconazole on phagocytic response of polymorphonuclear leukocytes in a rat model of acute sepsis. *Mediators Inflamm* [Internet]. 2005 Feb 24;2005(1):9–15 [cited 2024 May 29]. Available from: https://www.hindawi.com/journals/mi/2005/176179/
81. Shin JE, Kim JM, Bae EA, Hyun YJ, Kim DH. In vitro inhibitory effect of flavonoids on growth, infection and vacuolation of *Helicobacter pylori*. *Planta Med* [Internet]. 2005 Mar;71(3):197–201 [cited 2024 May 29]. Available from: http://www.thieme-connect.com/products/ejournals/html/10.1055/s-2005-837816
82. Mungall BA, Xu X, Klimov A. Surveillance of influenza isolates for susceptibility to neuraminidase inhibitors during the 2000–2002 influenza seasons. *Virus Res* [Internet]. 2004 Jul 1;103(1–2):195–7.
83. Punareewattana K, Smith BJ, Blaylock BL, Longstreth J, Snodgrass HL, Gogal RM, et al. Topical permethrin exposure inhibits antibody production and macrophage function in C57Bl/6N mice. *Food Chem Toxicol* [Internet]. 2001 Feb 1;39(2):133–9.
84. Sato K, Sato N, Shimizu H, Tsutiya T, Takahashi H, Kakizaki S, et al. Faropenem enhances superoxide anion production by human neutrophils in vitro. *J Antimicrob Chemother* [Internet]. 1999 Sep 1;44(3):337–41 [cited 2024 May 29]. Available from: https://dx.doi.org/10.1093/jac/44.3.337
85. Masihi KN, Brehmer W, Azuma I, Lange W, Müller S. Stimulation of chemiluminescence and resistance against aerogenic influenza virus infection by synthetic muramyl dipeptide combined with trehalose dimycolate. *Infect Immun* [Internet]. 1984;43(1):233–7 [cited 2024 May 29]. Available from: https://journals.asm.org/doi/10.1128/iai.43.1.233-237.1984
86. Hogan NA, Hill HR. Enhancement of neutrophil chemotaxis and alteration of levels of cellular cyclic nucleotides by levamisole. *J Infect Dis* [Internet]. 1978 Oct 1;138(4):437–44 [cited 2024 May 29]. Available from: https://dx.doi.org/10.1093/infdis/138.4.437
87. Ihm YK, Kang SY, Kim MH, Lee WI. Chemiluminescent assay versus immunoblotting for detection of positive reaction to allergens. *Lab Med* [Internet]. 2012 Apr 1;43(3):91–5 [cited 2024 May 30]. Available from: https://dx.doi.org/10.1309/LMK23OPMAVHH3XTI
88. Wang C, Wu J, Zong C, Xu J, Ju HX. Chemiluminescent immunoassay and its applications. *Chin J Anal Chem* [Internet]. 2012 Jan 1;40(1):3–10.
89. Yang Z, Fu Z, Yan F, Liu H, Ju H. A chemiluminescent immunosensor based on antibody immobilized carboxylic resin beads coupled with micro-bubble accelerated immunoreaction for fast flow-injection immunoassay. *Biosens Bioelectron* [Internet]. 2008 Sep 15;24(1):35–40 [cited 2024 May 30]. Available from: https://pubmed.ncbi.nlm.nih.gov/18430562/
90. Fu Z, Liu H, Ju H. Flow-through multianalyte chemiluminescent immunosensing system with designed substrate zone-resolved technique for sequential detection of tumor markers. *Anal Chem* [Internet]. 2006 Oct 1;78(19):6999–7005 [cited 2024 May 30]. Available from: https://pubmed.ncbi.nlm.nih.gov/17007526/
91. Liu H, Fu Z, Yang Z, Yan F, Ju H. Sampling-resolution strategy for one-way multiplexed immunoassay with sequential chemiluminescent detection. *Anal Chem* [Internet]. 2008 Jul 15;80(14):5654–9 [cited 2024 May 30]. Available from: https://pubmed.ncbi.nlm.nih.gov/18558775/
92. Urbanowska T, Mangialaio S, Zickler C, Cheevapruk S, Hasler P, Regenass S, et al. Protein microarray platform for the multiplex analysis of biomarkers in human sera. *J Immunol Methods* [Internet]. 2006 Oct 30;316(1–2):1–7 [cited 2024 May 30]. Available from: https://pubmed.ncbi.nlm.nih.gov/16996079/
93. Du L, Ji W, Zhang Y, Zhang C, Liu G, Wang S. An ultrasensitive detection of 17β-estradiol using a gold nanoparticle-based fluorescence immunoassay. *Analyst* [Internet]. 2015 Mar 21;140(6):2001–7 [cited 2024 May 30]. Available from: https://pubmed.ncbi.nlm.nih.gov/25672478/
94. Tao X, Jiang H, Yu X, Zhu J, Wang X, Wang Z, et al. An ultrasensitive chemiluminescence immunoassay of chloramphenicol based on gold nanoparticles and magnetic beads. *Drug Test Anal* [Internet]. 2013;5(5):346–52 [cited 2024 May 30]. Available from: https://pubmed.ncbi.nlm.nih.gov/23512826/

17

Next-Generation Sequencing: Current Trends and Challenges

Shama Mujawar, Aarohi Deshpande, Avni Bhambure, and Bhupendra Prajapati

17.1 Introduction

With the help of next-generation sequencing (NGS), hundreds of millions of deoxyribonucleic acid (DNA) sections can be instantly sequenced at once, offering extensive knowledge of the composition of the genome, mutations, gene activity patterns, and epigenetic variations. Due to the fact that DNA sequencing systems are so versatile, studies pertaining to rare genetic conditions, cancer genome studies, analysis of microbial communities, viral illnesses, and demographic genetics are currently being conducted. Furthermore, targeted therapeutics, personalized health strategies, and enhanced diagnostic techniques are among the innovations made conceivable by NGS technology [1]. NGS techniques have diversified into several generations, each distinguished by unique technological developments. Sanger sequencing has set the standard for first-generation DNA sequencing. Sanger's technique was utilized extensively thereby enabling instantaneous sequencing of both ribonucleic acid (RNA) and DNA that transformed the area of molecular biology. Sanger's technique employed capillary electrophoresis along with fluorescently marked dideoxynucleotides to accelerate the sequencing process, and this approach greatly boosted the speed and precision of the sequencing procedure. However, its cost-effectiveness and scalability were a challenge.

Second-generation sequencing systems, such as Illumina, altered genome sequencing by lowering per-base sequencing expense drastically and boosting performance. Due to its precision, it is frequently employed in professional and research programs, contributing to its widespread acceptance. The capacity for parallel sequencing of DNA makes this technique unique from the conventional Sanger sequencing methods. Roche's 454 sequencing approach, which uses pyrosequencing wherein the amino acid sequence is identified via determining the dissolution of a substance called pyrophosphate while nucleotides are incorporated into the DNA template is among the most prevalent second-generation sequencing tools that have developed. Ion Torrent sequencing is a different system that uses the detection of hydrogen ion discharge while creating DNA to ascertain the pattern of DNA. Reversing dye terminators serve as the foundation for the sequencing-by-synthesis technique adopted by the extensively used Illumina genome sequencing tool [1].

Third-generation DNA sequencing platforms, most particularly those from Oxford Nanopore Technologies (ONT) and Pacific Biosciences (PacBio), introduced the use of long-read sequencing features. Such platforms provide positive benefits in the investigation of convoluted genetic variations in structure and extended transcripts of RNA by enabling the genetic sequencing of longer portions of DNA. While precision was a problem for third-generation platforms early on, ongoing development has rendered them more valuable, particularly for tasks that demand deep genomic perspectives. The next-generation sequencing technologies from Illumina, especially the NovaSeq and HiSeq series, continue

DOI: 10.1201/9781003486909-17

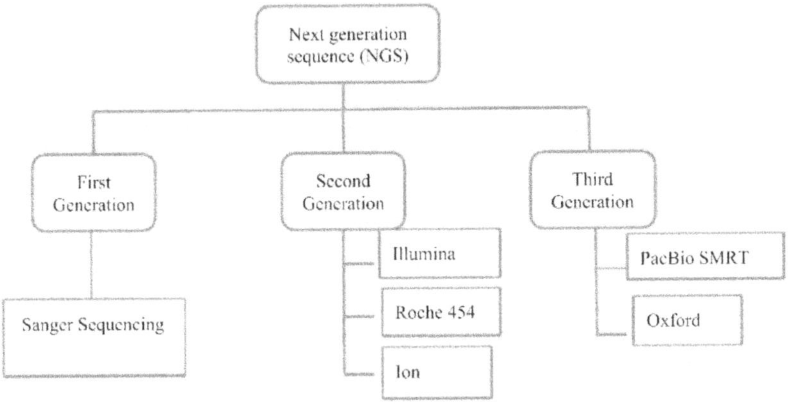

FIGURE 17.1 Evolution of next-generation sequencing (NGS) platforms.

to be increasingly popular across current generations and are currently being implemented in both medical and genome-wide research. Illumina is widely recognized for their preciseness, affordability, and significant throughput potential, thus serving as an indispensable part of DNA sequencing initiatives [1].

NGS techniques organize libraries for the sequencing of DNA or RNA within a system free of cells and without the need for a bacterial replication process. Furthermore, NGS methods simultaneously and concurrently sequence thousands of sequencing processes [2]. In addition, these contemporary technologies have given rise to novel research interests among young scientists. While NGS's potential is still unrealized, it is believed that it will soon overtake all other technologies as the go-to solution for medical research. The NGS platforms are summarized in Figure 17.1.

17.2 Current Trends in NGS Technologies

Over the years, there have been significant advances in NGS procedures that have successfully changed scientific research. These advances have presented unique resources that have relevant clinical utility. Some of these applications are also relevant in the field of molecular biology and genomics. Subsequent sub-sections of this chapter describe various aspects of NGS.

17.2.1 Single-Cell Sequencing

A revolutionary development in NGS is single-cell DNA sequencing, which allows scientists to investigate the genomic structure at a previously unattainable degree of resolution of individual cell types. This revolutionary technology sheds light on the biological processes underlying diseases, growth and development, and variation in cells. Several NGS-based approaches in the fields of transcriptomics, epigenomics, epigenetics, and genome sequencing are concentrating on characterizing specific cell types. By using single-cell analyses instead of mass population assessments, conventional characterization procedures will make it possible for investigators to make novel and possibly unforeseen biological advances. For instance, single-cell RNA sequencing (scRNA-seq) can trace the developmental trajectories of various cell generations as well as illustrate unusual intricate cell populations along with the regulatory associations between the genes. Growing evidence indicates the heterogeneity of gene activity.

Although every cell in our body has a remarkably similar gene makeup, the transcriptome information within each cell only represents a small portion of the total gene transcription. This means that more than half the genes and their respective expression profiles are yet to be established which can open up opportunities for disease treatments. However, most transcriptome assessment trials currently conducted base their findings on the idea that cells within a specific tissue are homogenous, which means that significant cell-to-cell variation happens to be overlooked in these research efforts. A better comprehension of the composition of the transcript genome in each cell will prove crucial for recognizing unpredictable biological events, as it will clarify its function within cell processes and clarify how the expression of genes can encourage advantageous or detrimental states [3].

Crucially, evaluating the variations in gene regulation among individual cells may reveal uncommon communities that might be invisible to the naked eye when analyzing a collection of cells. Deconvolution of extremely varied antibody cell groups in both normal and infected states has been recently made accessible by significant advancements in readily accessible research methods and computational biology. A substantial amount of individual cells must be profiled in order to perform a thorough transcriptome assessment. Previous approaches have concentrated on only the 5′ or 3′ ends of the transcripts in order to minimize the consequent sequencing expenses. This method efficiently eliminates polymerase chain reaction (PCR) bias, enhancing precision by assigning every single read to a distinct cell. These techniques make use of biological measurement and show greater uniformity than hidden molecular estimation with read-based sequencing terms [3]. Some notable tools employed for single-cell NGS sequencing include:

1) Drop-seq: Drop-seq performs a highly parallel analysis of mRNA transcripts from droplets of individual cells. A microfluidic device is used in this single-cell sequencing technique to divide droplets containing lysis buffer, a single cell, and a microbead coated in barcoded primers.
2) Smart-seq2: In this method, individual cells are lysed in a buffer containing free deoxyribonucleotide triphosphates (dNTPs) and oligo-deoxythymidine (dT)-tailed oligonucleotides with a universal 5′-anchor sequence. Its advantage includes improved coverage across transcripts and the level of mappable reads is high.
3) Single-cell ATAC-Seq (scATAC-Seq): Using microfluidics and molecular barcoding, scATAC-Seq is a technique that examines chromatin accessibility in individual nuclei derived from a single sample. Its applications include cell cluster and classification, and trajectory inference.
4) Mission Bio Tapestri platform: It is a single-cell sequencing solution which can be seamlessly integrated into an already established NGS workflow. Data on both genotype and phenotype from the same cell can be obtained. At the single-cell level, it can identify copy number variations (CNVs), single nucleotide variants (SNVs), and cell-surface proteins.
5) 10× Genomics Chromium System: The device breaks individual cells into tiny water droplets known as gel beads in emulsion (GEMs) using microfluidics. A single cell is included in each droplet, and each cell's RNA molecules are labeled with barcodes and ready for sequencing [4].

Some applications of single-cell sequencing include the assessment of cellular diversity, growth processes, disease progress, and nervous system structure.

17.2.1.1 Cellular Diversity

The intrinsic differences among single cells are hidden within the measured representation of cellular communities that conventional mass sequencing offers. Single-cell sequencing reveals formerly undiscovered details by enabling scientists to analyze and comprehend the genetic variations between tissues in a group of cells [3]. By focusing on a single cell to reveal the minute differences that add further to the greater complexity of cellular communities, this method acts as a potent microscope. Through the use of single-cell DNA sequencing, researchers can uncover details about variations in genes that were previously unknown. The method makes it possible to carefully examine and understand minute genomic variations among cells, revealing the complex genetic dynamics underlying cellular diversity. This process gives improved resolution which makes it easier to distinguish between different cell types and reveals the intricate pattern of variability in cells. Single-cell sequencing is especially important in areas like cancer studies, where identifying uncommon cell populations and comprehending their unique genetic characteristics can provide important information about tumor diversity, the course of the disease, and possible targets for therapy. Furthermore, single-cell sequencing enables researchers to investigate tissues at a finer scale, revealing genomic specifics that are crucial to the functions of biological structures and organs. Through analysis of the gene makeup of every single cell within connective tissues, researchers can identify minute differences that could have significant effects on growth, activity, and response of organs to outside stimuli [5, 6].

17.2.1.2 Growth Processes

Single-cell gene sequencing, which captures shifting patterns of transcription and networks of regulation at the single-cell level, is essential for understanding the steps in development. Connective tissue distinctions during embryogenesis and the growth of organs can be assessed with single-cell gene sequencing [3]. Again, single-cell sequencing plays a critical role in comprehending growth activities, and this is especially true for important biological events like bodily growth, tissue differentiation, and the development of embryos. Developing a better understanding of embryogenesis has been made possible partly by single-cell DNA sequencing. Researchers can follow the successive activation of DNA, detect cell and tissue generations, and understand the complex movements of cellular processes that conclude in the creation of a fully grown human being by closely examining the genetic patterns of each cell. This complete knowledge of embryogenesis is a background for future research into inherited diseases.

Scientists can examine the distinct genetic composition that cells possess in developing organs using single-cell gene sequencing, which offers new perspectives on tissue evolution, cell division, and the formation of functional frameworks. This information adds to the knowledge of organ functioning in both disease and health, as well as a basis for the discovery of the genetic signals governing the organogenesis process. The understanding of growth mechanisms provided by single-cell sequencing has implications for potential uses in regenerative medicine and illness. Such knowledge improves our fundamental grasp of biology and also creates opportunities for novel medical treatments and individualized strategies [7].

17.2.1.3 Disease Evaluation

Single-cell sequencing offers a great degree of detail for determining uncommon types of cells, monitoring cloned development, and revealing genetic variation within tumor microenvironment in disorders such as carcinoma. Often during these instances, variability within cells serves an integral part in the development of tumors and resistance to drugs [3]. Single-cell sequencing has proven to give the best results when identifying unusual and rare forms of cells in an infected tissue. Rare populations of cells that are frequently disregarded in large quantities of sequencing could contain essential data about disease subtypes, the possibility of metastasis, and the efficacy of pharmacotherapy. Single-cell sequencing makes it possible to track the growth of clones, providing insight into how particular cell populations change over time, proliferate, or develop resistance to therapy. Implementing tailored treatments that adjust to the disease's changing genetic surroundings will require the use of this technology. This involves working out immune system cell subtypes, comprehending the relationships between various cell populations, and identifying molecular structures that support cancer development and immunity evasion [8].

17.2.1.4 Neurology

Due to the intricacy of the nervous system, every single neuron and glial cell must be thoroughly understood. Single-cell sequencing is useful for connecting brain regions, elucidating the molecular underpinnings of neurological diseases, and revealing the variation within neuronal activity and its subtypes. Beyond its current uses, single-cell sequencing contributes to a better understanding of disease. Precision medicine methods have been rendered viable by the thorough understanding of cellular diversity. Customizing therapy according to the unique genetic composition of each cell has the potential to increase the effectiveness of treatment, reduce undesirable adverse effects, and boost clinical outcomes. This method is especially useful in estimating how genes are linked to specific diseases and locating possible treatment targets. One characteristic of the nervous system is variability found within neurological communities. Single-cell DNA sequencing reveals neuronal function and variants which in turn exhibit wide shifts leading to mental disorders. Scientists can classify distinct types of neurons via particular functions by recording individual gene transcription identities of each neuron. In some brain disorders, single-cell sequencing offers a more accurate approach in identifying precise cell types that are affected by a particular disease. It is anticipated that increased throughput, enhanced sensitivity, as well as the incorporation of multiomics techniques will augment our knowledge of the intricate functioning of the nervous system [9, 10].

17.2.2 High-Throughput Screening Techniques

Illumina NovaSeq and HiSeq series are two notable examples of high-throughput NGS systems, which mark a substantial growth in sequencing innovations. By significantly accelerating the rate and effectiveness of genome sequencing, these technologies have altered genome analysis and have had an enormous effect on several other areas of science. High-throughput processing is important since it enables the rapid creation of large quantities of sequencing information. High-throughput systems can handle several samples in a single run. This can be especially important during large-scale research or population-scale investigations that require comprehensive genome-wide assessment.

Illumina NovaSeq offers adaptability in relation to results and is built for scalability. Its various flow cell arrangements allow researchers to select the right magnitude for the requirements of particular projects. This is especially helpful for research on populations (large genome sequencing numbers) as well as other endeavors that call for comprehensive genome-wide coverage. The system's economical design strikes a compromise between the high costs of sequencing along with information output. This has opened it up to an extensive selection of investigations and educational facilities. NovaSeq is used in medical studies for tasks that need a thorough grasp of genome-wide analysis, such as finding variants linked to disease and researching the underlying genetics of disorders [11–13].

The combination of high throughput and adaptability is provided by the HiSeq series. It is appropriate for a number of investigations since it is capable of handling applications such as targeted sequencing, exome sequencing, and whole-genome sequencing. Large-scale population genome sequencing projects are the focus of the HiSeq X Ten. It additionally makes it possible to sequence many genomes of individuals at once, which aids in the attempt to comprehend genetic diversity. The HiSeq series is used to find mutations in genes linked to a number of diseases, which helps with patient diagnosis and tailored treatment. The HiSeq series is used by universities and other research organizations, including large-scale genome sequencing and fundamental molecular genetic studies. HiSeq series delivers adaptability for particular sequencing requirements, whereas NovaSeq's flexible flow cells as well as flexibility make it appropriate for larger projects. Due to its scalability, NovaSeq focuses on profitability and can be used for a number of project sizes. The decision between HiSeq and NovaSeq is influenced by several variables, including the size of the project, the required DNA sequencing, and financial constraints [14, 15].

Due to high-throughput sequencing's productivity in lowering cost per base, large amounts of genomic information can be accessed. Also, because sequencing is now affordable, academics and organizations can carry out goal-oriented experiments. With the emergence of novel instruments like droplet microfluidics, fluid-controlling structures, fluorescence-activated cell sorting (FACS), and community harvesters, the field of high-throughput screening has expanded significantly. Computerization of high-throughput screening avoids contamination and error by humans; lesser amounts of sample are needed for estimation; tiny portions in milliliters (in microplates) or as little as nanoliters (in drops) must be collected for measurement. Furthermore, labor expenses have been substantially decreased with the adoption of programmed operational systems deploying microplates as well as FACS which yields greater sensitivity and accuracy. New assay techniques have also led to quick and precise examination via detecting deviations associated with a desired metabolite. Both at the cellular and atomic levels, high-throughput screening is firmly established. It blends huge-scale statistical analysis via automated or micro-quantitative testing. Nowadays, high-throughput screening is employed throughout both basic and industrial microbiology, as well as research into biotechnology [16]. Some common clinical utility of high-throughput screening include research into whole genome, and cancer treatment alongside other branches of medicine.

17.2.2.1 Whole-Genome Sequencing

Whole-genome sequencing is especially appropriate for high-throughput channels, which allows for a complete analysis of whole biological composition. This has made it easy to find scarce modifications and alterations linked to certain diseases and to investigate the genomes across populations. Gene-coding or control area mutations can result in similar symptoms, providing the physician with potential answers for a particular ailment. NGS offers medical professionals a quick, economical, and comprehensive method for identifying the etiology of diseases. While it is feasible to sequence the human genome, scientists and medical professionals are usually interested in the areas (exome) that code for proteins. Since the exome only makes up slightly over 1% of the genome, sequencing it will be far less expensive than sequencing the full genome and will yield genome sequence information in the protein-coding zones. In the last few years, genome sequencing has grown and is commonly used throughout gene identification studies. Several investigations into genetic discovery led to an understanding of genomes associated with hereditary skin diseases. When the precise inherited cause of a transmissible appearance is unknown, exome sequencing can help identify gene mutations [17].

17.2.2.2 Medical Applications

High-throughput sequencing is becoming increasingly valuable in hospitals and clinics due to its rapid turnaround duration and affordability. It is employed in cancer treatment alongside other branches of medicine to guide individualized choices regarding therapy and to detect mutations in genes linked to a number of diseases. One of Illumina's flagship systems, NovaSeq, is renowned for its adaptability and flexibility. It is appropriate in a number of applications, including transcriptomics initiatives and whole-genome sequencing, due to its ability to produce enormous volumes of data for each run. Clinical genetic factors experienced a radical change as a result of high-throughput DNA sequencing, which has improved understanding of and capacity to address uncommon diseases in humans. Numerous cases exist where individuals have gained insight through a comprehensive, objective analysis of their genome. Prior to submitting reports, medical information of a patient must be verified. This is a significant burden on a genome-wide stage that can be occasionally mitigated by ranking calls according to call quality and/or pathogenicity. For Mendelian disorders, NGS whole-exome sequencing (WES) provides an evaluation rate of 25%, while whole-genome sequencing (WGS) encounters a marginally higher detection result (27%) for genetic conditions affecting children and adults [18].

Targeted NGS genetic sections, as opposed to WES and WGS, concentrate on portions of genetics, varying in number compared to multiple to thousands, contingent upon the nature of the individual diseases. NGS components have different diagnostic yields; the gestational skeletal abnormalities group has an expected diagnostic yield of 53%, whereas the acquired glycosylation illness group includes an estimated medical yield of about 14.8%. Targeted NGS genetic panels have the capacity to optimize coverage, sensitivity, and precision for genes of concern. Thus, compared to exome sequencing or genome sequencing, targeted NGS frequently yields greater evaluation. Nonetheless, a targeted NGS gene group may have an inferior diagnostic level in cases of high diagnostic unpredictability. Clinical studies come in two varieties: umbrella tests and bucket trials (sometimes referred to as basket tests). A single clinical trial can encompass multiple treatment approaches. Individuals with particular structural tumors are enrolled in an umbrella trial, and a therapy arm is assigned based on the genetic variants found within the cancer. Patients with various cancers who have a common genetic defect will participate in a basket trial to evaluate an experimental drug against the shared genetic mutation. NGS is performed on hundreds of thousands of malignant tumor specimens from individuals to find mutations that might react to particular therapies. Adaptive Biotechnology (Seattle, WA, USA) created the ClonoSEQ exam, an NGS-based test for people with multiple myeloma as well as B-cell leukemia with acute lymphoblastic leukemia, to measure and track minimal residual disease (MRD) [18].

17.2.3 NGS and MultiOmics

The breakthrough of NGS has not just quickened the rate of research in genomics but also has had a significant impact on the incorporation of information from multiple fields, including transcriptomics, metabolomics, and proteomics [19–21]. The advantages that NGS offers for scientists and how it impacts multiomics data are shown in Figure 17.2 and Table 17.1.

NGS-enabled multiomics analysis of data has significant consequences for personalized medicine. Investigators can find molecular fingerprints linked to diseases, forecast patient results, and customize treatments based on individual differences using genomics, transcriptomics, and various other omics data. This tailored strategy reduces side effects while increasing the effectiveness of therapeutic interventions.

NGS-driven multiomics research advances the discipline of system biology by providing a thorough comprehension of the complex nature of biological networks. Researchers can understand complex biological processes, interpret regulatory associations, and determine important mechanisms of signaling via the combination of genetic information with transcriptomics, epigenomics, and other fields.

Robust identification of biomarkers is facilitated by the application of multiomics data via NGS. Scientists can find novel biomarkers for disease identification, forecasting, and adverse drug reactions by establishing correlations between genetic variants, transcription trends, epigenetic alterations, and medical outcomes. This will have important ramifications for early disease assessment as well as monitoring.

The combination of multiomics data results in huge databases that call for sophisticated computing power and statistical analysis. The analysis of these intricate datasets necessitates the use of advanced machine learning techniques, online computing infrastructure, and advanced algorithms, highlighting the significance of mathematical developments in maximizing NGS-driven multiomics studies.

Each omics layer reveals key molecular findings, and their collective integration provides a comprehensive understanding of the intricate landscape of cancer biology. For instance, genomics identifies driver mutations, transcriptomics unveils dynamic gene expression patterns, and epigenomics highlights regulatory modifications. The "integrated insights" section synthesizes these multiomics findings, illustrating how a subset of cancer patients may exhibit specific genomic mutations, altered gene expression profiles, and distinct epigenetic signatures. This integrated approach offers a personalized view of cancer subtypes, fostering implications for prognosis and the development of targeted therapeutic strategies [28–30].

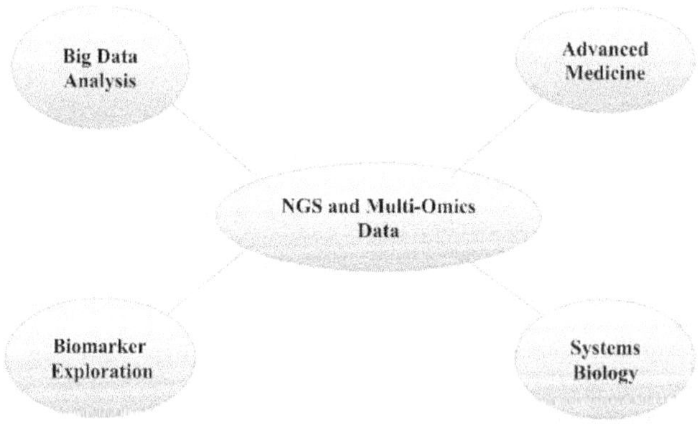

FIGURE 17.2 Advantages of NGS in MultiOmics Data

TABLE 17.1

Integration of genomics, transcriptomics, and epigenomics data in the context of cancer research

Omics layer	Key findings	Relevance to cancer research
Epigenomics	Hypermethylation of tumor suppressor gene promoters and altered histone modifications	Exploring epigenetic modifications influencing gene silencing and activation in cancer cells [22–24]
Genomics	Identification of key driver mutations in oncogenes and tumor suppressor genes	Understanding the genetic basis of cancer initiation and progression [25]
Transcriptomics	Elevated expression of specific oncogenes and dysregulation of tumor suppressor genes	Uncovering the dynamic gene expression patterns contributing to tumor phenotypes [26, 27]
Integrated insights	Identification of a subset of patients with specific genomic mutations, altered gene expression profiles, and distinct epigenetic signatures	Providing a personalized view of cancer subtypes with potential implications for prognosis and targeted therapies [28]

17.2.4 Long-Read Sequencing Technologies

Long-read sequencing (LRS) technologies, often known as third-generation sequencing technologies, have the ability to produce sequences larger than 10 kb straight from native DNA, in contrast to short-read sequencing methods which can produce reads of up to 600 bases. Although short-read sequencing is precise and cost-efficient, sequencing natural nucleic acid polymers which span eight orders of magnitude pose challenges in reconstructing and counting the original molecules. Long reads improve the detection of structural variants, transcript isoform recognition, mapping certainty, and de novo assembly. Moreover, base modifications in both DNA and RNA are preserved while amplification bias is removed using long-read sequencing [31].

Two primary long-read sequencing techniques, single-molecule real-time (SMRT) sequencing by Pacific Biosciences (PacBio), and nanopore sequencing by Oxford Nanopore Technologies Inc. (ONT) are common examples.

17.2.4.1 Single-Molecule Real-Time Sequencing

In this sequencing approach, DNA to be sequenced is a single-stranded circular template known as the SMRTbell template formed by ligating adaptors to the double-stranded DNA. Zero-mode waveguides (ZMW), tiny pores found in "SMRT Cell" chips, are used for sequencing. Each ZMW contains an individual immobilized DNA polymerase molecule that allows the sequencing of a single SMRTbell template. Fluorescent-labeled dNTPs are incorporated into the nascent strand by the polymerase as it processes the SMRTbell template during the sequencing step. The fluorophore is excited by a laser following each incorporation and the emission is captured on camera. The next dNTP is then integrated once the fluorophore has been separated from the nucleotide. The identity and sequence of every base in the template are revealed by repeating this procedure thousands of times [32, 33].

17.2.4.2 Nanopore Sequencing – Oxford Nanopore Technologies Inc.

Rather than circular DNA, the ONT long-read sequencing technique utilizes linear DNA molecules. Nanopore sequencing operates on the fundamental concept of transporting a single DNA strand through a membrane-embedded nanopore. Throughout the procedure, this nanopore, equipped with an attached enzyme, serves as a biosensor. The enzyme associated with the nanopore, which may be a polymerase or helicase, is firmly attached to the polynucleotide, regulating its movement through the pore. Real-time determination of the bases flowing through the pore is achieved by measuring and amplifying changes in the electrical signal across the membrane. ONT single-molecule readings are often longer than 10 kb, but some reads can be ultra-long, exceeding SMRT with lengths of more than 1 Mb [32, 33].

17.2.4.3 Application of Long-Read Sequencing

LRS has the ability to develop into a technology that is utilized to capture important genomic components that are challenging for traditional methods, in addition to producing high-quality genome assemblies (i.e., the platinum human reference genome). New research suggests that LRS technology may be crucial in identifying novel mutations in human disorders [32].

One of the notable areas where LRS technologies have already produced noteworthy outcomes and proven a great deal of clinical promise is cancer genomics. By employing long reads, numerous novel structural variants (SVs) can be found that would otherwise go undetected, such as in genes where other known variations were found to significantly raise the risk of cancer [34]. In one study, SVs in pancreatic cancer cell lines' CDKN2A and SMAD4 tumor suppressor genes were analyzed using MinION LRS [35]. The study identified loss-of-function variations in these tumor suppressor genes, represented by deletions, inversions, translocations, and combinations of inversions, from reads longer than 500 bp. Multilayer analysis of the epigenome and transcriptome is another application of LRS that has demonstrated considerable potential. Since LRS allows for complete coverage of transcript sequences, transcriptomics has profited from its use. Also, full-length complementary DNAs (cDNAs) may be sequenced to identify the structures of transcript isoforms.

In the realm of transplantation, long-read sequencing has shown to be an invaluable tool, especially when it comes to comprehending the intricate interactions between the immune systems of the donor and recipient. Human leukocyte antigen (HLA) typing has become extremely extensive and precise because of the development of PacBio and ONT LRS. LRS has been used to examine the variability of HLA in a cohort of transplant recipients, highlighting the significance of donor-recipient matching and its effect on outcomes following transplantation. Furthermore, the identification of the underlying causes of graft-versus-host disease (GVHD) has been greatly aided by LRS. An adverse effect of transplantation is called GVHD, in which the recipient's tissues are attacked by the donor's immune system.

According to the current research, LRS technology may be crucial in identifying mutations in human diseases that have an unidentified underlying genetic origin. Researchers at Stanford Medical School demonstrated the first LRS of the whole genome in the clinical setting in 2017. They utilized this technology to determine the genetic cause of the uncommon genetic condition known as Carney complex, which is related to multiple endocrine neoplasia syndromes. A 2.2-kb deletion in the PRKAR1 gene was shown to be the causative mutation. SMRT is also being employed to resolve SVs linked to Mendelian diseases. The identification of genetic disorders such as that affecting color vision is another exciting emerging application. The OPN1LW/OPN1MW gene cluster is associated with mild to severe issues affecting color vision.

LRS is finding significant use in the treatment of infectious diseases. LRS via ONT platforms can diagnose infectious pathogens in situ and can yield results in a matter of hours. It is a desirable alternative for supporting a possible quick response for the control and identification of disease causes and transfers. As a result, real-time genomic monitoring of pathogens has emerged as a novel tool to support challenging epidemiological inquiries and offer an environmental framework for newly developing infectious diseases. By using genetic information to investigate transmission networks, this may enhance the effectiveness of resource allocation and the efficiency of epidemiological studies.

17.2.5 Short-Read Sequencing Technologies

Second-generation sequencing, often known as short-read NGS, is the next development in sequencing technology following conventional first-generation Sanger sequencing. Massive sequencing of small (250–800 bp), clonally amplified DNA molecules sequenced in parallel is a frequent characteristic of short-read technology [36].

Clonal amplification and sequencing are the two consecutive components of short-read sequencing. Solid-phase amplification of DNA fragments is used in clonal amplification to provide potent, perceptible signals for sequencing. Single DNA fragments can anchor to flow cell surfaces (Illumina) or beads

(Thermofisher Ion Torrent) as the solid phase. Emulsion PCR (Ion Torrent) or "bridging" PCR (Illumina), depending on the sequencing platform, is employed for amplifying the attached DNA fragments into a million spatially dispersed template fragments. Both Illumina and Ion Torrent platforms work on the "sequencing-by-synthesis (SBS)" approach, which includes nucleotide incorporation on the extended DNA chain in a DNA polymerase-dependent manner [37].

17.2.5.1 Illumina

Illumina's NGS technology utilizes SBS coupled with a fluorescent-labeled reversible terminator method. With a fluorescent-labeled reversible terminator, Lumina's NGS approach builds upon SBS. Clonal amplification (cluster production) of DNA libraries is done before sequencing using "bridge amplification" PCR, which is done on the sequencing flow cell and managed by the sequencing instrument. For every sequencing cycle, a single fluorescently tagged reversible terminator-bound dNTP is inserted into the nucleic acid chain, and the resultant fluorescent signal is visualized. To allow the addition of the subsequently tagged dNTP, the terminator and fluorescent dye are detached from the integrated dNTP. With an error rate of 0.1%, Illumina reversible terminator technology combined with paired-end sequencing makes it the most precise base-by-base sequencing method available [36–38]

17.2.5.2 Ion Torrent

Ion Torrent stands out as the first method to develop semiconductor sequencing without the need for optical sensing. With reads ranging from 200 to 600 bp, this technique offers quick sequencing run durations between 2.5 and 4 hours. On the Ion Torrent platform, clonal amplification is accomplished by emulsion PCR, a bead-based technique using ion sphere particles in a micro-well. This procedure involves ligating adapter sequences to DNA fragments, which are trapped in a droplet of water-in-oil emulsion (micelle) along with a bead that has been covered in complementary adapters, primers, DNA polymerase, and dNTPs. Microwells are used to load micellas onto a semiconductor chip, which is then flooded with unmodified nucleotides in order of sequencing [36–38].

17.2.5.3 Application of Short-Read Sequencing

Across the entire genome, short-read genomic sequencing provides a less biased sampling strategy. This platform makes it easier to analyze both coding and noncoding variants and enables the identification of a broad range of variations that are clinically important. This enhances the detection of SVs like CNVs, copy-neutral events like inversions, and short tandem repeats (STRs), and permits the detection of coding variants in areas that are not sufficiently addressed by exome sequencing [39].

Due to the lack of information on SV population frequencies and a predicted phenotype from novel SVs that affect several genes, determining the potential for pathogenicity of SVs is difficult. Therefore, the present additional utility of short-read sequencing is tempered by different analytical and reporting techniques by clinical labs, despite the ability to capture a wider spectrum of pathogenic variance [39].

The characteristics of the cohort chosen, the quality of previous sequencing, the distinctive features of the phenotype under study, or the analytical methods employed to identify variations are some of the variables that can affect increasing diagnostic yields for short-read genome sequencing, which can differ among studies. Numerous studies have shown that short-read genome sequencing can result in an increase in diagnostic yield (from 5% to 20%) when performed after non-diagnostic ES [39]. For instance, pathogenic variants, involving a noncoding SNV and SVs, were successfully detected by short-read genome sequencing in a cohort of patients with Alagille syndrome that were previously undiagnosed by ES [40]. Diagnostic utility is expected to increase with the use of extensive variant calling pipelines by clinical labs along with larger variant databases, particularly with noncoding variation [39].

17.3 Whole-Genome Sequencing

Whole-genome sequencing has made it possible to analyze the entire genome. It has become an appealing approach for many reasons owing to extraordinary technological advancements and DNA sequencing cost reductions. While it is often associated with sequencing human genomes, its versatile and scalable nature makes it relevant for sequencing other species, such as agriculturally significant livestock, plants, or disease-associated microbes [41]. There are two types of whole-genome sequencing: de novo WGS and whole-genome resequencing (WGR).

17.3.1 De Novo Whole-Genome Sequencing

De novo WGS is the process of sequencing and assembling the complete genome of an organism for the first time. In order to prepare libraries, fragmentation of high-quality genomic DNA is performed which includes adding the sequencing adaptors to the fragments of DNA. In an effort to maximize genome coverage, high-throughput sequencing produces paired-end short reads (about 100 bp) from libraries with different insert sizes. A consensus sequence, which corresponds to a series of continuous scaffolds divided by gaps, is the end result of genome assembly [42].

17.3.2 Whole-Genome Resequencing

Whole-genome resequencing involves the comparison of variable sites among the genomes of individuals or populations. For accurate read mapping, this process necessitates the availability of the species genome sequence. To prepare a library, an individual's high-quality genomic DNA is fragmented with an insert size of around 350–500 bp. Using high-throughput sequencing, paired-end short reads (~100 bp) are extracted from the DNA library. Based on sequence similarity, short reads are mapped onto the reference genome of the species. The final outcome is a file containing the individual's variable sites [42].

17.3.3 Application of WGS

WGS can be used to establish the path of disease transmission within a population and provide information on the potential source. It also makes it easier to quickly and accurately identify the pathogen's virulence components during outbreak analysis. It was impossible to identify the "unique signature" of a deliberately engineered organism until WGS was used in forensics and bioterrorism. For instance, the microbiological characterization of the strains was performed by using WGS during the Amerithrax investigation into the 2001 shipment of anthrax spores. The *Bacillus anthracis* organisms employed in the attack were identified as the laboratory Ames strain after the relevant reference databases were compiled, and the material was further classified as a *Bacillus anthracis* Ames ancestor strain [43].

One of the main tenets of infection control, epidemiological surveillance of bacterial pathogens, has been made possible by the widespread use of WGS as a substitute for conventional bacterial typing. Mapping the epidemiology of multidrug-resistant diseases is essential in the era of rising antimicrobial resistance because it helps guide antibiotic prescribing practices and public health interventions. WGS not only enables the monitoring of resistant organisms but also the tracking of particular resistance mechanisms, such as motifs on mobile genetic components like plasmids and the clarification of gene transfer pathways. Several studies have documented the utilization of WGS to assist in hospital infection control protocols when pathogen transmission is suspected. Using WGS, researchers from the US National Institutes of Health (NIH) tracked a possible outbreak of carbapenem-resistant *Klebsiella pneumoniae* in 2012 and found that three separate transmission episodes were attributed to a single patient [44].

Largely through metagenomic investigations, WGS has been shown to be a helpful tool as a culture-independent technique of bacterial identification. Metagenomics is a technique that has yet to be utilized in regular diagnostics, but it entails sequencing the entire DNA in a clinical sample and then using bioinformatics analysis to separate the DNA of humans and non-pathogenic organisms in order to determine the causative source. Compared to high-diversity samples like feces, metagenomic investigations conducted on low-diversity sterile site samples are expected to offer higher yield due to the vast depth of sequencing necessary for species identification. For this application of WGS, high-quality samples with adequate genomic nucleic acid concentrations such as tissue or fluid aspirates are essential. The identification of new pathogens is another possible use for metagenomics, aside from the human microbiome studies [44].

17.4 Challenges with NGS

Although NGS has made tremendous strides, investigators still face several obstacles that affect the effectiveness and understanding of genomic information. It is important to overcome certain major obstacles that current research organizations face. While increasingly more testing facilities can conduct scRNA-seq experiments, there are still few computational and mathematical pipelines available for unprocessed records. Software applications like 10× Genomics and Fluidigm are offered by certain business entities, but the field is still young, and very few valuable resources have been created [3]. Rapid information processing, continuous transmission of data, and complex bioinformatics can be expensive. Laboratories have to account for the purchase of equipment and local or cloud-based storage, as well as for a significant rise in analysis of data or storage demands. Validating the whole NGS procedure from the extraction of DNA to carrying out analysis is essential. The sensitivity, precision, and consistency must be determined for NGS HLA typing, just like for any other medical lab test. It is important to make sure there are enough samples in the confirmation testing, at least 50 samples for each locus [45]. When NGS and WGS are compared, NGS dominates overall concerning labor expenses, read duration, and error percentage, but WGS which relies on Sanger sequencing remains the industry standard in the context of these metrics. When using information collected by capillary or Illumina, unique NGS methods may generate a variety of inaccuracies including substitutes, Indel (insertion/deletion), AT bias, and GC modifications [46].

Present-day NGS platforms produce a staggering amount of sequence information, including possibly as many as hundreds of millions of small reads (~50–150 bp) per process, owing to the severe decline in the sequencing duration and expenses. This presents significant computational biology problems such as NGS information storage, quality assurance, consistency, construction, and annotation. Currently, NGS platforms produce a staggering amount of sequence information, including possibly as many as hundreds of millions of small reads (~50–150 bp) per process, owing to the severe decline in the sequencing duration and expenses. This presents significant computational biology problems regarding NGS information storage, quality assurance, consistency, construction, and annotation [47].

While sequencing technologies are being developed, they are evolving rapidly and have a relatively brief period of generation. Correction efforts are ongoing, and third-generation DNA sequencing tools featuring actual-time single-molecule sequencing have become accessible. It appears that the fundamental disadvantage of third-generation sequencing platforms' narrow read size along with a high degree of error will soon become the past. While each of the various NGS innovations has benefits and drawbacks of its own, they are all characterized by affordable costs and massive data creation. Pyrosequencing established the primary causality; all the second-generation techniques will eventually be displaced by the rapidly improving current third-generation technological innovations. But when it comes to sequencing technologies, researchers in the biological sciences have a multitude of options [46].

Confidentiality, security of information, and moral challenges become more pressing as genome information grows and is more widely available. Teams conducting research must maneuver through intricate ethical and legal structures to guarantee the conscientious and safe management of genetic data. In numerous investigations, deriving significant insights from intricate genome data continues to be a challenge. It is still difficult to decipher the practical importance of discovered variants, particularly in noncoding sections of the human genome. Connecting genomic information to phenotypic results requires a full grasp of the physiological consequences of detected alterations or variations. Even though NGS has made great strides in multiomics research, information integration issues still exist. Accurate connection of diverse omics data necessitates the use of advanced bioinformatics resources due to their specific features and evidence of change. Creating reliable computer programs and unified techniques are continuing obstacles to maximizing the use of multiomics data.

Bioinformatics methods for data analysis have traditionally been verified for short-read sequencing data; thus, they must be modified for long reads. Furthermore, the cost of using LRS to analyze whole genomes is currently relatively high. Future applications will mostly depend on how much all NGS technologies cost, as well as how quickly short reads (i.e., the ~USD 100 genome) can be produced for even lower costs [26]. Since LRS throughput is extremely sensitive to molecular damage, high-quality, unnicked high molecular weight DNA is necessary for library preparation. To prepare libraries, it is crucial to accurately determine the size of high-molecular-weight DNA. This is because sequencing smaller, rapidly diffusing molecules using LRS technology might result in unequal read lengths because of loading biases. Furthermore, it is evident that proper diploid assembly and the detection of rare pathogenic variants depend on improvements in the read accuracy of specific LRS techniques. [48] The majority of the restrictions related to short-read sequencing are associated with the length of the produced reads. Reads may not be able to be mapped to the exact location in the reference genome because of their short length. In cases where reads cannot be aligned to the reference genome, they might be excluded, resulting in a gap in the sequencing data.

Gigabases of sequences are produced from a single run by the current short-read sequencing-by-synthesis and sequencing-by-ligation sequencing platforms like SoLiD, Ion Torrent, and Illumina. All of these platforms, however, have error rates that provide obstacles for the analysis of downstream bioinformatics. Substitution errors predominate on the Illumina and SoLiD platforms, while insertion/deletion errors predominate on the Ion Torrent platform [49, 50]. WGS data can yield extensive genomic information; however, this does not always translate to understanding transcription and gene expression. For instance, the occurrence of lukSF-PV does not always indicate the production of clinically severe infection with *Staphylococcus aureus* [44]. The absence of validation and utility comparisons in clinical trials is a significant drawback for WGS in clinical laboratories. Clinical efforts have customized sequencing techniques and data analytics around specific diseases, despite the regular publication of proof-of-concept studies [44].

17.5 Conclusion

NGS is an important breakthrough in the rapidly changing field of genomics, providing a new level of understanding of the complexity of a genome. By examining the constantly changing field of NGS, this chapter discussed the current trends and challenges associated with this technology. We explored a number of NGS methods, each advancing the limits of our knowledge and providing distinct advantages. Single-cell sequencing is an excellent demonstration of precision, providing previously unattainable resolution in the analysis of genetic heterogeneity. With this approach, genetic diversity may be thoroughly analyzed at an unparalleled resolution, yielding incredibly precise insights into individual cells. Additionally, scalability proves to be a crucial aspect for high-throughput screening techniques which empower researchers to swiftly analyze the vast datasets, leading to the acceleration of scientific discoveries. While investigating the sequencing technologies, the dichotomy between long-read sequencing and short-read sequencing becomes apparent. Due to long-read sequencing analyzing longer read lengths, a more comprehensive view of the genome is possible. Even so, short-read sequencing continues to be dependable and effective. These technologies continue to be essential in a number of genomic applications due to their rapidity and affordability. Additionally, this chapter highlights the challenges faced by NGS, despite its impressive advancements. Robust and efficient computing tools are necessary for the analysis and interpretation of the massive volume of data gathered. To manage the constantly expanding amount of NGS data and maintain accessibility for clinical and research applications, effective and secure storage solutions are essential. The ethical issues of informed consent, data privacy, and potential discrimination based on genetic information must be carefully considered. As the unresolved challenges are addressed, NGS will surely continue to be essential in deciphering life's complexities and influencing medical advancements.

REFERENCES

1. Satam H, Joshi K, Mangrolia U, Waghoo S, Zaidi G, Rawool S, et al. Next-generation sequencing technology: current trends and advancements. *Biology*. 2023;12(7):997.
2. Park ST, Kim J. Trends in next-generation sequencing and a new era for whole genome sequencing. *Int Neurourol J*. 2016;20(Suppl 2):S76–S83. https://doi.org/10.5213/inj.1632742.371
3. Hwang B, Lee JH, Bang D. Single-cell RNA sequencing technologies and bioinformatics pipelines. *Exp Mol Med*. 2018;50(8):1–14.
4. Jovic D, Liang X, Zeng H, Lin L, Xu F, Luo Y. Single-cell RNA sequencing technologies and applications: a brief overview. *Clin Transl Med*. 2022 Mar;12(3):e694. doi: 10.1002/ctm2.694. PMID: 35352511; PMCID: PMC8964935.
5. Medinger R, Nolte V, Pandey RV, Jost S, Ottenwälder B, Schlötterer C, Boenigk J. Diversity in a hidden world: potential and limitation of next-generation sequencing for surveys of molecular diversity of eukaryotic microorganisms. *Mol Ecol*. 2010;19:32–40.
6. Lavinder JJ, Horton AP, Georgiou G, Ippolito GC. Next-generation sequencing and protein mass spectrometry for the comprehensive analysis of human cellular and serum antibody repertoires. *Curr Opin Chem Biol*. 2015;24:112–20.
7. Ding PN, Becker T, Bray V, Chua W, Ma Y, Xu B, et al. Plasma next generation sequencing and droplet digital PCR-based detection of epidermal growth factor receptor (EGFR) mutations in patients with advanced lung cancer treated with subsequent-line osimertinib. *Thorac Cancer*. 2019;10(10):1879–84.
8. Joensen KG, Engsbro ALØ, Lukjancenko O, Kaas RS, Lund O, Westh H, Aarestrup FM. Evaluating next-generation sequencing for direct clinical diagnostics in diarrhoeal disease. *Eur J Clin Microbiol Infect Dis*. 2017;36:1325–38.
9. Jiang T, Tan MS, Tan L, Yu JT. Application of next-generation sequencing technologies in neurology. *Ann Transl Med*. 2014;2(12):125.
10. Rexach J, Lee H, Martinez-Agosto JA, Németh AH, Fogel BL. Clinical application of next-generation sequencing to the practice of neurology. *Lancet Neurol*. 2019;18(5):492–503.
11. Jeon SA, Park JL, Park SJ, Kim JH, Goh SH, Han JY, Kim SY. Comparison between MGI and Illumina sequencing platforms for whole genome sequencing. *Genes Genomics*. 2021;43:713–24.
12. Modi A, Vai S, Caramelli D, Lari M. The Illumina sequencing protocol and the NovaSeq 6000 system. *Methods Mol Biol*. 2021;2242:15–42.
13. Wu M, Wang Y, Wang Y, Wang X, Yu M, Liu G, Tang H. Study on the diversity of epiphytic bacteria on corn and alfalfa using Illumina MiSeq/NovaSeq high-throughput sequencing system. *Ann Microbiol*. 2021;71(1):1–11.
14. Ravi RK, Walton K, Khosroheidari M. MiSeq: a next generation sequencing platform for genomic analysis. *Methods Mol Biol*. 2018;1706:223–32.
15. Unno T. Bioinformatic suggestions on MiSeq-based microbial community analysis. *J Microbiol Biotechnol*. 2015;25(6):765–70.
16. Putatunda C. Microorganisms form the backbone of the fermentation industry: without a suitable one capable of producing a desired product. *Basic Biotechniques for Bioprocess and Bioentrepreneurship*. 2023 [updated 2023 Feb 27]. Available from: https://www.sciencedirect.com/science/article/abs/pii/B9780128161098000027.
17. Grada A, Weinbrecht K. Next-generation sequencing: methodology and application. *J Investig Dermatol*. 2013;133(8):1–4.
18. Chennagiri N, White EJ, Frieden A, Lopez E, Lieber DS, Nikiforov A, et al. Orthogonal NGS for high throughput clinical diagnostics. *Sci Rep*. 2016;6(1):24650.
19. Zhong Y, Xu F, Wu J, Schubert J, Li MM. Application of next generation sequencing in laboratory medicine. *Ann Lab Med*. 2021;41(1):25–43.
20. Yin Y, Butler C, Zhang Q. Challenges in the application of NGS in the clinical laboratory. *Human Immunol*. 2021;82(11):812–19.
21. Thakur V, Varshney RK. Challenges and strategies for next generation sequencing (NGS) data analysis. *J Comput Sci Syst Biol*. 2010;3(2):40–2.
22. Sandoval J, Esteller M. Cancer epigenomics: beyond genomics. *Curr Opin Genet Dev*. 2012;22(1):50–5.
23. Verma M. The role of epigenomics in the study of cancer biomarkers and in the development of diagnostic tools. *Adv Exp Med Biol*. 2015;867:59–80.

24. Ng HK, Roukos DH, Iacopetta B, Ku CS. Next-generation sequencing in cancer epigenomics and potential clinical applications. In: *Next generation sequencing in cancer research: volume 1: decoding the cancer genome.* Springer, New York. 2013. p. 31–53.
25. Luthra R, Chen H, Roy-Chowdhuri S, Singh RR. Next-generation sequencing in clinical molecular diagnostics of cancer: advantages and challenges. *Cancers.* 2015;7(4):2023–36.
26. Alkhateeb A, Rezaeian I, Singireddy S, Cavallo-Medved D, Porter LA, Rueda L. Transcriptomics signature from next-generation sequencing data reveals new transcriptomic biomarkers related to prostate cancer. *Cancer Informatics.* 2019;18:1176935119835522.
27. Supplitt S, Karpinski P, Sasiadek M, Laczmanska I. Current achievements and applications of transcriptomics in personalized cancer medicine. *Int J Mol Sci.* 2021;22(3):1422.
28. Pettini F, Visibelli A, Cicaloni V, Iovinelli D, Spiga O. Multi-omics model applied to cancer genetics. *Int J Mol Sci.* 2021;22(11):5751.
29. Yoo BC, Kim KH, Woo SM, Myung JK. Clinical multi-omics strategies for the effective cancer management. *J Proteomics.* 2018;188:97–106.
30. Menyhárt O, Győrffy B. Multi-omics approaches in cancer research with applications in tumor subtyping, prognosis, and diagnosis. *Comput Struct Biotechnol J.* 2021;19:949–60.
31. Amarasinghe SL, Su S, Dong X, et al. Opportunities and challenges in long-read sequencing data analysis. *Genome Biol.* 2020;21:30. https://doi.org/10.1186/s13059-020-1935-5
32. Mantere T, Kersten S, Hoischen A. Long-read sequencing emerging in medical genetics. *Front Genet.* 2019;10:426. doi:10.3389/fgene.2019.00426.
33. Logsdon GA, Vollger MR, Eichler EE. Long-read human genome sequencing and its applications. *Nat Rev Genet.* 2020 Oct;21(10):597–614. doi: 10.1038/s41576-020-0236-x.
34. Aganezov S, Goodwin S, Sherman RM, Sedlazeck FJ, Arun G, Bhatia S, et al. Comprehensive analysis of structural variants in breast cancer genomes using single-molecule sequencing. *Genome Res.* 2020;30(9):1258–73.
35. Oehler JB, Wright H, Stark Z, et al. The application of long-read sequencing in clinical settings. *Hum Genomics.* 2023;17:73. https://doi.org/10.1186/s40246-023-00522-3.
36. Hu T, Chitnis N, Monos D, Dinh A. Next-generation sequencing technologies: an overview. *Hum Immunol.* 2021. doi:10.1016/j.humimm.2021.02.012.
37. Slatko BE, Gardner AF, Ausubel FM. Overview of next-generation sequencing technologies. *Curr Protoc Mol Biol.* 2018 Apr;122(1):e59. doi: 10.1002/cpmb.59.
38. Kumar K, Cowley M, Davis R. Next-generation sequencing and emerging technologies. *Semin Thromb Hemost.* 2019. doi:10.1055/s-0039-1688446.
39. Wojcik MH, Reuter CM, Marwaha S, Mahmoud M, Duyzend MH, Barseghyan H, et al. Beyond the exome: what's next in diagnostic testing for Mendelian conditions. *ArXiv Preprint.* 2023 Jan 18:arXiv:2301.07363v1. Update in *Am J Hum Genet.* 2023 Aug 3;110(8):1229–48.
40. Rajagopalan R, Gilbert MA, McEldrew DA, Nassur JA, Loomes KM, Piccoli DA, et al. Genome sequencing increases diagnostic yield in clinically diagnosed Alagille syndrome patients with previously negative test results. *Genet Med.* 2021 Feb;23(2):323–30. doi: 10.1038/s41436-020-00989-8.
41. Chrystoja CC, Diamandis EP. Whole genome sequencing as a diagnostic test: challenges and opportunities. *Clin Chem.* 2014 May;60(5):724–33.
42. Fuentes-Pardo AP, Ruzzante DE. Whole-genome sequencing approaches for conservation biology: advantages, limitations and practical recommendations. *Mol Ecol.* 2017;26:5369–406.
43. Gilchrist CA, Turner SD, Riley MF, Petri WA, Hewlett EL. Whole-genome sequencing in outbreak analysis. *Clin Microbiol Rev.* 2015;28:1–36.
44. Kwong JC, McCallum N, Sintchenko V, Howden BP. Whole genome sequencing in clinical and public health microbiology. *Pathology.* 2015;47(3):199–210. doi:10.1097/PAT.0000000000000235.
45. Yin Y, Butler C, Zhang Q. Challenges in the application of NGS in the clinical laboratory. *Hum Immunol.* 2021;82(11):812–19.
46. Ambardar S, Gupta R, Trakroo D, Lal R, Vakhlu J. High throughput sequencing: an overview of sequencing chemistry. *Indian J Microbiol.* 2016;56:394–404.

47. Lavinder JJ, Horton AP, Georgiou G, Ippolito GC. Next-generation sequencing and protein mass spectrometry for the comprehensive analysis of human cellular and serum antibody repertoires. *Curr Opin Chem Biol.* 2015;24:112–20.
48. Warburton PE, Sebra RP. Long-read DNA sequencing: recent advances and remaining challenges. *Annu Rev Genom Hum Genet.* 2023;24:1–30.
49. Glenn TC. Field guide to next-generation DNA sequencers. *Mol Ecol Resour.* 2011;11(5):759–69.
50. Góngora-Castillo E, Buell CR. Bioinformatics challenges in de novo transcriptome assembly using short read sequences in the absence of a reference genome sequence. *Nat Prod Rep.* 2013;30(4):490–500.

18

Nanomedicine: Current Trends and Future Perspectives

Funmilola Adesodun Fisusi and Mansa Fredua-Agyeman

18.1 Nanomedicine

Nanomedicine can be defined broadly as the application of nanostructured materials in the prevention, diagnosis, treatment, and evaluation or monitoring of diseases and disease progression [1]. Although the definition of nanomedicine may appear intuitive, different authorities have different definitions for the term [2]. The British Society for Nanomedicine adopts a simple definition of nanomedicine as the application of nanotechnologies in a healthcare setting [3], while other bodies use more detailed or integrative definitions. For example, The European Science Foundation (ESF) defines the field of nanomedicine as "the science and technology of diagnosing, treating, and preventing disease and traumatic injury, of relieving pain, and of preserving and improving human health, using molecular tools and molecular knowledge of the human body". They describe the end goal of nanoscience as the achievement of medical benefits by applying engineered devices and nanostructures [4]. Another definition according to the National Institutes of Health (NIH) Roadmap for Medical Research describes nanomedicine as an offshoot of nanotechnology and that it is "highly specific medical intervention at the molecular level for curing disease or repairing damaged tissues, such as bone, muscle, or nerve" [5]. Although different organizations or authorities proffer different definitions for nanomedicine, they all acknowledge that it involves the application of nanomaterials in healthcare delivery.

18.2 Nanomaterials and Nanomedicine

Nanomedicine involves using nanomaterials or nanoparticles in healthcare delivery to produce the desired diagnostic, preventive, or therapeutic outcomes [3–5]. Nanomaterials are defined as "materials having at least one characteristic length scale in the range 1–100 nm, with at least one property being considerably different from that of the bulk counterpart as a result of the nanoscale dimensions" [6]. The application of nanomaterials in healthcare delivery is due to their possession of unique properties different from those of higher-size scale materials, and their higher surface area owing to their small size [7–9]. Nanomaterials form the mainstay of nanomedicine as they provide the platform for delivering the desired outcomes. Different types of nanomaterials have been employed in nanomedicine as therapeutic, diagnostic, or imaging/monitoring agents or delivery vehicles [9, 10]. These nanomaterials can be fabricated into nanostructures of varying length, shape, and surface characteristics to suit the desired purpose [9, 11]. The unique properties of nanostructure-based medicines (nanomedicines) aid in their use in the delivery of therapeutic agents. These include improved solubility and stability of loaded agents [12, 13], reduction in administered dose and dosing frequency, improved toxicity profile [12], and improved

DOI: 10.1201/9781003486909-18

pharmacokinetic profile [14]. They also provide the potential for functionalization with multiple ligands for enhanced transport and site-specific delivery [9]. Additionally, they offer the ability to incorporate and deliver comparatively large payload and for loading different classes of therapeutic and/or diagnostic agents into the same nanomedicine system, which can facilitate combination therapy [15]. These beneficial features of nanomedicines make them particularly useful in precision medicine as they can provide a platform for tailoring therapy to the patient's specific medical needs [16].

18.3 Clinical Utility in Nanomedicines

Although the use of nanomedicines in healthcare delivery is still an emerging area compared to conventional methods, it has shown considerable promise [17]. This is because nanomedicine has the potential of replicating Paul Erlich's magic bullet concept, that is, achieving optimum therapeutic outcomes by selectively producing toxic effects against disease-causing agents without harming humans [18, 19]. Therapeutics-loaded nanomedicines can be engineered to travel to and interact maximally with targets and release their payload exclusively at the desired site of action. These features can be achieved through surface functionalization with targeting ligands [20] and stimulus-responsive design, respectively [21]. Aside application of nanomedicines in the delivery of therapeutic molecules in disease treatment, they can also be used for the delivery of diagnostic materials [22] and for the co-delivery of both diagnostic and therapeutic molecules, simultaneously [23].

18.4 Nanomedicines in Targeted Delivery

One of the most important benefits of nanomedicines is their ability to achieve site-specific targeted drug delivery. This enables the nanomedicine to deliver its payload to the desired sites of action with minimal effect on other or surrounding areas [9, 17, 24]. Furthermore, the use of nanomedicines ensures maximum concentration of the loaded therapeutic agent at the site of action, thereby increasing efficacy and reducing off-target effects and toxicities [12, 24]. Targeted therapy using nanomedicines can be achieved by one of two strategies: passive targeting or active targeting (Figure 18.1).

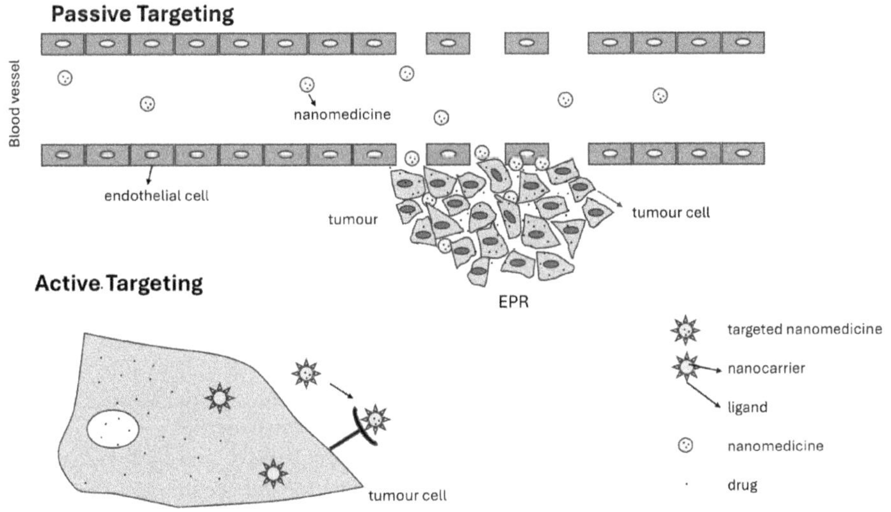

FIGURE 18.1 Strategies for targeted therapy at a tumor site using nanomedicines.

18.4.1 Passive Targeting of Nanomedicines

Passive targeting is the preferential accumulation of nanoparticles at sites of solid tumors [24, 25]. This is due to the enhanced permeability and retention (EPR) effect in solid tumors. This refers to the increased accumulation of the nanoparticles at the tumor site arising from rapid and "unorganized" angiogenesis which leads to defective (leaky) vasculature and poor lymphatic drainage [24–26]. The EPR effect results in vasculature with gaps up to 1μm in size, which can then permit the accumulation of nanoparticles [25 –27]. This provides an advantage over small-molecule agents which would not be retained in similar fashion but are more rapidly cleared from tumor sites [27]. Thus, passive targeting may provide an avenue for nanomedicines to deliver their payload to desired sites of action. Studies have demonstrated the application of passive targeting of nanomedicines for the efficient delivery of therapeutic agents to various tumor sites [28–31]. The EPR effect is also a feature of atherosclerosis, a chronic inflammatory disease of arterial walls, arising from disproportionate lipid levels in circulation. Atherosclerosis is also characterized by greater permeability of the vasculature which may be exploited for delivery of therapeutic agents using nanomedicines [24, 32–34].

Despite the seemingly obvious rationale for using passively targeted nanomedicines, this strategy does not always translate to the expected outcomes. This is due in part to the intra and inter-tumor heterogeneity, such as differences in the extent of disruption in the vasculature and perfusion and tumor micro and macro environment. A major limitation in the clinical translation of passively targeted nanomedicines is that preclinical animal tumor models do not possess the same features as human tumors. This makes it challenging to obtain the same level of success achieved in animal models in humans [25].

18.4.2 Active Targeting of Nanomedicines

Active targeting refers to the use of ligands (targeting ligands) to modify the surface of nanomedicines such that they can recognize specific disease targets. These may be used for targeting cell-surface proteins, receptors, cell features, or microenvironment changes that are disease-specific and absent in non-diseased cells or tissues. Targeting ligands may also be used to facilitate transport to the desired disease sites via endogenous transport systems [35, 36]. Actively targeted nanomedicines would still require the EPR effect to accumulate at disease sites, characterized by defective vasculature and lymphatic drainage. However, once present at the sites, cell recognition and uptake are facilitated by the targeting ligand [25, 36]. This enhances the therapeutic efficacy of the nanomedicines and reduces non-specific interaction with surrounding areas [27, 36]. Targeting ligands for nanomedicines include peptides, proteins, antibodies, sugars, vitamins, and nucleic acids, among others [26, 27].

18.5 Therapeutic Nanomedicines

The first therapeutic nanomedicine to be introduced into clinical practice was a stealth nanoliposome formulation of doxorubicin hydrochloride (Doxil®, Janssen) that received approval from the Food and Drug Administration (FDA) in 1995 [37–39]. This was more than 30 years after the discovery of liposomes – in 1964 [40]. Since the approval of Doxil®, several other nanomedicines have been approved, with scores at various stages of clinical development [37–39]. Most of these formulations have been developed for cancer therapy (more than 50%) and infections (about 14%), others have been developed for blood disorders, metabolic and endocrine diseases (about 9%), nervous system and mental disorders (about 5%), and cardiovascular diseases about (5%), among others. These formulations comprise different types of nanostructures such as liposomes and other lipid-based nanoparticles (33%), polymer-based nanoparticles (20%), antibody-drug conjugates (15%), nanocrystals (9%), and inorganic nanoparticles (3%). Other types include dendrimers, protein-based nanoparticles, viral vectors, and micelles [39].

18.6 Diagnostic Nanomedicines

Nanomedicines have applications as diagnostic agents (nanodiagnostics) to facilitate more sensitive and reliable detection and monitoring of disease progression and treatment efficacy [41]. Nanodiagnostics may be based on a number of nanomaterials and may be contrast agent-loaded or labeled nanomaterials or the nanomaterials themselves may serve as the diagnostic agents [42]. They are useful in facilitating the diagnosis of diseases such as cancers and atherosclerosis using magnetic resonance imaging (MRI) techniques to produce high-resolution images [22, 41, 43]. They can also be used for diagnosis of infectious diseases such as the coronavirus disease 2019 (COVID-19) [44, 45]. The concept of nanodiagnostics is not entirely new, as they have been used clinically for more than six decades [42]. Historic use of nanodiagnostics includes the use of colloidal sulfur radioisotopes such as Technetium-99m (^{99m}Tc) radiolabeled sulfur for planar scintigraphy and later for single-photon emission computed tomography (SPECT) imaging in the mid-1960s [46, 47]. Additionally, the use of gold nanoparticles for pregnancy tests since 1980 [47]. These nanoparticles are clinically used in present times. The former is used for lymphatic flow and identifying sentinel lymph nodes in tumors while the latter is used in influenza and COVID-19 rapid antigen tests [42].

Nanodiagnostics continue to have great potential in clinical application for early, highly sensitive and accurate disease diagnosis [48]. This is evidenced by the plethora of nanodiagnostics either already developed or at different stages of development for clinical applications [46, 49]. Due to the unique features associated with their nanoscale size, their application cuts across both anatomical and molecular imaging techniques [46, 49]. Nanodiagnostics provide certain benefits such as intense, stable, and reliable imaging signals and capabilities for site-specific targeting. Their benefits also include multimodal use (for different imaging techniques), multiplexing (detection of different molecular targets), and a high degree of interaction at the target site due to a large association constant arising from having multiple ligands per particle [49]. In addition, they are also amenable to being designed as theranostic agents, providing a platform for simultaneous use as diagnostic and therapeutic nanomedicines [41, 46, 49]. Ideal nanodiagnostics should be highly sensitive for early disease detection when only minimal changes have occurred. They should be highly specific, tunable for precision and personalized applications, and cost-effective [50].

Nanodiagnostics as with other nanomedicines has high potential for application in the setting of cancer and inflammatory diseases, which feature leaky vasculature and defective lymphatic drainage, thus benefiting from the EPR effect for facilitation of effective accumulation of nanoparticles [41, 49]. Although there have been many studies in the clinical development of potential nanodiagnostics, a relatively small number of these have been approved for clinical use [41, 46], and some have been discontinued or withdrawn [22]. This is not unconnected with the strict requirements for the pharmacokinetics of contrast agents such as rapid contrast enhancement and elimination after administration, which most preclinically used nanodiagnostics would not fulfill due to their slower accumulation and elimination patterns. Moreover, the toxicity and elimination patterns of many nanodiagnostics have not been clearly elucidated [41, 42, 50].

Various nanodiagnostics have been developed for clinical application. These can be carrier-facilitated agents such as radionuclides or contrast agent-loaded nanoparticles which require a carrier system such as organic nanoparticles (liposomes, dendrimers, micelles, or polymeric nanoparticles) for their delivery. Other types of nanodiagnostics such as inorganic nanoparticles serve as contrast agents due to their inherent molecular properties such as optical or magnetic. Examples include metallic and superparamagnetic nanoparticles [41, 46, 50].

18.6.1 Radionuclide Nanodiagnostics

Colloidal radioisotopes comprising Technetium-99m (^{99m}Tc) radiolabeled sulfur were the first clinically applied nanodiagnostics. These were used for planar scintigraphy and subsequently for SPECT imaging [46, 47]. Radioisotope nanodiagnostics find application in SPECT or positron emission tomography (PET). These imaging techniques provide advantages such as high sensitivity and specificity, accurate quantification, and greater tissue penetration over other techniques [11]. In current clinical practice, sulfur colloid ^{99m}Tc is the most frequently used colloidal radioisotope in the United States while albumin colloidal radioisotopes are favored in Europe because they produce higher labeling yield and smaller mean particle size [46, 49]. Stannous fluoride colloid radioisotopes (^{99m}Tc-SnF$_2$) have also been used, with others such as tin, rhenium, and polyvinylpyrrolidone carriers used to a much lesser extent [49]. Sulfur colloids have been used in the imaging algorithm for the staging of breast cancer and melanoma. However, they can also be used for other cancers such as prostate, cervical, and oral cavity cancers. They are used for the identification of sentinel lymph nodes and thus guide surgical interventions. For instance, subcutaneous injection (‹1 mL) of ^{99m}Tc-sulfur colloid nanoparticles near the breast tumor would help to identify affected lymph nodes to guide surgical removal. This would enable conservative rather than aggressive lymph node removals which can potentially lead to serious complications such as lymphoedema, which negatively impacts patients' quality of life.

Additionally, intravenous injection of colloids can be used for the evaluation of organs such as the liver, spleen, and bone marrow [46, 49, 51]. Stannous fluoride colloid radioisotopes can be applied in the assessment of infection and inflammation by using radiolabeled patients' leukocytes. Once injected back into the patients, the radiolabelled leukocytes (still intact and functional) would migrate to infection or inflammation sites for immune or inflammatory response, thereby producing a signal that can be recorded by SPECT. In addition, ^{99m}Tc-SnF$_2$ can also be used for distinguishing between inflammatory bowel disease and irritable bowel disease [49]. Furthermore, other radiolabeled nanoparticle systems such as liposomes, polymeric nanoparticles, dendrimers, metallic nanoparticles, and micelles have been developed for application as nanodiagnostics [11, 52, 53].

18.6.2 Carrier-Facilitated Nanodiagnostics

MRI is recognized as one of the most clinically useful diagnostic imaging techniques because it is non-invasive, generates high-resolution images, and does not involve the use of ionizing radiation [22, 54]. MRI techniques are used in applications such as cell tracking, investigation of perfusion, determining blood volume, capillary leakage, and for the detection of lymph node metastases [55, 56]. Contrast agents are used in MRI to enhance sensitivity and improve image resolution [22, 55]. These can be T_1 (positive) contrast agents such as gadolinium-based agents, which produce brighter MRI by accelerating longitudinal relaxation of protons. Alternatively, they can be T_2 (negative) contrast agents which shorten the protons' transverse relaxation time and produce darker images [54, 57]. Gadolinium-based contrast agents are the most clinically used MRI contrast agents [54].

While these agents have proven very useful in enhancing image quality, they suffer from drawbacks such as short duration of vascular enhancement caused by short residence time in the intravascular space and rapid blood clearance. Hence the need for development of agents with longer residence time in the intravascular space without extravasation into the interstitium. This can be achieved with the use of macromolecules which would not readily traverse into the extracellular space due to their size [54, 55]. In addition to adequate retention in the intravascular space and a suitable pharmacokinetic profile, a contrast agent should show high relaxivity for optimum performance [55, 58, 59]. Thus, various nanoparticle formulations of contrast agents have been developed including dendrimers [55] polymeric nanoparticles [58], nanoassembled capsules [59], micelles [60], and liposomes [61]. An example of a clinically used carrier-facilitated nanodiagnostic agent is Gadomer-17, which is a dendritic gadolinium (Gd) chelate bearing 24 Gd ions [55].

18.6.3 Metallic Nanodiagnostics

These are nanodiagnostics based on metal or metal oxides including nanoparticles of gold, silver, palladium, copper oxide, zinc oxide, and iron oxide, among others [62]. Advances in the development of various nanoparticles have produced nanodiagnostics, which play an important role in much-needed early disease diagnosis through molecular recognition of pathological markers in settings of various cancers and infections [62]. These nanoparticles can also be co-fabricated with other types of nanomaterials such as liposomes, proteins, polymers, or lipids to enhance molecular recognition, hence extending their diagnostic capabilities [63].

Gold nanoparticles have been used by many researchers as nanodiagnostics. This is due to the unique optical (localized surface plasmon resonance), electronic, and physicochemical properties of gold nanoparticles. They also exhibit tunability for shape and size, and ease of fabrication and functionalization [63–65]. Gold nanoparticles are important in point-of-care diagnosis and have been used in pregnancy test strips since the 1980s [47, 66, 67]. They also have applications in other diagnostic platforms including dark field microscopy, MRI, computed tomography, SPECT, and fluorescence imaging [63]. The localized surface plasmon resonance feature of gold nanoparticles has been particularly useful in the development of simple colorimetric tests [63, 65]. The size-dependent color changes following controlled aggregation have been used in different applications such as pregnancy tests, and the detection of various analytes and genes of interest [65]. Gold nanoparticles have also been developed for application in early cancer diagnosis [64, 68] and important point-of-care diagnostics such as biosensors for rapid detection of infections including COVID-19 [69–71]. Gold nanoparticles are recognized as one of those that hold the most promise in colorimetric analysis in terms of speed, simplicity, sensitivity, and cost-effectiveness [63]. They can also be combined with other materials [70] and surface functionalized using target-specific molecules for enhanced performance [63].

18.6.4 Superparamagnetic Nanodiagnostics

Magnetic nanoparticles such as iron oxide nanoparticles: superparamagnetic iron oxide (SPION) have found clinical application in imaging techniques like MRI due to their distinctive superparamagnetic properties [22, 72, 73]. They provide a very promising nano-platform for various applications because they are easy to synthesize, biocompatible, and amenable to surface functionalization and multifunctionality [73]. The SPIONs usually comprise iron oxide in the form of magnetite (Fe_3O_4) or maghemite (γ-Fe_2O_3) [73, 74]. SPIONs (20–150 nm diameter) are notable as T_2 contrast agents for MRI [22, 54]; however, more recently, it has been demonstrated that ultrasmall SPIONs (˂5 nm diameter) are excellent biocompatible T_1 contrast agents [54, 57]. The performance of SPIONs can be enhanced by surface coating with polymers such as polyethylene glycol [75], chitosan or chitosan derivatives [22, 73], dextran [76], polyvinyl alcohol, or polyvinyl pyrrolidone [73]. Despite the seeming potential of SPIONs, many previously used formulations have been discontinued or withdrawn [22, 73, 76] owing to safety and other concerns [73, 76]. Thus, there still exists a need for the development of safe and effective formulations for clinical use [76].

18.7 Theranostic Nanomedicines

Theranostic nanomedicines (nanotheranostics) are nanoparticle formulations that contain diagnostic and therapeutic payload. Nanotheranostics provides a platform for simultaneous disease detection/screening, treatment, and monitoring. This includes assessment of biodistribution, accumulation, and drug release at the desired site of action [41, 77–79]. They may be used to deliver a payload comprising any required combination of diagnostic agent(s), chemo/immune/gene therapeutic agent(s) and may be functionalized with the desired targeting ligands [77, 80]. Nanotheranostics offer the opportunity for timely assessment of the progress or otherwise achieved with therapeutic interventions, since the state of the disease can be monitored [80].

Perhaps the most important benefit of nanotheranostics is the bespoke potential for precision medicine applications as they can be tailored to suit specific patient population needs [80–82]. A great deal of research has been put into the development of various nano-platforms for application as theranostic nanomedicines including liposomes, micelles, polymeric nanoparticles, dendrimers, and inorganic nanoparticles [23, 80, 81]. These have been developed mostly for the therapy of different cancers including gastrointestinal [83, 84], breast [85, 86], brain [79, 87], and lung cancers [88, 89] and for cardiovascular diseases [90, 91].

18.8 Future Perspectives: Nanomedicines in Precision Medicine

According to the FDA, "precision medicine, sometimes referred to as personalized medicine is an innovative approach to tailoring disease prevention and treatment that takes into account differences in people's genes, environments, and lifestyles". Thus, the overall aim of precision medicine is to tailor the right treatments to the right patients at the right time [92]. This is very different from the approach of conventional medical treatment that relies on the use of medicines designed for the general population, assuming that "one-size-fits-all" [92–95]. Although the conventional approach works for some patients and has been the mainstay of medical diagnosis and treatment for decades, it is fraught with issues such as incidences of adverse reactions, treatment failures, and suboptimal outcomes in some patients [92, 95]. With the advent and continued development of precision medicine, it would be possible to design tailored preventive, diagnostic, and therapeutic management plans especially suited to patients and devoid of unwanted events [93]. Optimal therapeutic outcomes involve providing maximum therapeutic benefit to patients with little or no adverse effects. This desired outcome cannot be delivered by conventional therapies because of the generalized approach that is the main feature of such treatment strategies.

Precision medicine, which takes patient-specific factors into account to provide the most suitable options for patients has the potential to deliver desirable outcomes [94]. The unique features of nanomedicines place them in a pivotal position to facilitate precision medicine [82]. Specific advantages of nanomedicines over conventional medicines which provide the necessary platform for optimal outcomes in precision medicine include the potential to overcome challenges posed by physicochemical properties of drugs such as poor aqueous solubility and stability [12, 13]; the ability to alter pharmacokinetic and pharmacodynamic profile of drugs like half-life and toxicity profiles, respectively [12, 14]; ability to carry and deliver payload comprising different types of substances [15]; ability for modified and tunable release of payload; ability for surface functionalization and site-specific targeting [9, 79]. With the recent developments in theranostic nanomedicines, the "dream" of achieving precision or personalized medicine appears to be materializing. This is because this class of nanomedicines can be tailored to deliver the specific preventive and/or diagnostic plus therapeutic requirements for patients by using patient-specific characteristics [96]. Since these nanomedicines combine both diagnostic/monitoring (such as imaging) functionality with therapeutic capability, they provide a platform for simultaneous monitoring of disease and performance of the administered medicines. This would make it possible to continually review and adjust treatment modalities based on the progress/otherwise produced and adjust until desired optimum outcomes are achieved. Theranostic nanomedicines would play a very important role in realizing the goals of personalized medicine [82, 96].

18.9 Conclusion

Nanomedicine and precision medicine are emerging areas in the medical sciences. Although conventional therapy has been very useful and enjoyed great success in the past, it has since become imperative that there are certain limitations to this practice. Recent developments have brought about breakthroughs in medical research enabling technology for improved medical interventions. Areas such as precision medicine, nanotechnology, and improved diagnostic and treatment options have all taken medical care to a new height, which makes the future of medicine bright. Thus, personalized medicines can be envisioned to be actively targeted nanotheranostic formulations bearing multiple agents serving diverse/different (diagnostic, therapeutic, and prophylactic) purposes in disease management. Moreso, agents with different therapeutic modalities including genetic material, chemotherapeutic, and immunotherapeutic drugs can be incorporated within a single formulation.

REFERENCES

1. Soares S, Sousa J, Pais A, Vitorino C. Nanomedicine: principles, properties, and regulatory issues. *Front Chem.* 2018;6:360 .

2. Webster TJ. Nanomedicine: what's in a definition? *Int J Nanomedicine.* 2006;1(2):115–6.
3. Nanomedicine TBSf. *What is nanotechnology and what is nanomedicine?* The British Society for Nanomedicine; 2024. Available from: https://www.britishsocietynanomedicine.org/what-is-nanomedicine/.
4. European Science F, European Medical Research C. *Nanomedicine: an ESF-European Medical Research Councils (EMRC) forward look report.* Strasbourg: ESF; 2005. Available from: http://www.nanopharmaceuticals.org/files/nanomedicine.pdf.
5. Kantor LW. NIH Roadmap for medical research. *Alcohol Res Health.* 2008;31(1):12–13.
6. de Mello Donegá C. The nanoscience paradigm: "size matters!". In: de Mello Donegá C, editor. *Nanoparticles: workhorses of nanoscience.* Berlin, Heidelberg: Springer Berlin Heidelberg; 2014. p. 1–12.
7. Joudeh N, Linke D. Nanoparticle classification, physicochemical properties, characterization, and applications: a comprehensive review for biologists. *J Nanobiotechnol.* 2022;20(1):262.
8. Altammar KA. A Review on nanoparticles: characteristics, synthesis, applications, and challenges. *Front Microbiol.* 2023;14:1155622.
9. Zhu W, Wei Z, Han C, Weng X. Nanomaterials as promising theranostic tools in nanomedicine and their applications in clinical disease diagnosis and treatment. *Nanomaterials (Basel).* 2021;11(12):3346.
10. Khan MA, Singh D, Ahmad A, Siddique HR. Revisiting inorganic nanoparticles as promising therapeutic agents: a paradigm shift in oncological theranostics. *Eur J Pharm Sci.* 2021;164:105892.
11. de Barros AB, Tsourkas A, Saboury B, Cardoso VN, Alavi A. Emerging role of radiolabeled nanoparticles as an effective diagnostic technique. *EJNMMI Res.* 2012;2(1):39.
12. Su H, Wang Y, Gu Y, Bowman L, Zhao J, Ding M. Potential applications and human biosafety of nanomaterials used in nanomedicine. *J Appl Toxicol.* 2018;38(1):3–24.
13. Mitchell MJ, Billingsley MM, Haley RM, Wechsler ME, Peppas NA, Langer R. Engineering precision nanoparticles for drug delivery. *Nat Rev Drug Discov.* 2021;20(2):101–24.
14. Yuan D, He H, Wu Y, Fan J, Cao Y. Physiologically based pharmacokinetic modeling of nanoparticles. *J Pharm Sci.* 2019;108(1):58–72.
15. Chen D, Liu X, Lu X, Tian J. Nanoparticle drug delivery systems for synergistic delivery of tumor therapy. *Front Pharmacol.* 2023;14:1111991.
16. Alghamdi MA, Fallica AN, Virzì N, Kesharwani P, Pittalà V, Greish K. The promise of nanotechnology in personalized medicine. *J Pers Med.* 2022;12(5):673.
17. Patra JK, Das G, Fraceto LF, Campos EVR, Rodriguez-Torres MdP, Acosta-Torres LS, et al. Nano based drug delivery systems: recent developments and future prospects. *J Nanobiotechnol.* 2018;16(1):71.
18. Winau F, Westphal O, Winau R. Paul Ehrlich — in search of the magic bullet. *Microbes Infect.* 2004;6(8):786–9.
19. Williams KJ. The introduction of 'chemotherapy' using arsphenamine - the first magic bullet. *J R Soc Med.* 2009;102(8):343–8.
20. Majumder J, Taratula O, Minko T. Nanocarrier-based systems for targeted and site specific therapeutic delivery. *Adv Drug Deliv Rev.* 2019;144:57–77.
21. Pham SH, Choi Y, Choi J. Stimuli-responsive nanomaterials for application in antitumor therapy and drug delivery. *Pharmaceutics.* 2020;12(7):630.
22. Hobson NJ, Weng X, Siow B, Veiga C, Ashford M, Thanh NT, et al. Clustering superparamagnetic iron oxide nanoparticles produces organ-targeted high-contrast magnetic resonance images. *Nanomedicine (Lond).* 2019;14(9):1135–52.
23. Xue Y, Gao Y, Meng F, Luo L. Recent progress of nanotechnology-based theranostic systems in cancer treatments. *Cancer Biol Med.* 2021;18(2):336–51.
24. Narum SM, Le T, Le DP, Lee JC, Donahue ND, Yang W, et al. Chapter 4 - Passive targeting in nanomedicine: fundamental concepts, body interactions, and clinical potential. In: Chung EJ, Leon L, Rinaldi C, editors. *Nanoparticles for Biomedical Applications.* Elsevier; 2020. p. 37–53.
25. Ejigah V, Owoseni O, Bataille-Backer P, Ogundipe OD, Fisusi FA, Adesina SK. Approaches to improve macromolecule and nanoparticle accumulation in the tumor microenvironment by the enhanced permeability and retention effect. *Polymers (Basel).* 2022;14(13):2601.
26. Veiga N, Diesendruck Y, Peer D. Targeted nanomedicine: lessons learned and future directions. *J Control Release.* 2023;355:446–57.

27. Attia MF, Anton N, Wallyn J, Omran Z, Vandamme TF. An overview of active and passive targeting strategies to improve the nanocarriers efficiency to tumour sites. *J Pharm Pharmacol.* 2019;71(8):1185–98.
28. Wohlfart S, Khalansky AS, Gelperina S, Maksimenko O, Bernreuther C, Glatzel M, et al. Efficient chemotherapy of rat glioblastoma using doxorubicin-loaded PLGA nanoparticles with different stabilizers. *PLoS One.* 2011;6(5):e19121.
29. Qian L, Zheng J, Wang K, Tang Y, Zhang X, Zhang H, et al. Cationic core-shell nanoparticles with carmustine contained within O^6-benzylguanine shell for glioma therapy. *Biomaterials.* 2013;34(35):8968–78.
30. Fisusi FA, Siew A, Chooi KW, Okubanjo O, Garrett N, Lalatsa K, et al. Lomustine nanoparticles enable both bone marrow sparing and high brain drug levels - a strategy for brain cancer treatments. *Pharm Res.* 2016;33(5):1289–303.
31. Abd Kadir E, Uchegbu IF, Schätzlein AG. High-Capacity glycol chitosan-based nanoemulsion for efficient delivery of disulfiram. *Int J Pharm.* 2023;640:123036.
32. Perera B, Wu Y, Nguyen NT, Ta HT. Advances in drug delivery to atherosclerosis: investigating the efficiency of different nanomaterials employed for different types of drugs. *Mater Today Bio.* 2023;22:100767.
33. Kim Y, Lobatto ME, Kawahara T, Lee Chung B, Mieszawska AJ, Sanchez-Gaytan BL, et al. Probing nanoparticle translocation across the permeable endothelium in experimental atherosclerosis. *Proc Natl Acad Sci U S A.* 2014;111(3):1078–83.
34. Barua S, Mitragotri S. Challenges associated with penetration of nanoparticles across cell and tissue barriers: a review of current status and future prospects. *Nano Today.* 2014;9(2):223–43.
35. Clemons TD, Singh R, Sorolla A, Chaudhari N, Hubbard A, Iyer KS. Distinction between active and passive targeting of nanoparticles dictate their overall therapeutic efficacy. *Langmuir.* 2018;34(50):15343–9.
36. Pérez-Herrero E, Fernández-Medarde A. Advanced targeted therapies in cancer: drug nanocarriers, the future of chemotherapy. *Eur J Pharm Biopharm.* 2015;93:52–79.
37. Ventola CL. Progress in nanomedicine: approved and investigational nanodrugs. *Pharmacy and Therapeutics.* 2017;42(12):742–55.
38. Shan X, Gong X, Li J, Wen J, Li Y, Zhang Z. Current approaches of nanomedicines in the market and various stages of clinical translation. *Acta Pharm Sin B.* 2022;12(7):3028–48.
39. Thapa RK, Kim JO. Nanomedicine-based commercial formulations: current developments and future prospects. *J Pharm Investig.* 2023;53(1):19–33.
40. Madni A, Sarfraz M, Rehman M, Ahmad M, Akhtar N, Ahmad S, et al. Liposomal drug delivery: a versatile platform for challenging clinical applications. *J Pharm Pharm Sci.* 2014;17(3):401–26.
41. Rizzo LY, Theek B, Storm G, Kiessling F, Lammers T. Recent progress in nanomedicine: therapeutic, diagnostic and theranostic applications. *Curr Opin Biotechnol.* 2013;24(6):1159–66.
42. Pallares RM, Kiessling F, Lammers T. Bridging the gap between lab and clinic for nanodiagnostics. *Nanomedicine (Lond).* 2023;18(5):413–6.
43. Cheng J, Huang H, Chen Y, Wu R. Nanomedicine for diagnosis and treatment of atherosclerosis. *Adv Sci.* 2023;10(36):2304294.
44. Wang Y, Yu L, Kong X, Sun L. Application of nanodiagnostics in point-of-care tests for infectious diseases. *Int J Nanomedicine.* 2017;12:4789–803.
45. Rosati G, Idili A, Parolo C, Fuentes-Chust C, Calucho E, Hu L, et al. Nanodiagnostics to face SARS-CoV-2 and future pandemics: from an idea to the market and beyond. *ACS Nano.* 2021;15(11):17137–49.
46. Pallares RM, Mottaghy FM, Schulz V, Kiessling F, Lammers T. Nanoparticle diagnostics and theranostics in the clinic. *J Nucl Med.* 2022;63(12):1802–8.
47. Rivas L, Escosura-Muñiz Adl, Pons J, Merkoçi A. Chapter 14 - Lateral flow biosensors based on gold nanoparticles. In: Valcárcel M, López-Lorente ÁI, editors. *Comprehensive analytical chemistry.* Elsevier, Amsterdam; 2014. Vol. 66, p. 569–605.
48. Alharbi KK, Al-Sheikh YA. Role and implications of nanodiagnostics in the changing trends of clinical diagnosis. *Saudi J Biol Sci.* 2014;21(2):109–17.
49. Thakor AS, Jokerst JV, Ghanouni P, Campbell JL, Mittra E, Gambhir SS. Clinically approved nanoparticle imaging agents. *J Nucl Med.* 2016;57(12):1833–7.
50. Park SM, Aalipour A, Vermesh O, Yu JH, Gambhir SS. Towards clinically translatable in vivo nanodiagnostics. *Nat Rev Mater.* 2017;2(5):17014.
51. Newman EA, Newman LA. Lymphatic mapping techniques and sentinel lymph node biopsy in breast cancer. *Surg Clin North Am.* 2007;87(2):353–64, viii.

52. Wu S, Helal-Neto E, Matos A, Jafari A, Kozempel J, Silva YJA, et al. Radioactive polymeric nanoparticles for biomedical application. *Drug Deliv.* 2020;27(1):1544–61.
53. Dams ET, Oyen WJ, Boerman OC, Storm G, Laverman P, Kok PJ, et al. 99mTc-PEG liposomes for the scintigraphic detection of infection and inflammation: clinical evaluation. *J Nucl Med.* 2000;41(4):622–30.
54. Chen C, Ge J, Gao Y, Chen L, Cui J, Zeng J, et al. Ultrasmall superparamagnetic iron oxide nanoparticles: a next generation contrast agent for magnetic resonance imaging. *Wiley Interdiscip Rev Nanomed Nanobiotechnol.* 2022;14(1):e1740.
55. Misselwitz B, Schmitt-Willich H, Ebert W, Frenzel T, Weinmann H-J. Pharmacokinetics of gadomer-17, a new dendritic magnetic resonance contrast agent. *Magn Reson Mater Phys Biol Med.* 2001;12(2):128–34.
56. Kim J, Chhour P, Hsu J, Litt HI, Ferrari VA, Popovtzer R, et al. Use of nanoparticle contrast agents for cell tracking with computed tomography. *Bioconjug Chem.* 2017;28(6):1581–97.
57. Oberdick SD, Jordanova KV, Lundstrom JT, Parigi G, Poorman ME, Zabow G, et al. Iron oxide nanoparticles as positive t1 contrast agents for low-field magnetic resonance imaging at 64 mT. *Sci Rep.* 2023;13(1):11520.
58. Reynolds CH, Annan N, Beshah K, Huber JH, Shaber SH, Lenkinski RE, et al. Gadolinium-loaded nanoparticles: new contrast agents for magnetic resonance imaging. *J Am Chem Soc.* 2000;122(37):8940–5.
59. Plush SE, Woods M, Zhou Y-F, Kadali SB, Wong MS, Sherry AD. Nanoassembled capsules as delivery vehicles for large payloads of high relaxivity Gd3+ agents. *J Am Chem Soc.* 2009;131(43):15918–23.
60. Cormode DP, Naha PC, Fayad ZA. Nanoparticle contrast agents for computed tomography: a focus on micelles. *Contrast Media Mol Imaging.* 2014;9(1):37–52.
61. Šimečková P, Hubatka F, Kotouček J, Turánek Knötigová P, Mašek J, Slavík J, et al. Gadolinium labelled nanoliposomes as the platform for MRI theranostics: in vitro safety study in liver cells and macrophages. *Sci Rep.* 2020;10(1):4780.
62. Jouyandeh M, Sajadi SM, Seidi F, Habibzadeh S, Munir MT, Abida O, et al. Metal nanoparticles-assisted early diagnosis of diseases. *OpenNano.* 2022;8:100104.
63. Oliveira BB, Ferreira D, Fernandes AR, Baptista PV. Engineering gold nanoparticles for molecular diagnostics and biosensing. *Wiley Interdiscip Rev Nanomed Nanobiotechnol.* 2023;15(1):e1836.
64. Baptista PV. Could gold nanoprobes be an important tool in cancer diagnostics? *Expert Rev Mol Diagn.* 2012;12(6):541–3.
65. Aldewachi H, Chalati T, Woodroofe MN, Bricklebank N, Sharrack B, Gardiner P. Gold nanoparticle-based colorimetric biosensors. *Nanoscale.* 2017;10(1):18–33.
66. Wilson R. The use of gold nanoparticles in diagnostics and detection. *Chem Soc Rev.* 2008;37(9):2028–45.
67. Luo G, Zhang J, Sun Y, Wang Y, Wang H, Cheng B, et al. Nanoplatforms for sepsis management: rapid detection/warning, pathogen elimination and restoring immune homeostasis. *Nano-Micro Lett.* 2021;13(1):88.
68. Singh P, Pandit S, Mokkapati V, Garg A, Ravikumar V, Mijakovic I. Gold nanoparticles in diagnostics and therapeutics for human cancer. *Int J Mol Sci.* 2018;19(7):1979.
69. Dinnes J, Deeks JJ, Adriano A, Berhane S, Davenport C, Dittrich S, et al. Rapid, point-of-care antigen and molecular-based tests for diagnosis of SARS-CoV-2 infection. *Cochrane Database Syst Rev.* 2020;8(8):Cd013705.
70. Beduk T, Beduk D, de Oliveira Filho JI, Zihnioglu F, Cicek C, Sertoz R, et al. Rapid point-of-care COVID-19 diagnosis with a gold-nanoarchitecture-assisted laser-scribed graphene biosensor. *Anal Chem.* 2021;93(24):8585–94.
71. Khan J, Rasmi Y, Kırboğa KK, Ali A, Rudrapal M, Patekar RR. Development of gold nanoparticle-based biosensors for COVID-19 diagnosis. *Beni Suef Univ J Basic Appl Sci.* 2022;11(1):111.
72. Mody VV, Siwale R, Singh A, Mody HR. Introduction to metallic nanoparticles. *J Pharm Bioallied Sci.* 2010;2(4):282–9.
73. Dulińska-Litewka J, Łazarczyk A, Hałubiec P, Szafrański O, Karnas K, Karewicz A. Superparamagnetic iron oxide nanoparticles-current and prospective medical applications. *Materials (Basel).* 2019;12(4):617.
74. Dadfar SM, Camozzi D, Darguzyte M, Roemhild K, Varvarà P, Metselaar J, et al. Size-isolation of superparamagnetic iron oxide nanoparticles improves MRI, MPI and hyperthermia performance. *J Nanobiotechnology.* 2020;18(1):22.
75. Lassenberger A, Scheberl A, Stadlbauer A, Stiglbauer A, Helbich T, Reimhult E. Individually stabilized, superparamagnetic nanoparticles with controlled shell and size leading to exceptional stealth properties and high relaxivities. *ACS Appl Mater Interfaces.* 2017;9(4):3343–53.

76. Unterweger H, Dézsi L, Matuszak J, Janko C, Poettler M, Jordan J, et al. Dextran-coated superparamagnetic iron oxide nanoparticles for magnetic resonance imaging: evaluation of size-dependent imaging properties, storage stability and safety. *Int J Nanomedicine.* 2018;13:1899–915.
77. Chen X, Gambhir SS. Theranostic nanomedicine. *Acc Chem Res.* 2011;44(10):841–9.
78. Singh D, Dilnawaz F, Sahoo SK. Challenges of moving theranostic nanomedicine into the clinic. *Nanomedicine.* 2020;15(2):111–4.
79. d'Angelo M, Castelli V, Benedetti E, Antonosante A, Catanesi M, Dominguez-Benot R, et al. Theranostic nanomedicine for malignant gliomas. *Front Bioeng Biotechnol.* 2019;7:325.
80. Shete MB, Patil TS, Deshpande AS, Saraogi G, Vasdev N, Deshpande M, et al. Current trends in theranostic nanomedicines. *J Drug Deliv Sci Technol.* 2022;71:103280.
81. Janjic JM, Bai M. Design and development of theranostic nanomedicines. In: Berezin MY. *Nanotechnology for biomedical imaging and diagnostics.* John Wiley & Sons, Inc., New Jersey. 2014. p. 429–65.
82. Jo SD, Ku SH, Won Y-Y, Kim SH, Kwon IC. Targeted nanotheranostics for future personalized medicine: recent progress in cancer therapy. *Theranostics.* 2016;6(9):1362–77.
83. Lodhi MS, Khan MT, Aftab S, Samra ZQ, Wang H, Wei DQ. A novel formulation of theranostic nanomedicine for targeting drug delivery to gastrointestinal tract cancer. *Cancer Nanotechnology.* 2021;12(1):26.
84. Zha Y, Xue C, Liu Y, Ni J, De La Fuente JM, Cui D. Artificial intelligence in theranostics of gastric cancer, a review. *Med Rev.* 2023;3(3):214–29.
85. Kim MW, Jeong HY, Kang SJ, Jeong IH, Choi MJ, You YM, et al. Anti-EGF receptor aptamer-guided co-delivery of anti-cancer siRNAs and quantum dots for theranostics of triple-negative breast cancer. *Theranostics.* 2019;9(3):837–52.
86. Thakur V, Kutty RV. Recent advances in nanotheranostics for triple negative breast cancer treatment. *J Exp Clin Cancer Res.* 2019;38(1):430.
87. Chakraborty P, Das SS, Dey A, Chakraborty A, Bhattacharyya C, Kandimalla R, et al. Quantum dots: the cutting-edge nanotheranostics in brain cancer management. *J Control Release.* 2022;350:698–715.
88. Yin X, Cui Y, Kim RS, Stiles WR, Park SH, Wang H, et al. Image-guided drug delivery of nanotheranostics for targeted lung cancer therapy. *Theranostics.* 2022;12(9):4147–62.
89. Tang J, Zheng F, Zhao J, Zhao J. Self-assembled multifunctional nanotheranostics loading GEM for targeted lung cancer therapy. *Mater Sci Eng C.* 2020;112:110786.
90. Manners N, Priya V, Mehata AK, Rawat M, Mohan S, Makeen HA, et al. Theranostic nanomedicines for the treatment of cardiovascular and related diseases: current strategies and future perspectives. *Pharmaceutics (Basel).* 2022;15(4):441.
91. Wu Y, Vazquez-Prada KX, Liu Y, Whittaker AK, Zhang R, Ta HT. Recent advances in the development of theranostic nanoparticles for cardiovascular diseases. *Nanotheranostics.* 2021;5(4):499–514.
92. U.S. Food & Drug Administration. Precision medicine. 2018 [updated 2018 Sept 27]. Accessed 2024 May 30. Available from: https://www.fda.gov/medical-devices/in-vitro-diagnostics/precision-medicine.
93. Blau R, Krivitsky A, Epshtein Y, Satchi-Fainaro R. Are nanotheranostics and nanodiagnostics-guided drug delivery stepping stones towards precision medicine? *Drug Resist Updates.* 2016;27:39–58.
94. NHS England. Precision medicine. 2020 [updated 24 August 2020]. Accessed 2024 May 30. Available from: https://transform.england.nhs.uk/ai-lab/explore-all-resources/understand-ai/precision-medicine/.
95. Wang Y, Sun S, Zhang Z, Shi D. Nanomaterials for cancer precision medicine. *Adv Mater.* 2018;30(17):e1705660.
96. Puccetti M, Pariano M, Schoubben A, Giovagnoli S, Ricci M. Biologics, theranostics, and personalized medicine in drug delivery systems. *Pharmacol Res.* 2024;201:107086.

19

Immunohistochemistry Application in Laboratory Medicine: Current Approaches and Challenges

Mawusi Adepa Mawuli

19.1 Introduction

19.1.1 Immunohistochemistry

Immunohistochemistry (IHC) is a medical laboratory assay used to demonstrate antigens in tissues using antibodies that bind specifically to the antigens. It is a valuable tool in histologic diagnosis and a treatment/management decision-making tool. The method is affected by several factors, such as differences in tumor biology, specimen processing and staining, and observation and interpretation of results [1]. The process must be standardized for efficient use, ultimately improving patient care.

The fluorescence-labeled antibody method is the oldest IHC method. The use of enzyme-labeled antibodies was adapted to mitigate problems with the use of fluorescence-labeled antibodies, including lack of end-product permanency (due to photobleaching), autofluorescence of nearby tissues, and the need for a fluorescence microscope. Enzyme-labeled antibody products are permanent and can be visualized using conventional light or electron microscopes. Acid phosphatase and peroxidase are the two most common enzyme conjugates; however, the latter has the advantage of being more stable and having a longer storage life. Demonstration of antigens using ultrathin sections is useful for electron microscopy. Ultrathin sections enable easy access of immunolabels to antigens. Demonstrating antigens in frozen sections has provided valuable information that other techniques could not address [2].

For sections that require fixation, one key issue is how to "unmask" the antigens to allow binding to immunolabels. Since its discovery, 10% formalin (3.7–4% formaldehyde) has been widely used in histopathology as it provides the best preservation of detailed tissue morphology. Formalin fixation, however, was shown to affect a lot of antigens adversely [3].

These effects were, however, mitigated by some technical developments, such as the use of particular monoclonal antibodies and antigen retrieval methods. The development of antigen retrieval (AR) techniques proved that formalin cross-linkages with antigens (proteins) could be reversed. Early study of the chemical reaction between formalin and proteins indicated that these reactions were limited to certain imidazole and indol amino acid side chains and that they were reversible by heat treatment (120°C) or alkane treatment, a process known as antigen retrieval.

19.1.2 Developments in Antigen Retrieval Methods

Effect of temperature at retrieval: Studies show that high temperature is the most critical factor affecting antigens retrieval from formalin-fixed paraffin wax-embedded tissues (FFPE). Optimal results for an AR-IHC are correlated with the product of the heating temperature (T) and time (t) of heating AR treatment, where "T" and "t" are the heating conditions. In essence, heating at a lower temperature will require more heating time to attain optimal antigen retrieval than heating at a higher temperature.

DOI: 10.1201/9781003486909-19

Effect of pH on retrieval: The pH of the AR solution has been reported to influence the quality of IHC staining. For some antigens, the quality of IHC staining remains the same over a range of pH of AR solution. On the other hand, some antigens show significant variation in staining over a range of pH solutions. Studies have shown that for any AR solution, the pH of the solution is more important than the chemical composition of the retrieval solution [4].

Effect of molarity: A report by Shi et al. [4] indicates that the molarity of the solution is not key for citrate and other buffers used in AR. Some salts, such as aluminum chloride, have been shown to be effective for AR in demonstrating vimentin in FFPEs. This shows that for some antigens, AR may require the use of solutions with peculiar molarity.

Effect of metal ions: Earlier studies showed that metal salts were applied in AR-IHC due to zinc-formalin fixation, which resulted in better quality immunostaining than pure water. Subsequently, a study conducted by Siitonen et al. showed that immunostaining of PCNA (proliferating cell nuclear antigen) monoclonal antibodies (19A2 and PC10) in breast carcinoma was best demonstrated using lead thiocyanate as AR retrieval solution [5]. A significant drawback, however, with the use of lead in AR solution is its toxicity. Presently, an improvement on this is the development of alternatives such as citrate and Tris buffers, urea, ethylenediaminetetraacetic acid (EDTA) or ethylene glycol-bis (β-aminoethyl ether (EGTA), and glycine-HCl buffer.

Antigen retrieval: applications

a) AR has proven to be a useful tool in surgical pathology with increased sensitivity in demonstrating antigens in archival specimens. AR made it possible to demonstrate several antigens, including Ki67 and thrombospondin-1, which were otherwise not demonstrable using IHC, even when other unmasking methods were used. At present, AR on archival specimens has replaced frozen sections, which was previously the gold standard for IHC.
b) Anatomical morphology: AR-IHC is useful in analytical morphology, demonstrating antigens relevant to the central nervous system (CNS). Some of these developments were shown in studies where celloidin-embedded human brain tissue sections were used to trace the auditory axonal formation and maturity of the CNS, using monoclonal antibodies (MAb) to neurofilament and microtubule-associated protein (MAP2). Subsequently, the results of these studies were shown to correlate with the results of another study that proved a correlation between epitope mapping of MAP2 using western blotting.

Additionally, the microwave (MW) AR technique has aided in the demonstration of the androgen receptor in prostate cancer for both diagnostic and prognostic purposes.

Further advancement in the MW AR method includes its applications in double immunostaining, triple immunostaining, and immunoelectron microscopy.

Tissue microarray: The concept of the tissue microarray was introduced by Kononen in the late nineties [6]. A tissue microarray comprises several pieces of tissues obtained from donor blocks that have been organized into a single tissue block. Sections from the block can be taken and subsequently stained (IHC) to allow simultaneous detection and examination of antigens and gene expression profiling. The technology includes samples from different tumor types (multi-tumor), samples from one organ at different tumor stages (progression), clinical cases with follow-up samples (prognosis), and frozen samples for RNA detection (cry microarray) In this era of digitization, the tissue microarray would significantly increase the efficiency of IHC. Additional information can also be obtained from consecutive sections from the microarray tissue block for diagnosis, prognosis, and identification of drug targets. The tissue microarray can serve as a valuable material for optimization of reagents and quality control. The method, however, requires highly technical skills in preparation for the microarray. There is also difficulty with selecting tissue due to its small size. Heterogeneity in tumors, which could be a potential concern in preparing tissue microarrays, can be overcome by taking at least 2 cores per tumor specimen. Currently, the tissue microarray can be produced using an automated tissue array.

Multiplex immunostaining chip (MI chip): This technology involves the detection of several antigens in a single sample. A chip made of silicon rubber is embedded with 50 different antibodies. The size of the chip is the same as the size of a glass slide. Each antibody resides in a 2 mm well. The technology involves clamping the chip to a tissue section to allow the tissue to be stained. This allows for the differential diagnosis of tumors. The method is very cost-effective and efficient.

19.2 Factors Affecting IHC Performance

Multiple factors affect the performance of an IHC. Discussing these is important in ensuring that the results of an IHC are reliable and reproducible. These factors will be categorized under preanalytical, analytical, and post-analytical.

19.3 Preanalytical

Fixation: Fixation is the first step in processing tissue samples for histopathological evaluation. The fixative's importance is to preserve and stabilize all cellular materials (e.g., proteins) and components, permit conventional staining, and perform other procedures, such as IHC. This process has been identified as an essential initial step in ensuring optimal results of an IHC stain.

Fixation must be done within 30–60 minutes of surgical specimen removal. Specimens must be fixed in a specimen with a fixative volume of at least 1:10. All fixed specimens must be processed within 48 hours after fixation. Larger samples, such as mastectomy and uterus, may require slicing and longer fixation times to ensure that the core of the organs is adequately fixed. Fixatives can be categorized into denaturating and cross-linking fixatives. For example, fixatives containing aldehyde groups are cross-linking fixatives, while alcoholic fixatives are denaturating/coagulating fixatives. Coagulating fixatives work by breaking hydrogen bonds and precipitating proteins without causing cross-linkages. Formaldehyde is the oldest and most frequent fixative used in histopathology. Formaldehyde preserves the general structure of cellular organelles and molecules such as nucleic acids, peptides, and lipids, but seldom carbohydrates. Formalin works by forming formalin bridges/cross-links with proteins in the tissues.

The longer the fixation time, the more cross-links are formed, and vice versa. These cross-links are reversible with antigen retrieval methods. Ethanol, a denaturation fixative, may not adequately preserve cellular components, leading to a possible shift in intracellular immunoreactivity. Compared to formaldehyde; however, ethanol does not have as much deleterious effect on tissues: Its low molecular weight allows for easy penetration into tissues. No one fixative is suitable for all antigens. The use of a particular fixative depends on the type of antigens and recommendations from manufacturers of antibodies for IHC staining. Note: inadequate fixation will cause autolysis or putrefaction. Immunohistochemical reactions could be altered due to reduced/increased fixation times, leading to a weak staining reaction, false negative results, increased background staining, and non-specific staining.

The fixation time (in formalin) for routine cases submitted from different facilities to a histopathology lab is unmonitored. Therefore, the issue arises as to how to ensure that all specimens submitted to the histopathology lab are treated in such a manner as to obtain the actual results needed. The antigen retrieval method ensures that at least these inherent differences in fixation times do not adversely affect IHC results. The method also adds to the advantage of archived formalin-fixed paraffin wax-embedded tissue over frozen sections.

Effect of decalcification on IHC: All bony specimens must be decalcified before processing for histology, immunohistochemistry, or molecular analysis. Decalcifying solutions are either acids or chelating agents. Examples of acids include hydrochloric acid (inorganic) and formic acid (organic). Ethylenediaminetetraacetic acid (EDTA) is a common chelating agent used for decalcification. Decalcification may alter proteins and nucleic acids, which can negatively affect IHC. It is important to choose a suitable decalcifying solution for the antigen of interest and control the decalcification process. Control can be done by varying the number of cycles and duration of decalcification.

Effect of processing solutions and incubation buffers: Tissues are taken through "processing" following fixation. Processing involves dehydration, clearing, and infiltration of tissues. Dehydration is done using changes of increasing grades of alcohol (70, 85, 95, and absolute). Clearing is done using xylene. Infiltration is done with molten paraffin (60°C). Solutions used for processing tissues can affect IHC because non-polar solvents used in paraffin wax embedding can modify the conformations of antigens (Ags). Inadequately processed tissue will be poorly infiltrated with molten paraffin wax, resulting in poorly embedded tissues. Inadequate processing may result from insufficient incubation times, the use of processing solutions several times without changing, inadequate volumes of processing solutions, and inappropriate solutions like ethanol. Very high temperatures of processing solutions (molten paraffin wax) will result in dry and brittle tissues that will be difficult to embed and section. An automatic tissue processor is available to process tissues.

Embedding, sectioning/microtomy, mounting of sections onto slides, and drying/heating of sections prior to actual IHC staining: Embedding involves the formation of a tissue block using molten paraffin wax by adequately orienting the tissue in a mold. When the molten wax is cooled, the embedded block can be sectioned. It is essential to ensure the correct orientation for the tissue type is done. This ensures that histology and subsequent IHC can be adequately reported.

Sectioning/microtomy involves cutting thin sections from the embedded tissue block using a microtome (2–4 μm). Sections >4 μm will be difficult to observe under the light microscope for proper IHC reporting. It is important to avoid folds and scattering of sections during microtomy as these will obscure the general tissue structure and make reporting difficult. For example, DAB may be trapped in folds in tissue and will appear as brown patches or spots. It is also important to avoid "wasting" of the tissue block during sectioning. This is particularly important for tiny biopsies where there is the most likely chance of losing the tissue. For more extensive biopsies, wasting may result in the loss of tumor areas, mainly if these areas are small within the tissue. In some cases, wasting may also result in the loss of antigens as one cuts more profoundly into the tissue. Carryovers from previous sections must be avoided at all times. Carryovers can lead to misdiagnosis of cases. Clean adhesive /coated/charged slides must be used. Unclean slides can cause backgrounds that will obscure staining. Using uncharged or coated slides will cause disengagement of sections from the slides during the IHC staining procedure. Last, slides must be labeled appropriately with the sample ID and the specific IHC stain to be run. Sections on slides must be dried by placing the slides in an upright position on a piece of tissue paper. This is to ensure adequate adherence to sections on slides. Further incubation of the section in an oven (60°C) for at least 30 minutes is done to ensure further adherence of sections onto slides before IHC staining. Sections/slides must be stained immediately after they are ready. Storage of sections may negatively affect IHC staining. For example, a study showed that for some cases, there was loss of p53 staining when sections of previously positive (controls) were stored at room temperature for up to two months, as compared to freshly sectioned cases [7]. For most antigens, however, an overnight incubation at 65°C is enough to maintain the antigens' immuno reactivity and ensure the sections do not wash off during the IHC staining.

19.4 Analytical

The IHC staining proper: The first step is to hydrate the sections (that is, bring the sections down to water). This involves taking the sections through xylene (clearing), decreasing alcohol concentrations, and finally to water. Hydration allows the sections to take up the reagents of the IHC staining procedure, which are mainly water-based. Inadequate hydration will prevent adequate permeation of staining solutions/reagents. Following the hydration of tissues, antigen retrieval is done on samples that have been fixed. Frozen sections do not require antigen retrieval. The most widely used AR method is heat-induced epitope retrieval (HIER). The heat source could be either a water bath, pressure cooker, microwave oven, heating plate, or autoclave. Temperature for heating plate and water bath: the temperature of the retrieval solution is usually at 100°C, and the incubation time is 10 minutes. Enzymes such as trypsin or proteases for epitope retrieval apply to some antigens such as the cytokeratin and Igs, where sections are incubated for 10 minutes at 37°C. Overall, the best antigen retrieval method and retrieval solution for each antigen/antibody must be obtained as part of optimizing the IHC procedure. The primary aim of AR is to "release" formalin cross-links with antigens.

Protein and indigenous peroxidase blocking: To prevent background staining and non-specific binding in IHC, endogenous proteins and peroxidases in tissues must be blocked. Proteins can be blocked using either milk protein, serum from the animal from whom the secondary antibody was raised, or egg white. Peroxidases in blood cells are usually blocked using 3–5% hydrogen peroxide solution. This is particularly important for tissues with many blood cells, such as the liver. Inadequate blocking would result in staining artifacts that could be misreported as positive staining.

Antibody incubation: Incubation in antibodies follows the blocking step. The temperature and incubation time of the antibody must be optimized for each test. This also applies to all new batches of antibodies procured for IHC use. Storage of antibodies is also essential. It is not advisable to freeze-thaw antibodies all the time, as this can enhance degradation of the antibody. Prediluted antibodies can be stored in the refrigerator at 4–8°C. While dilutions can be prepared from concentrated antibodies and the stock frozen at –20°C. The use of expired antibodies must also be avoided.

Biochemistry of antigen/antibody interactions; hydrophobic – it involves amino acids that have surface tension lower than that of water such as phenylalanine, tryptophan, and tyrosine; electrostatic – it involves oppositely charged portions of Abs and Ags between carboxyl and amino terminal ends; Van der Walls – is an example of a weak electrostatic interaction; hydrogen bonding – involves bonds between OH and C=OO; NH and C=OO and OH and NH groups – a precise fit is needed for this to happen.

Affinity: describes the thermodynamic expression of the bonding energy of an Ab to an epitope/antigenic determinant.

Isoforms: describes the different structures an Ag can take. This is mainly due to alternate splicing of the primary transcript to different mature transcripts that can lead to the formation of proteins that vary slightly and post-translational modifications such as glycosylation, phosphorylation, and proteolytic processes that add to the proteins' complexity.

Immunogens used in IHC: There are two broad sources of immunogens: synthetic peptides and purified proteins [8]. Synthetic peptides have known amino acid sequences. For purified proteins, it is challenging to obtain "pure" or homogenous proteins from cells or tissues. The amino acid sequence of purified proteins. Table 19.1 shows some advantages and disadvantages of synthetic and purified proteins as immunogens.

Monoclonal and polyclonal antibodies: An antibody is a protein that is produced in response to specific immunogens. Structurally, antibodies are Y-shaped and made of two light chains and two heavy chains. For both heavy and light chains, there is a constant region as well as a variable region. The constant region of the heavy chain (Fc) determines the antibody's class and its biological function. The variable regions of both heavy and light chains constitute the antigen binding site or paratope. (In IHC, the paratope binds to epitopes in cells/tissues; the Fc portion is a binding site for either a secondary antibody or a tag). Different animal species can be used, such as mice, rabbits, goats, horses, and chickens. Antibodies are the primary reagents that are used in IHC. Antibodies could be either monoclonal or polyclonal. Monoclonal antibodies are produced against a single epitope/antigenic determinant. It is mainly compared to polyclonal

TABLE 19.1

Advantages and disadvantages of synthetic and purified proteins

	Advantages	Disadvantages
Synthetic peptides	Known amino acid sequence, hence easy to predict which protein it can bind to, as well as the possibility of cross-reactive proteins	The normal three-dimensional structure of the native protein may be lost; hence may vary in immunogenicity The presence of other proteins that can be closely associated with the synthetic peptide in vivo can lead to the masking of the epitope leading to false negative results In vivo, post-translational modifications may occur, and this could result in differences between the native protein and synthetic proteins
Purified proteins	The immunogenicity of purified proteins is stable	Purification can be technically difficult Contamination can readily occur, leading to increased immunogenicity The targeted protein may contain epitopes that are not specific to the antigen. If these epitopes are highly immunogenic, this can be problematic. Same post-translational modifications for different proteins

antibodies. However, monoclonal antibodies are not as sensitive as polyclonal antibodies. Polyclonal antibodies are produced in multiple species and are directed against different epitopes of an antigen. Commercially available antibodies can be obtained from other manufacturers. It is essential to get antibodies from the most reliable source. Antibodies obtained for research purposes must produce the same results when the experiment is repeated (reproducible results). Failure in this regard will lead to the publication of false data, negatively impacting research. Quality control of antibodies cannot be underestimated in this regard.

- Each new batch of antibodies must be validated because there may be variations between batches, and some of the existing information about the antibody may not apply to a new batch.

The manufacturer must provide important information about the antibody, including the species in which the Ab was raised, the Ab concentration, suitability of the Ab for IHC (FFPE/frozen sections), prediluted/concentrated, staining pattern, storage temperature, immunogen used, species reactivity, and recommended control tissue.

Secondary antibody + detection system: this has enabled the detection of small amounts of proteins on FFPE with little or no background staining. The detection systems include the use of enzymes and fluorophores. The horse radish peroxidase (HRP) and the alkaline phosphatase are the earliest and most common enzymes used. The DAB is the substrate for the HRP and the fast red. The HRP/DAB detection system is the most commonly used. Advancement in the HRP detection system has resulted in the use of the polymer (dextran) based and the Envision antibody complex [9].

Detection: DAB must not be exposed to light as it can cause oxidation of the dye before its use.

Counterstaining with Hx: filtering of solution before use creates a purple-black precipitate on the slide.

Mounting: improper dehydration causes a hazy look on the slide due to a mixture of water, xylene, and mountant.

Reporting and interpretation of results: All IHC test results must be reported in a positive and negative control context. This is to prevent the reportage of false positive or false negative results. The interpretation and reporting of an IHC stain is dependent on factors such as the amount of tissue available (biopsy or resections), amount of antigen present in the available tissue, staining pattern (focal/localized or diffuse), localization of the target antigen (nuclear, cytoplasmic, or membranous), and staining intensity (weak, moderate, or strong). A 5% staining is usually reported as a positive staining for diagnostic markers. Some available scoring systems have been adopted to report some IHC tests. An example is the Allred system for reporting ER and PR. The expertise of the individual reporting the IHC stain is crucial. Sometimes, individuals may report different things, such as staining intensity.

Quality assurance: All IHC laboratories require certification. As with other medical laboratories, an IHC laboratory must have the ISO 15189 certification. A certified IHC laboratory is necessary because it assures that IHC testing is done considering all the quality management practices. Overall, the assurance is given that an IHC result reflects the patient's status.

Qualification of laboratory staff and pathologists, modern IHC equipment, quality-controlled test methods, and documentation of IHC processes are all relevant to quality assurance practices.

Some programs have been developed to ensure quality IHC testing. For example, The College of American Pathologists (CAP)/National Society for Histotechnology HistoQIP–IHC (program code HQIHC), is designed to improve the preparation of IHC slides. The HHQIHC program requires all participants to submit IHC slides on gastrointestinal, skin, and genitourinary biopsies to be reviewed by a panel of experts (proficiency testing/External Quality Assessment (EQA). Some other programs include PM2 (ER/PR), HER2 (breast), GHER2 (gastric HER2), and MK (general IHC).

Controls: Both positive and control tissues validate an IHC procedure. A positive control is tissue customarily expected to show immunoreactivity to a particular antibody. Controls must be used for every run of IHC. Usually, a control tissue is placed at one end of a slide, while the test tissue occupies the other end on the same slide. Several controls can be assembled into a tissue array and used for validation. Figure 19.1 shows a sample IHC worksheet. This is helpful as a tool for quality assurance.

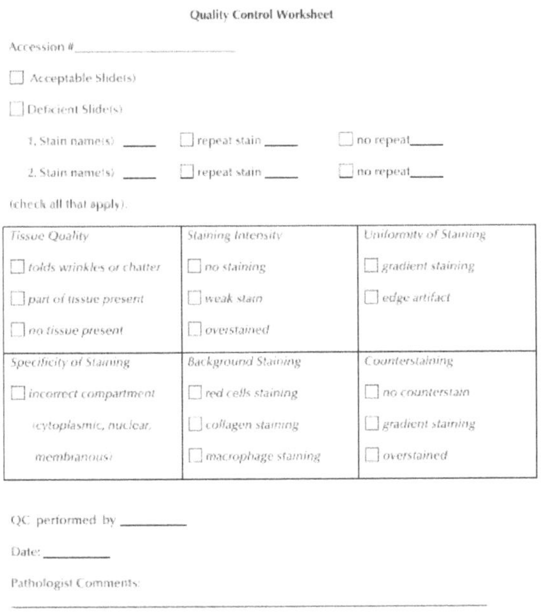

Quality Control Worksheet

Accession #__________

☐ Acceptable Slide(s)

☐ Deficient Slide(s)

1. Stain name(s) ____ ☐ repeat stain ____ ☐ no repeat____

2. Stain name(s) ____ ☐ repeat stain ____ ☐ no repeat____

(check all that apply).

Tissue Quality	*Staining Intensity*	*Uniformity of Staining*
☐ *folds wrinkles or chatter*	☐ *no staining*	☐ *gradient staining*
☐ *part of tissue present*	☐ *weak stain*	☐ *edge artifact*
☐ *no tissue present*	☐ *overstained*	
Specificity of Staining	*Background Staining*	*Counterstaining*
☐ *incorrect compartment*	☐ *red cells staining*	☐ *no counterstain*
(cytoplasmic, nuclear,	☐ *collagen staining*	☐ *gradient staining*
membranous)	☐ *macrophage staining*	☐ *overstained*

QC performed by ________

Date: ________

Pathologist Comments:

chemistry Laboratory Quality Control Worksheet. Abbreviation: QC, quality control.

FIGURE 19.1 Quality control worksheet.

REFERENCES

1. Bussolati G, Leonardo E. Technical pitfalls potentially affecting diagnoses in immunohistochemistry. *J Clin Pathol.* 2008;61(11):1184–92.
2. Ramos-Vara J, Miller M. When tissue antigens and antibodies get along: revisiting the technical aspects of immunohistochemistry—the red, brown, and blue technique. *Vet Pathol.* 2014;51(1):42–87.
3. Grigorev I, Korzhevskii D. Current technologies for fixation of biological material for immunohistochemical analysis. *Sovrem Tekhnol Med.* 2018;10(2 (eng)):156–64.
4. Shi S-R, Cote RJ, Taylor CR. Antigen retrieval immunohistochemistry: past, present, and future. *J Histochem Cytochem.* 1997;45(3):327–43.
5. Siitonen SM, Kallioniemi O-P, Isola JJ. Proliferating cell nuclear antigen immunohistochemistry using monoclonal antibody 19A2 and a new antigen retrieval technique has prognostic impact in archival paraffin-embedded node-negative breast cancer. *Am J Pathol.* 1993;142(4):1081.
6. Kononen J, et al. Tissue microarrays for high-throughput molecular profiling of tumor specimens. *Nat Med.* 1998;4(7):844–7.
7. Prioleau J, Schnitt SJ. p53 antigen loss in stored paraffin slides. *N Engl J Med.* 1995;332(22):1521–2.
8. Mighell A, Hume W, Robinson P. An overview of the complexities and subtleties of immunohistochemistry. *Oral Dis.* 1998;4(3):217–23.
9. Kämmerer U, et al. A new rapid immunohistochemical staining technique using the EnVision antibody complex. *J Histochem Cytochem.* 2001;49(5):623–30.

20

Health Diagnosis: Future Perspectives

Emmanuel Kwaku Ofori, Seth Kwabena Amponsah, and Yashwant V. Pathak

20.1 Introduction

Health diagnostics is poised for a dramatic transition driven by the rapid advancement of technology and a deeper understanding of disease dynamics. Healthcare professionals frequently face novel challenges stemming from increased duties and recurrent interruptions in the healthcare system. Furthermore, diagnostics might be an exceedingly challenging process. The diagnostic process may employ several techniques, including imaging modalities like X-rays, magnetic resonance imaging (MRI), computed tomography (CT) scans, blood tests, and biopsy procedures. The outcomes of these assessments aid healthcare professionals in identifying the most effective treatment strategy for their patients [1, 2].

The global emphasis on improving healthcare service efficacy using information technology has emerged due to an aging patient demographic and a need for more medical professionals. Artificial Intelligence (AI) is a domain of algorithmic software that empowers machines to utilize knowledge for problem-solving. It can potentially emulate human cognitive processes and intellectual endeavors [3]. AI generally denotes a machine's capacity to perform mental functions linked to human intelligence, encompassing sensing, reasoning, learning, environmental interaction, problem-solving, decision-making, and creative expression. AI is often utilized in the healthcare sector and can assist in developing novel therapies in the information era. The capacity of AI in disease diagnosis has elicited significant interest. AI has the potential to discover specific medications for complex diseases, enhance the management of chronic conditions, and reduce medical errors [4]. The ability of integrative AI to identify malignant cells is significantly augmented by employing many algorithms rather than a singular one, resulting in better diagnostic precision. AI methodologies also assist in predicting the recurrence of various cancer kinds [5].

This chapter will explore the future perspectives of health diagnosis, examining the potential benefits and difficulties associated with introducing new technology. By analyzing the current trends and making predictions about future developments, our objective is to provide a comprehensive perspective of the shifting landscape of diagnostic technology. In addition, we will discuss the significance of ensuring that everyone has equitable access to new diagnostic technology and the ethical issues that must be considered.

20.2 Artificial Intelligence and Machine Learning in Diagnostics

20.2.1 AI and ML in Radiology

The area of radiology has demonstrated a great deal of potential for implementing AI and ML, both of which can enhance the accuracy and efficiency of image processing. Using deep learning (DL), computers can process vast amounts of imaging data to identify patterns and anomalies that human radiologists would miss. They recognize and localize complicated patterns from various radiological imaging modalities [6]. Imaging acquisition inventions, such as CT and MRI, as well as the development of

DOI: 10.1201/9781003486909-20

digitized picture archiving and communication systems (PACSs), are among the early milestones in the history of computer technology [7]. These complex patterns have achieved performance equivalent to human decision-making in recent applications.

AI systems that are effective and efficient can assist radiologists in reducing their workloads while simultaneously increasing their accuracy and consistency. It may eventually alter the workflow of radiology for specific jobs. Concerns have been voiced by several authors and researchers over the impending demise of radiology as a field of study because growing advancements in AI will eventually replace human radiologists. This is not the case.

AI essentially functions as a source of innovation that will improve radiology's impact on patient outcomes, boosting the importance of the discipline [8]. Radiologists will increasingly be expected to be data or information managers rather than spend all their time memorizing and recognizing patterns and differential diagnoses. To comprehend the implementation of AI in clinical settings, having a foundational understanding of imaging informatics is essential. Those who are in training and radiologists should have an understanding of the informatics infrastructure that is required to support the seamless integration and complicated interplay of AI tools.

Ethical concerns have been raised concerning the use of AI in healthcare. Biases can arise from datasets that either over-represent, under-represent, or entirely exclude key characteristics pertinent to the operation. There is also the possibility of "automation bias", which refers to the phenomenon in which people tend to rely only on the work of a computer rather than employing their critical judgment and inspection. In addition, AI entails collecting personal health information, which raises concerns over data protection and privacy. Concerns around meaningful permission and adequate anonymization and de-identification of data continue to be of high priority [9, 10]. The AI algorithms must be sufficiently transparent and understandable for healthcare providers to monitor AI's reasoning and effects and explain AI's workings to patients and other relevant parties. This is necessary to protect against the harm that could be caused by technology.

20.2.2 Interpretative Uses of AI in Radiology

The digital mammography technique is the imaging modality that is utilized the most frequently for screening for breast cancer. However, this technique has a low sensitivity (especially in dense breasts) and a relatively large frequency of false positives. As a result of these factors, there has been a significant amount of interest throughout history in the creation of computer-assisted tools capable of assisting radiologists in the process of identifying early malignant lesions. These AI algorithms are more accurate than human professionals. In addition to improving accuracy, diagnostic tools powered by AI also reduce the time required for picture processing. This is very important in situations of emergency, where it is of the utmost need to arrive at a diagnosis as swiftly as possible. The workflow in radiology departments can be optimized with the help of AI, which can also assist in triaging patients and prioritizing those patients who require immediate treatment. In most cases, radiologists are the ones who develop study protocols by basing them on particular clinical factors. This may take a lot of time. Research has demonstrated that ML algorithms can determine clinical procedures for studies using MRI scans of the brain, musculoskeletal system, and the entire body.

20.3 AI in Pathology

The study of pathology is another area in which AI and ML are significantly advancing. Within the realm of digital pathology, the digitization of biopsy samples is an indispensable component. It is anticipated that the discipline of pathology and laboratory medicine will play an even more significant and pivotal role as the applications of AI and ML spread across a broader range of healthcare settings [11, 12]. Pathology laboratories have been using information technology tools for a considerable time to accomplish automated tissue processing, staining, and the preparation of synoptic reports. The development of digitalized whole slide image (WSI) technology, on the other hand, has garnered the most interest from physicians and pathologists, and the utilization of digital pathology (DP) is currently developing into a standard practice [13].

However, image analysis and AI require a digital pathology process to realize their full promise in pathology. Pathologists are thus provided with considerable alternatives to their initial diagnosis due to these algorithms' ability to identify malignant cells and other abnormalities with high precision. An example of this would be that systems based on AI have demonstrated a high degree of accuracy in the diagnosis of prostate cancer, which has resulted in more reliability and consistency [14, 15]. Through AI, digital slides can be shared with specialists worldwide. This makes it possible for patients who live in historically underserved areas to gain access to specialized knowledge and improves their diagnostic outcomes.

The advantages of digital pathology are clearly stated in terms of quality, efficiency, and delivering resilience to services, and the adoption of this technology is increasing [16]. AI can identify essential elements in slides, advancing work efficiency and diagnostic practice reliability compared to pathologists. AI can also recognize small cell changes on histological and cytological images that pathologists cannot identify. Specific mutations can also be predicted within cancer cells based on these changes.

In pathology, applications of AI may also involve diagnosing uncommon and complicated cases, which are frequently difficult for regular pathologists to deal with since they are so unusual. Searching for photos that are comparable to query photographs from extensive histopathology databases is something that AI is capable of doing. This is incredibly helpful in the pathological diagnosis process since it increases the likelihood of arriving at an accurate diagnosis for challenging cases. This is accomplished by rapidly collecting similar examples from pathological image databases that are easily accessible and contain uncommon and complicated situations. Automated quantification of immunohistochemistry (IHC) staining intensity, receptors, and other indicators scoring in the breast and other tissue is gaining much interest [17]. More recently, efforts have been made to predict breast cancer biomarkers directly from the H&E slides.

The ability to forecast patient prognosis and responsiveness to specific therapy only based on morphological characteristics is one of the most significant potential uses of AI in the field of pathology. Pathologists only use a small number of morphological discoveries on tissue sections to define the histological type and grade of the tumor specimen. This is not only based on the association with the outcome but also on their capacity and skills in visual identification and their ability to recognize these qualities and reach an acceptable level of concordance. Incorporating many other components, such as the microenvironment, is also essential. Image-based AI tools have the potential to provide a novel classification system that is based on clinical relevance according to outcome and response to therapy. These tools can also correlate features related to the morphology, architecture, stroma, and microenvironment of tumor cells and lymphovascular invasion [18].

Among the potential advantages that AI applications could bring to pathology services are the following: a reduction in the number of errors caused by humans during the handling and processing of specimens, faster turnaround times, management of workload, quality assurance measures, and automatic reporting. Regarding staining quality, tissue representation on the slide, processing mistakes, quality of staining of the external and on-slide control samples, and even the quality of tissue fixation, AI technologies can identify the spectrum of faults that might occur on scanned slides. Regarding workflow management, AI may assist in triaging cases into high or low priority, sorting and classifying cases to ensure that urgent cases are always evaluated first, and matching slides and identity cards. The necessity to double diagnostically subjective report cases can be reduced using AI techniques. AI and pathologists working together can produce results that are superior to those made by humans in terms of accuracy, consistency, timeliness, and utility. By examining the features of tumor cells, the structural alterations of lesions, and the expression patterns of biomarkers, these models assist pathologists in the disease diagnosis process.

20.4 AI in Genomics

The field of genomics is advancing thanks to the application of AI and ML, making it feasible to evaluate complex genetic data. These technologies, which can identify genetic changes associated with various diseases, can be used to design personalized therapy regimens. In oncology, for example, genetic research that AI drives is used to identify mutations that particular medications can target, boosting cancer treatment's effectiveness [19]. AI also helps to disclose genetic predispositions to diseases such as Alzheimer's and cardiovascular diseases. AI is assisting in analyzing whole-genome sequencing data, which is helping to reveal these disorders. By combining genetic data with clinical and lifestyle information, AI can provide comprehensive insights into an individual's health risks. The provision of proactive and preventive care is made possible as a result of this.

Our understanding of the genetic basis of diseases has been fundamentally revolutionized due to recent breakthroughs in genomic sequencing, in particular next-generation sequencing (NGS). In addition to providing accurate insights into genetic polymorphisms and their associated diseases, NGS makes it possible to sequence entire genomes speedily and cost-effectively [20]. It has been demonstrated that sequencing the genome has been groundbreaking in cancer diagnosis. Because of this, oncologists can deliver individualized drugs that are more successful than typical therapies and have fewer harmful effects. Identifying genetic abnormalities present within cancerous tumors is necessary to accomplish this.

As an illustration, the identification of the HER2 mutation in breast cancer patients has led to the development of targeted drugs such as trastuzumab, which has resulted in a significant improvement in the outcomes for patients [21]. In addition, genomic sequencing is applied in liquid biopsy, a diagnostic tool used to discover circulating tumor DNA (ctDNA) in blood samples [22]. This method offers a comprehensive perspective of the patient's condition by, among other things, facilitating the early detection of cancer, monitoring the progression of the disease, and evaluating the patient's reaction to treatment.

20.5 Pharmacogenomics

Pharmacogenomics, the study of how genetic variations influence how an individual reacts to prescribed pharmaceuticals, is one of the critical components of personalized medicine. When specialists in the medical field have a comprehensive understanding of these hereditary traits, they can better modify prescription regimens to enhance effectiveness while effectively limiting undesired consequences. Patients are likely to respond favorably to specific antidepressants or those at risk of experiencing significant side effects from particular medicines can be identified through genetic testing. Furthermore, pharmacogenomics enhances the effectiveness and safety of medications for treating chronic conditions such as diabetes and cardiovascular illnesses. It has been established that genetic testing can guide the selection of drugs and dosages in chronic metabolic ailments, thereby reducing the risk of adverse reactions and increasing the likelihood of improving patient outcomes.

There is a wide range of responses to medications among individuals, and the effects of pharmaceuticals can sometimes be unpredictable. There is a large amount of variance in the reactions of individuals that can be attributed to differences in DNA sequences that modify the production or function of proteins targeted by medicines. There are still a lot of obstacles that we need to conquer to properly comprehend the role of genetic polymorphisms in the disparities in pharmacological effects between individuals and to put this newly acquired information into clinical practice. Monogenic (single gene) features affecting drug metabolism are currently the most well-known examples of genetic polymorphisms that alter human drug response [23]. Genomics can be utilized to uncover new targets by finding genes that are either under or overexpressed in cancer cells that are vulnerable to anticancer medicines compared to those that are resistant to these agents. Inhibitors that could reverse the drug resistance phenotype could potentially target the products of such overexpressed genes, which are plausible targets for such inhibitors. Another application is the use of gene expression in target tissues (for example, cancer cells) to determine the effects of chemotherapy and how cells react to treatment with single medications or drug combinations [24]. This kind of application is also known as gene expression analysis. One commonly used method involves retrospectively searching for genetic variants that predispose a small proportion of patients to severe toxicities. This method consists of obtaining genomic DNA from patients participating in large clinical trials of a novel medication.

These trials are recommended to contain exhaustive and rigorous pharmacogenomic studies and preclinical, experimental models that reinforce clinical relationships. The application of pharmacogenomics has the potential to make this process easier by enabling the translation of knowledge regarding the variability of the human genome into more effective treatments.

20.6 Wearable Technology and Continuous Health Monitoring

As a result of its capacity to offer continuous health monitoring, wearable devices are gaining growing popularity. Smartwatches and fitness trackers are examples of wearable technology that can monitor vital signs, patterns of physical activity, and sleep patterns. This provides patients and healthcare practitioners with valuable information that can be used to improve their health. Because these devices are fitted with sensors that can monitor the user's heart rate, blood pressure, and oxygen saturation levels, they make it possible to detect potential health issues earlier.

As an illustration, wearable ECG monitors can detect anomalies in the heart, such as atrial fibrillation (AFib), which prompts customers to seek medical care as soon as feasible [25]. Wearable technology has also been developed to monitor biochemical indicators such as glucose levels, lactate levels, and your present hydration level. These cutting-edge sensors can produce continuous health data, which may be exploited for real-time diagnostics and the development of tailored health remedies. Continuous glucose monitors (CGMs) have been a game-changer in diabetes management. These devices provide glucose readings in real-time and make it possible to control better glycemic levels. This information can be transmitted to healthcare providers promptly, permitting rapid interventions and adjustments to treatment programs. In addition to monitoring, wearable technologies can provide tailored feedback and recommendations based on the gathered data. For example, wearables might advise patients regarding changes to their lifestyle, such as increasing the amount of physical exercise they get or making alterations to the food they eat, to aid patients in better managing their conditions.

20.7 Telemedicine and Remote Diagnostics

Telemedicine, which uses various telecommunication technologies, makes it feasible to perform remote consultations, diagnostics, and treatment plans, thereby improving the availability of medical care. This strategy is advantageous for patients who require access to healthcare institutions located in remote or impoverished areas.

Through conferencing and electronic health records (EHRs), these platforms make it feasible for healthcare providers to make decisions founded on reliable information. Telemedicine has expanded its scope beyond consultations to include diagnostic procedures. Digital stethoscopes and portable ultrasound machines are two examples of gadgets that fall under this category. Telemedicine is a highly significant component in managing chronic diseases through remote monitoring. For people with conditions such as diabetes, hypertension, metabolic syndrome, and heart disease, the use of devices that continuously monitor their health metrics can be of great benefit [26]. This makes intervening and adjusting treatment regimens possible at the appropriate time. The primary equipment required for remote consultation work is computer mainframes, monitors, high-definition cameras, printers, speakers, microphones, and other computer accessories. This type of labor depends on the technology within the internet. County-level physicians can contact specialists at higher-level medical institutions through the system's remote consultation capability. Consultation specialists can also query the patient's electronic medical record within the system, which allows them to completely comprehend the patient's primary complaint, medical history, prior history, physical examination, and different auxiliary examination information. County-level hospitals obtain imagery by utilizing the imaging equipment already present in the hospital and then the images are uploaded to a cloud server. The remote imaging function allows medical professionals in higher-level hospitals to see the photos directly stored on the cloud server. Some patients in critical condition and whose need for medical services cannot be satisfied by the institutions at the grassroots level are transferred to hospitals at higher levels so that they can continue receiving treatment.

Some patients with limited access to medical resources may find that remote appointments provide a more convenient option for receiving medical care at their convenience. The number of people who use telemedicine is not particularly widespread, and there is still much space for advancement in this field.

20.8 Integrating Big Data in Diagnostics

The healthcare industry consistently generates a significant amount of data, including patient records, medical imaging, genomic data, and data from wearable devices. Synthesizing this information through big data analytics can ultimately lead to more accurate diagnoses and greater individualization in medical care. By examining patient data, predictive models can identify individuals at a high risk of getting particular conditions. The provision of early intervention and preventative care is made possible by the acquisition of this information. The accuracy of diagnosis and treatment efficacy is improved due to these systems, which perform data analysis on patients and provide suggestions supported by evidence. Accordingly, these systems can alert healthcare providers about the likelihood of drug interactions, provide recommendations for alternative therapies, and identify individuals who would benefit from a particular treatment.

20.9 Ethical and Societal Considerations

The digitization of diagnostic data and various medical records has made data privacy and security protection of the utmost importance. The digital gap continues to be a barrier to equitably distributing diagnostic technologies. People who live in rural locations and areas with low socioeconomic status may have restricted access to new diagnostic technology, which can exacerbate the health disparities that already exist [27, 28]. Healthcare providers must comply with rules such as the Health Insurance Portability and Accountability Act to prevent breaches and illegal access to patient information. In addition, it is of the utmost importance to install robust cybersecurity measures and comply with the legislation requirements.

Encryption, secure access controls, and continuous monitoring of data systems are all essential components for protecting sensitive health information. AI systems could inherit biases present in the training data, leading to variations in diagnosis accuracy between different classes of people. Therefore, it is essential to ensure that training datasets are varied. This will help limit the impacts of bias and make diagnostics more egalitarian. When addressing biases, developing transparent AI systems that explain their decision-making processes can be helpful. By understanding how AI algorithms arrive at specific diagnoses, healthcare staff can identify and correct potential biases, ultimately leading to more equitable diagnostic outcomes.

20.10 Future Directions

The seamless incorporation of a wide range of technological advancements is essential to the progression of diagnostic care in the future. AI, telemedicine, wearable technology, and genetics have the potential to develop a comprehensive healthcare model centered on the patient. The next step in the progression of AI-driven diagnostics is to develop diagnostic tools that can integrate a large number of data sources and produce diagnostic insights that are both comprehensive and aware of context. When imaging data, genetic information, and clinical history should all be combined to arrive at diagnoses that are more accurate and specific to the individual. The future generation of wearable technology may be capable of continually monitoring a broader range of health markers. Future wearables are projected to incorporate sensors that identify biomarkers for various ailments. This would make it possible to diagnose health problems earlier and personalize treatment regimens for each patient to improve their health. Some of the potential uses of wearable biosensors include the monitoring of inflammation markers, the prediction of flare-ups in autoimmune disorders, and the facilitation of prophylactic medicine.

Some variables, such as advancements in internet connectivity and the development of increasingly advanced remote diagnostic instruments, contribute to telemedicine's expansion. Telemedicine systems may combine virtual reality (VR) and augmented reality (AR) to give equally immersive and engaging consultations [29, 30]. This would further alleviate the gap between in-person and remote therapy. The area of genomics is making remarkable gains, with an increased emphasis on epigenetics. Combining genetic information with epigenetic data can improve our understanding of disease mechanisms, resulting in more precise diagnostic and treatment approaches.

20.11 Conclusion

The application of technology in diagnostic treatment is producing a shift in the healthcare landscape, which is currently going through a significant upheaval. Big data analytics is helping to improve the management of illnesses, and AI and ML are helping to improve diagnostic accuracy. Telemedicine is helping to make healthcare more accessible, while wearable technology provides continuous health monitoring. Genomics is helping to pave the way for personalized medicine. Despite these achievements, some obstacles remain to overcome, including discrimination based on algorithmic bias, concerns over data privacy, and issues around equitable access to technology.

REFERENCES

1. Abhisheka B, et al. Recent trend in medical imaging modalities and their applications in disease diagnosis: a review. *Multimed Tools Appl.* 2024;83(14):43035–70.
2. Kumar D, et al. A comparative study of medical imaging modalities. *Int J Radiol Sci.* 2021;3:9–16.
3. Fazal MI, et al. The past, present and future role of artificial intelligence in imaging. *Eur J Radiol.* 2018;105:246–50.
4. Ahmed Z, et al. Artificial intelligence with multi-functional machine learning platform development for better healthcare and precision medicine. *Database.* 2020;2020:baaa010.
5. Kumar Y, et al. A systematic review of artificial intelligence techniques in cancer prediction and diagnosis. *Arch Comput Methods Eng.* 2022;29(4):2043–70.
6. Saba L, et al. The present and future of deep learning in radiology. *Eur J Radiol.* 2019;114:14–24.
7. Najjar R. Redefining radiology: a review of artificial intelligence integration in medical imaging. *Diagnostics (Basel).* 2023;13(17).
8. Zhang Z, Sejdić E. Radiological images and machine learning: trends, perspectives, and prospects. *Comput Biol Med.* 2019;108:354–70.
9. Li F, Ruijs N, Lu Y. Ethics & AI: a systematic review on ethical concerns and related strategies for designing with AI in healthcare. *Ai.* 2022;4(1):28–53.
10. Naik N, et al. Legal and ethical consideration in artificial intelligence in healthcare: who takes responsibility? *Front Surg.* 2022;9:862322.
11. Kim I, et al. Application of artificial intelligence in pathology: trends and challenges. *Diagnostics (Basel).* 2022;12(11).
12. Alowais SA, et al. Revolutionizing healthcare: the role of artificial intelligence in clinical practice. *BMC Med Educ.* 2023;23(1):689.
13. Jain E, et al. Whole slide imaging technology and its applications: current and emerging perspectives. *Int J Surg Pathol.* 2024;32(3):433–48.
14. Ström P, et al. Artificial intelligence for diagnosis and grading of prostate cancer in biopsies: a population-based, diagnostic study. *Lancet Oncol.* 2020;21(2):222–32.
15. Agrawal S, Vagha S. A comprehensive review of artificial intelligence in prostate cancer care: state-of-the-art diagnostic tools and future outlook. *Cureus.* 2024;16(8).
16. Betmouni S. Diagnostic digital pathology implementation: learning from the digital health experience. *Digit Health.* 2021;7:20552076211020240.

17. Priego-Torres BM, et al. Deep learning-based instance segmentation for the precise automated quantification of digital breast cancer immunohistochemistry images. *Expert Syst Appl.* 2022;193:116471.
18. Roxanis I, et al. The significance of tumour microarchitectural features in breast cancer prognosis: a digital image analysis. *Breast Cancer Res.* 2018;20:1–11.
19. Dlamini Z, et al. Artificial intelligence (AI) and big data in cancer and precision oncology. *Comput Struct Biotechnol J.* 2020;18:2300–11.
20. Yadav D, et al. Next-Generation sequencing transforming clinical practice and precision medicine. *Clin Chim Acta.* 2023:117568.
21. Oh D-Y, Bang Y-J. HER2-targeted therapies—a role beyond breast cancer. *Nat Rev Clin Oncol.* 2020;17(1):33–48.
22. Abou Daya S, Mahfouz R. Circulating tumor DNA, liquid biopsy, and next generation sequencing: a comprehensive technical and clinical applications review. *Meta Gene.* 2018;17:192–201.
23. Desta Z, Flockhart DA. Pharmacogenetics of drug metabolism, in clinical and translational science. 2017, Elsevier. p. 327–45.
24. Chawla S, et al. Gene expression based inference of cancer drug sensitivity. *Nat Commun.* 2022;13(1):5680.
25. Simonson JK, et al. Characterizing real-world implementation of consumer wearables for the detection of undiagnosed atrial fibrillation in clinical practice: targeted literature review. *JMIR Cardio.* 2023;7:e47292.
26. Keshet A, et al. Wearable and digital devices to monitor and treat metabolic diseases. *Nat Metab.* 2023;5(4):563–71.
27. Chen X, et al. Differences in rural and urban health information access and use. *J Rural Health.* 2019;35(3):405–17.
28. Haimi M. The tragic paradoxical effect of telemedicine on healthcare disparities- a time for redemption: a narrative review. *BMC Med Inform Decis Mak.* 2023;23(1):95.
29. Hilty DM, et al. A review of telepresence, virtual reality, and augmented reality applied to clinical care. *J Technol Behav Sci.* 2020;5:178–205.
30. Worlikar H, et al. Mixed reality platforms in telehealth delivery: scoping review. *JMIR Biomed Eng.* 2023;8:e42709.

Index

For Product Safety Concerns and Information please contact our EU
representative GPSR@taylorandfrancis.com
Taylor & Francis Verlag GmbH, Kaufingerstraße 24, 80331 München, Germany

www.ingramcontent.com/pod-product-compliance
Ingram Content Group UK Ltd.
Pitfield, Milton Keynes, MK11 3LW, UK
UKHW050353071126
477531UK00011B/598

* 9 7 8 1 0 3 2 7 8 2 3 2 4 *